Neurological Differential Diagnosis

Neurological Differential Diagnosis

an illustrated approach
with 288 figures

JOHN PATTEN

HAROLD STARKE LIMITED
LONDON

SPRINGER-VERLAG
NEW YORK · HEIDELBERG · BERLIN

First published October 1977
Revised reprint November 1978
Second reprint January 1980
Third reprint 1981
Fourth reprint 1982
© John Patten 1977

John P. Patten, BSc., M.B., M.R.C.P., is Consultant Neurologist at the Regional
Neurological Unit, Guildford, Surrey; formerly Resident Medical Officer, The National
Hospital for Nervous Diseases, London; and has been Visiting Assistant Professor of
Neurology in the University of Texas Medical Branch, Galveston, Texas

Library of Congress Cataloging in Publication Data

Patten, John, 1935–
    Neurological differential diagnosis.

    Includes index.
    1. Nervous system—Diseases—Diagnosis.
    2. Diagnosis, Differential. I. Title

RC348.P37   616.8′04′75   77–6897
ISBN 0–387–90264–3 (Springer)

ISBN 0–287–66988–2 Harold Starke Ltd., United Kingdom
ISBN 0–387–90264–3 Springer-Verlag New York Inc.
ISBN 3–540–90264–3 Springer-Verlag Berlin Heidelberg

Harold Starke Limited, Pegasus House, 116–120 Golden Lane, London EC1Y 0TL, England
Springer-Verlag New York Inc., 175 Fifth Avenue, New York 10010, U.S.A.
Springer-Verlag Heidelberger Platz 3, D-1000 Berlin 33, Germany
Springer-Verlag D-6900 Heidelberg 1, FRG.

Printed in Great Britain at the Whitefriars Press Ltd, London and Tonbridge

CONTENTS

PREFACE

The majority of doctors are ill at ease when confronted by a patient with a neurological problem. Candidates for qualifying examinations and higher diplomas dread that they will be allocated a neurological "long case".

This is a serious reflection on the adequacy of training in neurology. It is still possible in some medical schools for a student to go through his entire clinical course without an attachment to the neurological unit. Increasing competition for teaching time has led to the situation where in most U.S. medical schools and at least one new medical school in the U.K., a two-week clinical attachment to the neurology service is considered adequate. Those fortunate enough to attend a post-graduate course find a minimum of three months' intensive training is necessary before any confidence in tackling a neurological problem is achieved.

Unfortunately, neurological textbooks seldom seem to recognise the intensely practical nature of the subject. There are many short texts that achieve brevity by the exclusion of explanatory material; these are difficult to read and digest. At the opposite extreme are the neurological compendia, often unbalanced by excessive coverage of rare diseases and all based on the assumption that patients announce on arrival that they have a demyelinating, heredofamilial, neoplastic, etc., etc., disorder. These texts are useful only to those who already have a good working knowledge of neurological diseases.

Patients present with symptoms that need careful evaluation before physical examination which in turn should be firmly based on the diagnostic possibilities suggested by the history. Understanding neurological symptoms and signs requires a good knowledge of the gross anatomy of the nervous system, its blood supply and supporting tissues; and yet an almost universal feature of neurological texts is the paucity of instructive diagrams. Most students readily admit that this is an insoluble problem as their poorly remembered neurological anatomy is often both inadequate and inappropriate to the clinical situation.

The present text is a personal approach to this complex and fascinating subject and basically reflects the way the author coped with this difficulty. The subject matter is dealt with in two ways:

(1) A symptomatic, regional anatomical basis for those areas where local anatomy determines symptoms and signs, allowing what might otherwise be regarded as "small print" anatomy to be understood and appreciated.

(2) A full discussion of the historical diagnostic clues in those conditions that are diagnosed almost exclusively on symptoms such as headache, face pain and loss of consciousness.

Throughout, an attempt has been made to preserve the "common things are common" approach which is widely rumoured to be the secret of passing examinations, and is also the basis of good clinical practice. Rare disorders are discussed briefly, but it is important that beginners realise that rare diseases are usually diagnosed when it becomes apparent that the disorder does *not* fit into any of the common clinical pictures. The first aim therefore should be to gain a very good grasp of the common disorders rather than attempting to learn long lists of very rare diseases.

The text is profusely illustrated by the author and although anatomical accuracy has been preserved, artistic licence has been taken whenever necessary to illustrate an important point. Each diagram is drawn from a special angle of view that enables the reader to visualise the area under discussion *in situ* in the patient. It is easy to construct a "diagram" so remote from actual anatomy that it becomes incomprehensible. It is hoped that this problem has been avoided.

Neurological terms are defined whenever they occur and neurological "jargon" is explained, although the beginner is well advised to keep to factual statements until he is very sure of himself. As an example of the incorrect use of jargon the following is abstracted from a report by a physician. The patient actually had a left sixth nerve palsy and a mild hemiparesis due to cerebal metastases.

He has the spastic dystonic gait of the multiple sclerotic. Also he has a third nerve paraplegia with ocular movements to the left and with nystagmus. He has cogwheel rigidity of the upper extremities and an absence of patellar reflexes. His speech is beginning to slur and there is the mask facies of the multiple sclerotic . . . I do not believe . . . further studies to be necessary as the clinical signs are all too obvious!

Specific references are not given; this book is intended for the novice who wishes to develop a "feel" for the subject and in the author's opinion references are unnecessary. This is not intended to indicate that the writer claims originality for all the information provided. The knowledge contained in this text is a distillate of wisdom gained from many teachers and, indeed, generations of teachers who have passed on their own observations. The personal part of this text is the attempt to organise this information around the anatomy of the nervous system to reinforce this knowledge and make the subject less intimidating to the beginner. In particular I would like to acknowledge my debt to my first teacher, Dr. Swithin Meadows, who aroused my enthusiasm for the subject and then inspired me to attempt to emulate his skill as a clinical neurologist.

I am also indebted to many undergraduate students at Westminster Medical School, University College Hospital and the University of Texas Medical Branch, and post-graduates at the National Hospital for Nervous Diseases whose questions, suggestions and enthusiasm originally encouraged me to bring this approach to a wider audience.

Dr. John R. Calverley, M.D., Associate Professor of Neurology in the University of Texas Medical Branch at Galveston, provided enormous encouragement in the early development of this project and allowed me to try the format on several generations of post-graduate students in his Department.

I would like to express my thanks to him and his colleagues for making my stay in his Department so in-structive and enjoyable. Dr. M. J. Harrison read the original manuscript and made many useful suggestions which have been incorporated into the text. I am very grateful for his help and encouragement.

I would like to thank my wife and family for their continued support during the years this text has been in preparation and Miss Gillian Taylor for typing the often illegible manuscript.

John Patten

Guildford, 1977

Chapter 1

HISTORY-TAKING AND PHYSICAL EXAMINATION

By tradition the first chapter in any textbook of C.N.S. diseases deals with history-taking, and this necessity appears inescapable. Yet in neurology the history is so critical, in indicating both the site and the nature of the lesion, that adequate coverage is impossible in a single chapter. The features of the clinical history appropriate to each region will form a major part of each of the subsequent chapters. At this stage discussion will be confined to some broad generalisations.

The secret of good history-taking is to be a good listener. However rushed the doctor may be, it is vital that the patient feels that he has the whole of the doctor's time and attention during the interview. The doctor must also be constantly aware that the majority of patients are extremely frightened, even though their actual behaviour may range from tongue-tied, tremulous anxiety to the blustering type of patient who insists that he came only because his wife was worried about him! The patient requiring most care, attention and caution is the one who is self-effacing and apologetic for wasting your time; with remarkable regularity these are the patients who have a serious disease.

Every effort should be made to put the patient at ease. Several minutes spent discussing inconsequential subjects such as the weather may seem to be time-wasting to the uninitiated but the relaxation and the insight gained into the patient's mood, his reaction to his disease and his intellectual ability is often greater than one can obtain with several minutes of formal testing, or more direct questioning.

As soon as the patient is talking freely the subject of his symptoms should be introduced. Although a referring letter may be of help in guiding the questioning, it is always important to ask the patient to relate the *entire* history again. Otherwise, half-digested views expressed by other doctors, relatives or workmates may intrude into the history as facts rather than supposition. The importance of cross-checking the history with a relative or friend is vital. In diseases affecting the patient's consciousness or intellect the history may be confused or impossible to obtain without the help of a third party. In other conditions patients frequently understate the duration and severity of their disability and again a completely different story may emerge from enquiries made of a relative. In general these supplementary interviews are best conducted in another room while the patient is undress-ing, particularly in the case of epileptic attacks in children, where the parents are often loath to reveal any of the details of ictal behaviour in front of the child. Peculiar behaviour traits at any age clearly cannot be discussed easily in front of the patient and a private interview with relatives, fellow-employees and others in contact with the patient is vital.

In all cases an accurate history of the entire course of the illness is essential. The diagnostic differences between weakness of an arm coming on overnight, over a week or over several months are so important that vague statements such as "gradually" should not be accepted at face value. A clerk with a radial nerve palsy present on waking one Sunday morning was cautiously asked if he had been drinking. With considerable reluctance, anxiety and embarrassment he admitted that he had become drunk for the first time in his life the night before. Yet with a single question one could exclude a stroke (the diagnosis made elsewhere) and explain both the aetiology and excellent prognosis of a "Saturday night radial nerve palsy" to the relieved patient.

In many patients bizarre historical events may be deliberately concealed for fear of embarrassment or of moral judgements made by the doctor. The onset of symptoms during sexual activity or alcohol indulgence are frequently suppressed for this reason. The family of an elderly patient with periodic confusion and amnesia (who had been extensively investigated elsewhere) were asked about her drinking habits. An initial angry denial was later retracted following a family conference, with the admission that her wardrobe was full of empty sherry bottles! Considerable tact is called for in these instances and yet the matter must be pursued if unnecessary investigations and incorrect diagnoses are to be avoided.

In neurological medicine, in addition to the importance of making the diagnosis, in many instances the doctor's subsequent role will be to help the patient accept and cope with what may prove to be a lifelong disability. The establishment of an easy confident relationship at the first interview will help ensure a useful supportive role in the future.

When one sees the comment "hopeless historian" on the notes it is really as much a comment on the doctor taking the history! The doctor must tailor the interview to suit the patient and the skill to do this can only be acquired; it cannot be taught. The ability to sit back and listen does not come easily to many, but it is only the eventual realisation that one cannot force the pace of an interview without losing much of value that leads to the ability to take a good history.

The circumlocutory historian and the patient who insists on including irrelevant detail can be the most trying of all. Any attempt to alter the line of questioning will start another sequence of irrelevances. It is best to sit and listen and wait for the useful pieces of information to emerge. These are often the facts regarded as the least important by the patient! Considering how infinitely variable symptoms could be, it is amazing how often patients eventually describe their feelings and symptoms in almost identical phrases. The diagnosis of several classical syndromes depends on typical symptom descriptions. For example, the "red hot needle" jabs of pain in tic douloureux; the feeling of "déjà vu" often associated with temporal lobe attacks, or the "icy cold bandage around the waist or legs" described by patients with spinal cord lesions. Some of the feelings are so bizarre that the patient hesitates to describe them for fear of being accused of imagining things. A useful rule in neurology is that the more bizarre and unusual a symptom, the more likely it is to be organic. An arrogant approach—assuming that a symptom which is not known to the examiner must be functional or imaginary—is very likely to lead to mis-diagnosis. It is dangerous to presume universal knowledge.

The above suggestions may not appeal to those who think that a doctor ought not to adopt a passive role and who see themselves as too busy and too important to be slowed down by vague patients. Such a person would be ill advised to embark on a career in neurology.

The usual sequence of a medical consultation is that the history leads on to the physical examination. It is only at this stage that the full value of the history becomes apparent. If a *full* neurological examination were performed on each patient it would take up to an hour for its completion and would prove extremely boring. The history serves to indicate those parts of the examination that should be performed with special care, skill and finesse. Few would perform exactly the same physical examination on a patient with headache as they would on a patient with pain in the leg, and yet the ability to tailor the examination to the situation is based entirely on the history. If a confident diagnosis of the site and probable nature of the lesion has not been made by the completion of the history it is very unlikely that the diagnosis will suddenly become apparent during the physical examination.

Having made a provisional diagnosis based on the history, the physical examination should be performed in the same relaxed way. A warm room with reasonable privacy is essential for a neurological examination. Although the doctor is accustomed to the sight of a tendon hammer and tuning fork, he must remember that the patient may not have seen either previously. He should always explain what he is about to do *before* doing it. Suddenly flashing a light in the patient's eyes or sticking a pin into a limb without warning hardly inspires patient confidence or patient co-operation. When attempting to elicit the plantar responses the examiner should warn the patient that it will hurt. Patients will tolerate considerable discomfort if invited to do so, but do not take kindly to unannounced aggression! Elicitation of both the supinator and ankle jerks is quite painful for the patient and yet one sees doctors repeatedly striking the tendon and wondering why the patient will not relax. Notes such as "patient will not relax" or "plantars impossible" can usually be regarded as due to poor examination technique rather than an adverse comment on the patient's co-operation.

The correct method of performing the various parts of the neurological examination will be detailed in the following chapters. This will always be in the setting of diseases that actually cause abnormalities.

In the author's view the only way to understand the mechanism and correct elicitation of physical signs is in relation to the situation where correct technique actually matters. For example, in a patient with backache, correct testing of the corneal response may not be critical, but in a patient with a giddy attack, facial weakness or face pain, the sign must be understood and elicited correctly, as the depression or absence of a corneal response may be the only physical sign of an underlying lesion in the cerebello-pontine angle.

Throughout this book the emphasis is on the recognition of the diagnostic features in the history, and the planning of the clinical examination to confirm or refute the provisional diagnosis *at the bedside*. The ultimate objective is to arrive at the correct diagnosis in the least number of moves and at the least risk to the patient; this must always be the overriding consideration.

Chapter 2

THE PUPILS AND THEIR REACTIONS

Due to the long intracranial and extracranial courses of the nerve pathways controlling the size and reactions of the pupils, lesions in many areas may cause pupillary abnormalities. Important differential diagnostic information may easily be overlooked by a cursory examination of the pupils or unnecessary investigations may be performed when a physiological inequality in pupil size is mistaken for a physical sign. In the unconscious patient the size and reactions of the pupils are of paramount importance in both diagnosis and minute-to-minute management of the patient.

BASIC EXAMINATION TECHNIQUE

1. The size, shape and symmetry of the pupils in moderate lighting conditions should be noted.

2. The direct and indirect responses of the pupils to a bright light should be elicited. An inadequate light source is the most frequent cause of absence of the light reflexes. The direct light reflex is the constriction of the pupil that occurs when it is directly illuminated. The indirect response or consensual light reflex is the simultaneous constriction of the opposite pupil.

3. The accommodation reaction should be tested. This reaction is the constriction of the pupil that automatically occurs as the patient attempts to converge the eyes. Failure to elicit this response is usually due to the patient's failure to converge the eyes. Convergence is most easily achieved if the patient tries to look at the end of his own nose, or at the examiner's finger brought in from below the line of the nose. The majority of people find it much easier to converge while looking downwards. It is helpful if the examiner holds the patient's eyelids up so that the pupils can be easily observed.

General Considerations

1. It is essential to establish whether any drops have been put in the patient's eyes. Many patients have been investigated for what later proved to be pharmacological pupillary inequality because of a failure to observe this simple rule.

2. If the pupils are unequal it is important to decide *which* is abnormal. A frequent mistake is to investigate for the cause of a dilated pupil on one side when the patient actually has a constricted pupil on the other side due to a Horner's syndrome!

3. If the pupils are unequal in size there are two additional features that may help establish the cause. If there is ptosis of the eyelid on the side of the *small* pupil the patient has a Horner's syndrome on that side. If there is ptosis on the side of the *large* pupil the patient has a partial third nerve lesion on that side. The light reflex and accommodation reflexes will be normal in Horner's syndrome and impaired in a partial third nerve lesion. In the absence of ptosis if both pupils react normally to light and accommodation the patient has "physiological anisocoria" (i.e. he has probably always had pupillary inequality). Many normal people have slight asymmetry in the size of the pupils.

4. Whenever a patient is found to have a widely dilated pupil that is fixed to light and accommodation without ptosis, the possibility that the patient has deliberately instilled atropine drops into the eye should always be considered. The writer has encountered this situation twice; both the patients were nurses.

5. Pupils are usually small in infancy, become larger in adolescence and are "normal" size in adulthood. In old age they again become small and the light reaction is accordingly difficult to see. Many elderly patients are incorrectly suspected of having Argyll–Robertson pupils because of this normal change in pupil size with age which is called "senile miosis" (miosis—pupillary constriction; mydriasis—pupillary dilation).

6. The pupils of many patients show a phasic constriction and dilation to light of constant intensity. This phenomenon is called "hippus" and has no definite pathological significance.

PUPIL SIZE AND REACTIONS

Pupil size is controlled by a ring of constrictor fibres innervated by the parasympathetic nervous system and a ring of radially arranged dilator fibres controlled by the sympathetic nervous system.

The resting size of the pupil is governed by the amount of light falling on either eye and depends on the integrity of the parasympathetic nerves. Increased activity in the sympathetic is reflected in slight pupillary dilation as occurs in an anxiety state. It is unusual for changes in pupil size to affect vision so that the majority of pupillary abnormalities are asymptomatic.

Parasympathetic Pathways (Figure 2.1)

The intensity of light falling on the retina is conveyed in the optic nerve to the optic chiasm. The impulses are then split and conveyed in *both* optic tracts to *both* lateral geniculate bodies. Some ten per cent of the fibres reaching the geniculate bodies subserve the light reflex and are relayed in the periaqueductal grey to both Edinger–Westphal nuclei and therefore light falling on *either* eye inevitably excites *both* nuclei and causes constriction of *both* pupils—the anatomical basis of the consensual light reflex.

The Edinger–Westphal nuclei are also stimulated by activity in the adjacent third nerve nuclear mass which controls the medial rectus muscles. therefore when both medial rectus muscles are activated in an attempt to converge the eyes, the Edinger–Westphal nuclei become active and constrict the pupils, this being the suggested basis of the accommodation reflex.

The parasympathetic fibres are carried in the third nerve to the orbit; and lie in a superficial and dorsal position which may explain the variable abnormalities of the pupil in third nerve palsies to be discussed later (Figure 2.1A).

The final relay of the pathway is in the ciliary ganglion in the posterior orbit, which gives origin to eight to ten short ciliary nerves, which sub-divide into sixteen to twenty branches, that pass around the eye to reach the constrictor muscle of the pupil.

Clinical Lesions affecting the Parasympathetic Control of the Pupil

1. The light reflex and the resting size of the pupil depend on adequate light perception by at least one eye. There is *no* direct light reaction in a completely blind eye, but the resting pupil size will be the same as the pupil size in the intact eye. If both eyes are blind both pupils will be dilated and fixed to light *if* the cause is located anterior to the lateral geniculate bodies. If, however, bilateral blindness is the result of destruction of the occipital cortex the light reflex pathways will be intact. Therefore, it is possible for a patient to be completely blind with preserved light reflexes in both eyes. Furthermore, if there is *any* perception of light in an eye that is for practical purposes blind, the light reaction may well be intact.

Lesions in the retina, optic nerve and chiasm and the optic tract of minimal degree, in particular optic nerve damage due to multiple sclerosis, cause what is known as an "afferent pathway lesion". This results in an abnormal pupillary

response known as the Marcus Gunn pupil. When the normal eye is stimulated by a bright light there is no abnormality. When the affected eye is stimulated the reaction is slower, less complete, and so brief that the pupil may start to dilate again (the pupillary escape phenomena). The reaction is best seen if the light is rapidly alternated from one eye to the other, each stimulus lasting about a second with two or three seconds between. The reaction is thought to be due to a reduction in the number of fibres subserving the light reflex on the affected side.

2. A lesion of one optic tract does not affect the resting size of the pupil due to the consensual light reflex. In this situation a better light reflex may be seen if the light is shone on the intact half of the retina (see Chapter 3 for details of the field defect). This is called the Wernicke pupil reaction. It is very difficult to elicit this sign due to dispersion of light in the eye.

3. Lesions compressing or infiltrating the tectum of the mid-brain (the area of the superior collicular bodies) will interfere with the decussating light reflex fibres in the periaqueductal area. This results in pupils that are dilated and fixed to light. This is often coupled with loss of upward gaze and is known as the Parinaud syndrome (see Chapter 7).

4. The Argyll–Robertson pupil is also traditionally ascribed to damage in the periaqueductal area. The typical Argyll–Robertson pupil is small, irregular and fixed to light, but reacts to accommodation. It is the latter feature that suggests that the light pathways leading to the Edinger–Westphal nuclei are damaged, but this cannot explain the small size of the pupil or its irregularity. It is also worth noting that accommodation is a much stronger stimulus to pupillo-constriction than light and the apparent dissociation may merely reflect very minimal pupil reactivity. It has been suggested that a local lesion of the iris must be responsible. (The Argyll–Robertson pupil reaction is a classical sign of meningo-vascular syphilis.) Other causes of Argyll–Robertson pupils are pinealomas, diabetes and brain stem encephalitis. These conditions usually cause fixed *dilated* pupils; a *small* irregular fixed pupil is usually due to neurosyphilis. The Argyll–Robertson pupil cannot be dilated by atropine (Figure 2.2). Other causes of small pupils that are apparently fixed to light include senile miosis and the instillation of pilocarpine drops in the treatment of glaucoma.

5. Epidemic encephalitis lethargica, which last occurred in the 1920s, caused many cases of Parkinsonism associated with loss of the ability to converge the eyes. This disability produced pupils that reacted to light but not to accommodation. This "reversed" Argyll–Robertson pupil has become a clinical rarity.

Figure 2.1. The Parasympathetic Control of the Pupil

Aqueduct (note the pathways relaying around the peri-aqueductal area)

Superior colliculus

Edinger–Westphal nuclei

Lateral geniculate body

Convergence centre

Figure 2.1A. Enlarged section of third nerve

Blood vessel on pia mater (supply surface of the nerve including pupillary fibres)

Fibres to pupil (lie dorsal and peripheral)

Vasa nervorum

III nerve

III nerve

Pial sheath of nerve

Vasa nervorum supplies central part of nerve

Optic chiasm

Ciliary ganglion (on branch to the inferior oblique muscle)

Short ciliary nerves (18–20 in all)

Sphincter pupillae

THE PHARMACOLOGY OF ABNORMAL PUPILS

Figure 2.2. Argyll—Robertson Pupil

Note. Ptosis, pupil is small, irregular, does not react to light, but does to accommodation

1% atropine solution in both eyes
No effect on A—R pupil   Wide dilatation of the normal pupil

(for illustrative purposes only, left pupil is shown as normal. A—R pupils are usually bilateral although they can be asymmetrical)

Figure 2.3. Holmes—Adie Pupil

Note. No ptosis, pupil is large, regular, does not react to light (other than prolonged exposure) but may show some response to accommodation

2.5% methacholine (mecholyl) in both eyes
The sensitised H—A pupil   No effect on the
promptly constricts   normal pupil

(Holmes—Adie pupils are usually unilateral—another feature to distinguish them from the A—R pupil)

6. Lesions affecting the third nerve may or may not involve the pupillary fibres. This is of great differential diagnostic value and will be discussed in detail in Chapter 5. At this point it is sufficient to note that if the nerve trunk is infarcted the superficial pupillary fibres may well be spared. As a general rule, if the pupil is affected the cause is surgical (i.e. compressive); and, if spared, the cause is medical (either diabetes, meningovascular syphilis or arteriosclerosis). The whole investigative approach to the patient with a third nerve lesion is influenced by the state of the pupil.

7. Degeneration of the nerve cells in the ciliary ganglion causes a Holmes—Adie or "tonic" pupil. The cause of this condition is unknown but it is often associated with loss of knee jerks and impairment of sweating. The Holmes—Adie pupil is a widely dilated, circular pupil that may react very slowly to very bright light, and shows a more definite response to accommodation. This dissociation again probably demonstrates the greater constrictive effect of accommodation. Both reactions are minimal and thought to be produced by slow inhibition of the sympathetic and *not* by any residual parasympathetic activity. The Holmes—Adie pupil is usually unilateral and more frequently found in females. It is often unnecessarily confused with Argyll—Robertson pupils which are small, irregular and usually bilateral. Congenital syphilis can cause fixed dilated pupils, but these are bilateral and other signs of congenital neurosyphilis will usually be found.

Confirmation of the diagnosis is best made by the pupillary response to $2\frac{1}{2}$ per cent methacholine drops. This chemical is too rapidly hydrolysed by acetylcholine-esterase to have any effect in the normal eye. In the denervated pupil, post-denervation hypersensitivity (due to enzyme depletion) allows the pupillo-constrictor effect to be seen. It has recently been shown that 80 per cent of diabetic patients react to methacholine in this way and 8 per cent of normal subjects also show a response. Therefore the test cannot be regarded as entirely specific for the Holmes—Adie pupil (Figure 2.3).

8. Blunt trauma to the iris may disrupt the fine short ciliary nerve filaments in the sclera causing an irregularly dilated pupil with impairment of the light reaction. A history of trauma is diagnostic. This is called post-traumatic iridoplegia (paralysis of the iris).

9. Diphtheria is a rare cause of pupillary dilatation due to damage to the ciliary nerves. It usually occurs in the second and third weeks of the illness and is often combined with the palatal paralysis. The pupillary abnormality usually recovers.

Sympathetic Pathway

The course of the cervical sympathetic pathway is shown in Figure 2.4. Although the pathway apparently starts in the hypothalamus there is a considerable degree of *ipsilateral* cortical control (see Chapter 10). A lesion anywhere in the pathway on the right side will affect the right pupil. There are three neurones. The first passes from the hypothalamus to the lateral grey in the thoracic spinal cord; the second from the spinal cord to the superior cervical ganglion and the third from the superior cervical ganglion to the pupil and blood vessels of the eye.

Figure 2.4. Horner's Syndrome

(showing the complete course of the sympathetic and pathological lesions and their sites of occurrence)

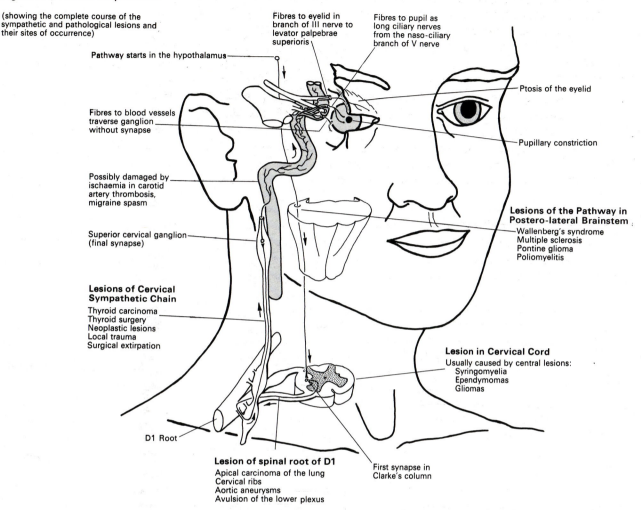

Fibres to eyelid in branch of III nerve to levator palpebrae superioris

Fibres to pupil as long ciliary nerves from the naso-ciliary branch of V nerve

Pathway starts in the hypothalamus

Ptosis of the eyelid

Fibres to blood vessels traverse ganglion without synapse

Pupillary constriction

Possibly damaged by ischaemia in carotid artery thrombosis, migraine spasm

Lesions of the Pathway in Postero-lateral Brainstem
Wallenberg's syndrome
Multiple sclerosis
Pontine glioma
Poliomyelitis

Superior cervical ganglion (final synapse)

Lesions of Cervical Sympathetic Chain

Thyroid carcinoma
Thyroid surgery
Neoplastic lesions
Local trauma
Surgical extirpation

Lesion in Cervical Cord
Usually caused by central lesions:
    Syringomyelia
    Ependymomas
    Gliomas

D1 Root

Lesion of spinal root of D1
Apical carcinoma of the lung
Cervical ribs
Aortic aneurysms
Avulsion of the lower plexus

First synapse in Clarke's column

The third neurone enters the cranial cavity on the surface of the carotid artery and reaches the eye and eyelid as follows:

1. Fibres carried in the third nerve innervate the levator muscle of the eyelid.
2. Fibres in the nasociliary nerve traverse the ciliary ganglion without synapse to supply the blood vessels of the eye.
3. Other fibres branch from the nasociliary nerve as the long ciliary nerves to innervate the pupil by passing around the eye.

Abnormalities of the Sympathetic Pathway

Wherever the site of the lesion, a single physical sign results from damage to the sympathetic pathway and is known as Horner's syndrome. Associated physical signs allow the location of the causative lesion to be identified in some cases.

Horner's syndrome can be extremely subtle and the sign is easily overlooked by the less than obsessional examiner.

The features are as follows:

1. The affected pupil is slightly smaller than its fellow, due to reduced pupillodilator activity. This asymmetry is minimal in a bright light and exaggerated in darkness. The pupil reacts *normally* to light and accommodation but over a reduced range.
2. There is a variable degree of ptosis of the eyelid. In severe cases the lid may reach to the edge of the pupil, in other patients the ptosis may be barely detectable; and may vary from time to time during the day.

3. The conjunctiva may be slightly bloodshot (loss of vasoconstrictor activity).
4. Sweating over the forehead may be impaired, depending on the site of the lesion (see later).
5. In congenital Horner's syndrome the iris on the affected side fails to become pigmented and remains a blue-grey colour.
6. Enopthalmos (sunken eye) is not an easily detected feature of Horner's syndrome in man.

Causes of Horner's Syndrome

1. *Hemisphere Lesions*

Hemispherectomy or massive infarction of one hemisphere may cause a Horner's syndrome on the same side.

2. *Brain Stem Lesions*

The sympathetic pathways in the brain stem lie adjacent to the spinothalamic tract throughout its course. Hence Horner's syndrome due to a brain stem lesion is often associated with pain and temperature loss on the opposite side of the body. Vascular lesions, multiple sclerosis, pontine gliomas, and brain stem encephalitis may all cause a Horner's syndrome at this level (see Chapter 11).

3. *Cervical Cord Lesions*

Due to the central position of the pathway in the lateral column at D1 level the sympathetic is often involved in central cord lesions. Syringomyelia, cord gliomas or ependymomas will usually cause loss of pain sensation in the arms, loss of arm reflexes and often a *bilateral* Horner's syndrome. This can be very hard to detect as it is only the ptosis that draws attention to the condition—the pupils being small, but symmetrical and reactive! (see Chapter 15).

4. *D1 Root Lesions*

The D1 root is rarely affected by simple disc lesions, or degenerative disc disease. The root lies on the apical pleura where it may be damaged by primary or metastatic malignant disease. The classical syndrome of Pancoast, usually due to a cancer of the lung apex, consists of pain in the axilla, wasting of the small hand muscles and a Horner's syndrome, all on the same side. Other causes include cervical rib (usually in young females) and avulsion of the lower brachial plexus (Klumpke's paralysis). (See Chapter 18.)

5. *The Sympathetic Chain*

Throughout its course in the neck the sympathetic may be damaged by neoplastic infiltration, during surgical procedures on the larynx or thyroid, or surgically extirpated for a

Figure 2.5. Horner's Syndrome

Note. Slight ptosis. Small but normally reacting pupil

Peripheral Lesion (above superior cervical ganglion)

Cocaine 4% in both eyes

No effect as amine oxidase depleted due to post-ganglionic denervation

Dilates the normal pupil

Central Lesion (below superior cervical ganglion)

Cocaine 4% in both eyes

Dilates the pupil as amine-oxidase NOT depleted by pre-ganglionic lesion

Dilates the normal pupil

Adrenaline 1:1000 in both eyes

Marked effect as adrenaline is not destroyed by amine-oxidase. Even the lid will elevate

Too rapidly destroyed by amine-oxidase to have any effect

Adrenaline 1:1000 in both eyes

No effect as normal amine-oxidase levels still present

No effect on the normal pupil

number of indications. Malignant disease in the jugular foramen at the skull base causes various combinations of Horner's syndrome and lesions of cranial nerves IX, X, XI and XII (see Chapter 6).

6. *Miscellaneous*

Congenital Horner's syndrome is not rare and has been mentioned previously. Horner's syndrome may occur during migraine headache. Lesions in the cavernous sinus or orbit usually damage both the sympathetic and the parasympathetic leading to a semi-dilated pupil that is fixed to light combined with other extra-ocular nerve palsies (see Chapter 5).

Other Features of Horner's Syndrome

The associated physical signs or history usually leave little doubt as to the site and cause of Horner's syndrome. There are some other useful diagnostic pointers.

Central lesions usually affect sweating over the entire head, neck, arm and upper trunk on the same side. Lesions in the lower neck affect sweating over the entire face. Lesions above the superior cervical ganglion may not affect sweating at all, as the main outflow to the facial blood vessels and sweat glands is below the superior-cervical ganglion.

The presence of three neurones in the pathway leads to some useful pharmacological tests based on the phenomenon of denervation hypersensitivity.

The decrease in amine-oxidase caused by a lesion at or beyond the superior cervical ganglion, sensitises the pupil to adrenaline 1:1,000, which has no effect on the normal pupil.

Conversely, the effect of cocaine on the pupil *depends* on its blocking effect on amine-oxidase, therefore cocaine has no effect on a distally denervated pupil. It will only dilate the pupil in a Horner's syndrome if the lesion is below the superior cervical ganglion and there is amine-oxidase at the nerve endings for it to block.

These tests may be useful in the absence of other localising neurological signs in indicating the approximate site of the lesion. The pattern of responses are summarised in Figure 2.5.

PUPILLARY ABNORMALITIES IN THE UNCONSCIOUS PATIENT

The management of head injuries and the unconscious patient are discussed in Chapter 23.

1. *Normally Reacting Equal Pupils*

In an unconscious patient normal pupils are a reassuring sign indicating that no immediate surgical action is necessary. In the absence of a history of head trauma an immediate search for metabolic causes of coma should be initiated. Seventy per cent of unconscious patients have *not* had an intra-cranial catastrophe, but are in diabetic coma, hypoglycaemic coma, other metabolic coma, or have taken a drug overdose. Normal pupillary reactions are an important pointer to these possibilities. Only glutethamide and amphetamine (dilated pupils) or opiates (constricted pupils) cause misleading pupillary changes.

Table 1

PUPILLARY ABNORMALITIES

Reaction to Light	Small Pupils	Large Pupils
Non-reactive	A–R pupil	Holmes—Adie pupil
	Pontine	Post-traumatic
	haemorrhage	iridoplegia
	Opiates	Mydriatic drops
	Pilocarpine drops	Glutethamide overdose
		Cerebral death
		Atropine poisoning
		Amphetamine overdose
Reactive	Old age	Childhood
	Horner's	Anxiety
	syndrome	Physiological anisocoria

2. *Unequal Pupils*

This is the single most important physical sign in the unconscious patient. Until proved otherwise a dilated pupil indicates that a herniated temporal lobe is stretching the third nerve on that side and prompt surgical action is required. Problems occur if the eye was directly damaged in the injury, or if someone has put mydriatic drops in the eye in the pointless search for papilloedema (pointless because patients with acute head injury will die long before papilloedema can appear).

3. *Bilateral Dilated Pupils*

The final stage of progressive tentorial herniation is heralded by progressive dilatation of the previously unaffected pupil. The chances of the patient recovering from this stage are remote. This is also used as one of the signs of irreversible cerebral damage in cardiac arrest. Glutethamide, atropine (mushroom) and amphetamine poisoning are the only metabolic causes of bilateral dilated pupils.

4. *Bilateral Pin-point Pupils*

This situation is the hall-mark of another lethal neurological situation; a massive intra-pontine haemorrhage which is usually accompanied by pin-point pupils, deep coma and a spastic tetraparesis with brisk reflexes. Opiates produce similar pupillary abnormalities but depressed reflexes. In the elderly unconscious patient the possibility that pilocarpine drops have been instilled for glaucoma should be considered in view of the hopeless prognosis if intrapontine haemorrhage has occurred. Other causes of coma should be rapidly excluded if this is the case.

The pupils should always be examined with the special problems of that particular patient in mind. In this way there is less risk of a subtle abnormality being overlooked and the risk of unnecessary investigation of physiological variations is greatly reduced.

Chapter 3

THE VISUAL FIELDS

The visual pathways extend from the retina to the occipital pole. Part of their course is extra-cerebral and part in the substance of the hemisphere.

Due to the complex but constant decussations and rotations of nerve fibres in the visual pathways, visual field defects can provide very accurate localising information.

Patients tend to notice abrupt visual deterioration and may present with a detailed description of their defect whereas defects of slow onset may develop unnoticed by the patient. A routine examination of the optic fundus, visual acuity and visual fields should be made in all patients with neurological disease. It is unwise to assume that the patient's visual fields are normal because he has no visual symptoms. At the opposite extreme patients with seriously impaired vision require very careful field testing however difficult this may be to perform.

Often in the neurological examination signs are more easily detected if the examiner has some idea as to what he might find, or what he must exclude. The technique and use of confrontation field testing at the bedside is described in detail in relation to the various clinical situations in which field defects may be encountered.

CONFRONTATION TESTING OF THE VISUAL FIELDS

The results of confrontation testing are often recorded in clinical notes somewhat disparagingly as 'fields grossly normal'; as if the test were a poor substitute for more accurate testing. In skilled hands confrontation testing can be as accurate as screen or perimeter testing and in some situations may be the only way that the fields can be tested.

These situations include the examination of patients with a seriously disturbed mental state, physical disability preventing the patient from sitting at the apparatus or a dense central field defect that prevents the patient fixing his eyes on a target object, which is necessary to keep the eye still during testing.

In patients with greatly reduced visual acuity qualitative tests of the fields using hand movements and finger counting can only be performed by confrontation methods.

The Technique (Figure 3.1)

For accurate field testing red and white hatpins of 2 mm. and 5 mm. diameter should be used. Routine screening is usually performed with a 5 mm. white pin. The smaller pins are useful for detecting small scotomata (small field defects in the centre of the visual fields). The red pins are especially useful in testing the visual fields where a compressive lesion of the optic nerve, optic chiasm or optic tract is suspected. In these situations the ability to count fingers (marked CF on a field chart) and to detect hand movements (marked HM on the chart) are also of value.

1. The examiner should sit opposite the patient, ideally in a chair but where circumstances demand one may lean across the bed in front of the patient. Each eye is tested individually and if the examiner routinely holds the patient's other eye shut with his hand held at arm's length, a constant examiner-patient distance is established. An idea of the size of the normal field at this distance is easily acquired and skill in detecting early peripheral field defects is quickly achieved.

2. Throughout the test the patient is asked to look straight at the examiner's eye (the right eye when testing the patient's left eye and vice versa). This ensures that the patient holds his eye still during testing. If the patient cannot see the examiner's eye, he is asked to stare in the direction of the examiner's face while an assessment of the peripheral visual field is made. The examiner is in an ideal position to see if the patient has to move his eye to find the test object.

3. The test pin (usually the 5 mm. white) is brought in along a series of arcs to a point some 18 inches in front of the patient's eye. If an arc from behind were not used the patient's temporal field would extend to infinity if the test object was large enough. The pin should be brought in from "round the corner" of the patient's field—from four directions, NE., SE., SW. and NW. This will be bound to pick up any field defect in either the upper or lower temporal or nasal fields.

4. The close control that the examiner has over the whole proceedings enables quick repeat testing to be performed and "pseudo" field defects due to bushy eyebrows or a large nose are quickly detected. Quite often field defects due to these problems are accidentally recorded on a standard perimeter. Merely tilting the patient's head from the line of the obstructing organ will solve the problem.

5. If any defect is difficult to interpret, on an organic basis, as a cross check on the patient's reliability the patient's blind spot should be found and compared with the examiner's own blind spot.

Figure 3.1. Visual Field Testing by Confrontation

Bring object in from this position in an arc, and on same arc from the nasal side as shown

Subject

Hand holds eye closed, steadies subject's head and determines distance

Fixation point

Subject co-operation may be checked by comparison of blind spots

Examiner

The results should be recorded *as seen by the patient* which means reversing the defect as seen by the examiner during confrontation testing. To further avoid confusion the right and left fields should be clearly indicated and a factual note added as to the nature of the field defect made; i.e. right homonymous hemianopia, or bitemporal upper quadrantic hemianopia etc. The different terms are illustrated in Figure 3.2.

APPLICATION OF CONFRONTATION TESTING TO SPECIFIC CLINICAL SITUATIONS

1. The Patient who has Noticed a "Hole" in his Vision

Small scotomas are often noticed by accident while the patient is reading a notice or looking at a clock (a scotoma is a small patch of visual loss in the visual field). The onset always appears to be abrupt as it is invariably *noticed* suddenly by the patient. An exception occurs when an embolus impacts in the central retinal artery and then moves peripherally. Abrupt blindness followed by a diminishing

deficit can usually be described on a minute-to-minute basis by an intelligent patient and leaves no doubt as to both the acuteness of onset and the nature of the problem.

Faced with this symptom it is best to allow the patient to find the defect himself by moving the white pin about in his own visual field. Once the position is found the size and shape of the defect can be established by moving the pin in and out of the blind area. Special attention should be paid to whether: (1) the defect crosses the horizontal meridian (retinal lesions due to a vascular occlusion do not do so), (2) the defect extends to the blind spot (defects due to B_{12} deficiency, toxins, or glaucoma usually extend into it), (3) the defect crosses the vertical meridian (organic visual field defects due to pathway damage usually show a sharp vertical edge).

2. The Patient with "Blurred Vision in One Eye"

The examiner should ask the patient to look in the general direction of his eye if the patient's visual acuity is too poor to actually see it. Then, working outwards from the defect with a 5 mm. white pin, the examiner should try to establish the size and shape of the scotoma. If the pin is not seen at all, two

Figure 3.2. Field Defect Nomenclature

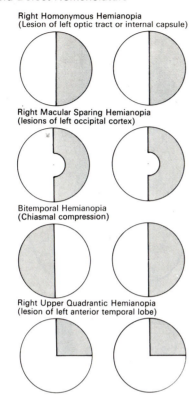

Right Homonymous Hemianopia
(Lesion of left optic tract or internal capsule)

Right Macular Sparing Hemianopia
(lesions of left occipital cortex)

Bitemporal Hemianopia
(Chiasmal compression)

Right Upper Quadrantic Hemianopia
(lesion of left anterior temporal lobe)

deterioration occurs in the course of an ongoing visual failure ophthalmoscopy will often reveal the presence of optic atrophy. If optic atrophy is found, however poor the visual acuity, the fields *must* be tested. Chiasmal compression may be misdiagnosed as retrobulbar neuritis or tobacco amblyopia if the fields are *not* tested. Patients with chiasmal compression often develop severe but unrecognised bitemporal field defects and seek advice only when central vision becomes acutely impaired. If a bitemporal field defect is detected urgent investigation to exclude a lesion compressing the optic chiasm is mandatory.

CASE REPORT

A 36-year-old patient had been investigated for infertility and subsequently became pregnant following the use of Clomiphen. During the pregnancy she became toxaemic with a blood pressure as high as 200/120. In the 34th week she developed rapidly progressive visual failure initially thought to be due to the hypertension. On neurological examination both optic discs were pale but there was no suspicion of papillaedema or haemorrhage into the maculae. Although visual acuity was less than 6/60, using hand movements and finger counting it was obvious that she had a dense bitemporal hemianopia due to chiasmal compression. The child was delivered by caesarean section immediately and the chiasm explored the next day. The remnants of a pituitary tumour were found admixed with blood clots. Following this her vision became normal and the premature infant developed normally. Any delay in recognition of the clinical situation could have resulted in permanent blindness.

Testing for a bitemporal field defect involves the standard routine except that the red pin is particularly helpful. The typical defect resulting from damage to the chiasm is a bitemporal hemianopia. In the early stages this may be a defect to a *red* object only. The patient may describe the red pin as appearing to be grey in the affected half field changing to red as it crosses into the intact nasal half field. Many normal people notice that the red pin is a duller red in the temporal field and that it is appreciably brighter in the nasal field; this is a physiological variation without significance. Later in the course of the disease the defect extends to cause complete loss of recognition of a white pin in the temporal fields and finally finger and even hand movements will not be detected as the defect becomes complete.

Even at this late stage if the chiasm is compressed from below, (by a pituitary lesion) the upper half of the temporal field may be completely lost but some hand movements may be detected in the lower half field, or vice versa in the case of chiasmal compression from above and behind (by a craniopharyngioma), (see Figures 3.6 and 3.13 for explanation).

or three fingers held still should be tried and finally, if all else fails, a moving hand should be brought in from the periphery. If the examiner can establish that there is a rim of intact peripheral vision, however poor it is, then the patient has a central scotoma, usually implying either retrobulbar neuritis or optic nerve compression (see below). Once a central scotoma in one eye is detected it is essential to test the peripheral field of the *good* eye, looking for a defect in the upper temporal field. If such a defect is present, it is highly likely that the optic nerve is compressed, (see Figure 3.11 for explanation). This is known as a junctional scotoma.

3. The Patient with Sudden Visual Deterioration in Both Eyes

Acute *bilateral* inflammation of the optic nerve (retrobulbar neuritis) may occur but is unusual. The two important conditions to be excluded are severe bilateral papilloedema due to any cause or the rapidly progressive phase of visual deterioration in a patient with optic chiasmal compression.

Papilloedema alone does not affect central vision but when a haemorrhage or exudate occurs into the macula area of the retina rapid visual failure will occur. This possibility can be readily excluded by fundal examination. If sudden

Figure 3.11. Intracranial Optic Nerve Compression

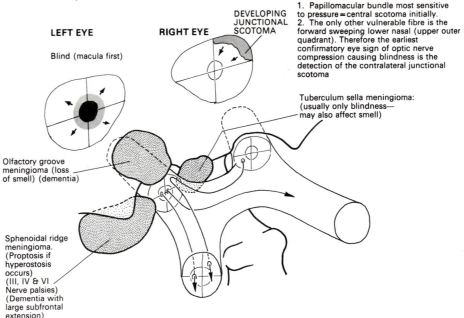

LEFT EYE

Blind (macula first)

RIGHT EYE

DEVELOPING JUNCTIONAL SCOTOMA

Olfactory groove meningioma (loss of smell) (dementia)

Sphenoidal ridge meningioma. (Proptosis if hyperostosis occurs) (III, IV & VI Nerve palsies) (Dementia with large subfrontal extension)

Tuberculum sella meningioma: (usually only blindness— may also affect smell)

Features:
1. Papillomacular bundle most sensitive to pressure = central scotoma initially.
2. The only other vulnerable fibre is the forward sweeping lower nasal (upper outer quadrant). Therefore the earliest confirmatory eye sign of optic nerve compression causing blindness is the detection of the contralateral junctional scotoma

up to his eye and discovered he could not see. He had accidentally discovered he had become blind in the right eye. This proved to be due to optic nerve compression by a meningioma.

Any central scotoma that is discovered accidentally or any "acute retrobulbar neuritis" that does not recover should be regarded as due to optic nerve compression until proved otherwise.

An important part of the initial and follow-up examinations is a search for an early field cut in the opposite eye due to damage to the decussating fibres that loop forward into the optic nerve. This is known as the anterior chiasmal Syndrome of Traquir.

In all cases the sense of smell and the functioning of cranial nerves III, V, VI and the corneal reflex should be carefully tested.

c. *Optic Nerve Glioma*

Malignant gliomas in the optic nerve, optic chiasm or optic tract mainly occur in children or in patients with neurofibromatosis. The visual defect produced by a glioma in the optic nerve is usually a "hole" in vision which may occur anywhere in the field. Optic atrophy is usually well established by the time that the defect is noticed and x-rays may reveal evidence of enlargement of one or both optic foraminae. Gliomas in the optic chiasm or optic tract produce the typical field defects of lesions in these areas.

d. *Metastatic Disease*

The optic nerve may be secondarily involved by local or remote malignant disease including the malignant lymphomas.

4. Optic Chiasm Lesions

The anatomy of the chiasm has already been indicated in detail in Figure 3.6. From a practical point of view four anatomical features are important.

a. The optic chiasm does not lie on the tuberculum sellae as is often thought but is usually situated above and behind the pituitary gland and the dorsum sellae (Figure 3.12). There is some anatomical variation in the exact position which may cause variations in the field defect. The position described and discussed is that most frequently reported.

b. The central papillo-macular bundle is less vulnerable to compression in the chiasm and visual defects usually spread in from the periphery to involve macular vision late in the course of the disease.

c. The lower nasal fibres (upper temporal fields) cross low and anteriorly in the chiasm and are damaged by lesions arising in the pituitary fossa.

d. The upper nasal fibres (lower temporal fields) cross high and posteriorly in the chiasm and are damaged by lesions damaging the chiasm above and behind— notably craniopharyngiomas.

a. *Anterior Chiasmal Lesions* (Figure 3.11)

The junction of the optic nerve and the chiasm may be damaged from any direction. Meningiomas commonly arise from the densely adherent dura mater in this region and cause progressive visual failure in one eye with loss of sense of smell and/or lesions of cranial nerves III, IV, V and VI. The visual field loss includes a peripheral defect in the opposite eye (the anterior chiasmal syndrome of Traquir).

b. *Chiasmal Lesions*

The basic field defect is a bitemporal hemianopia—the patient is in effect wearing "blinkers". The defect may develop very insidiously with later abrupt visual failure as the presenting symptom. In both sexes endocrine dysfunction usually antedates visual symptoms by many years. In the male impotence and in the female secondary amenorrhoea are the main endocrine symptoms.

In addition to chromophobe adenomas (non-functioning pituitary tumours), eosinophil adenomas (secreting growth hormone and causing acromegaly), aneurysms of the carotid syphon, and chordomas arising from notochord remnants in the dorsum sella may all produce identical syndromes. It is always wise to perform full plain x-rays, angiography and pneumo-encephalography *before* surgical exploration to exclude these other lesions. All cause a bitemporal hemianopia, that spreads down from *upper* field into the lower field (Figure 3.13).

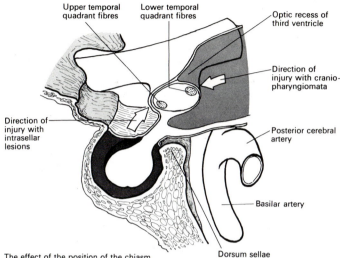

Figure 3.12. Relationship of the Optic Chiasm to the Third Ventricle and Hypophysis Cerebri

The effect of the position of the chiasm and the decussating fibres in it lead to three general points of great clinical importance:
1. Pressure causes bitemporal defects in vision
2. Lesions arising in the sella cause a defect starting in upper quadrants
3. Lesions arising behind or above the sella cause defects starting in lower quadrants

Figure 3.13. Chiasmal Compression from below

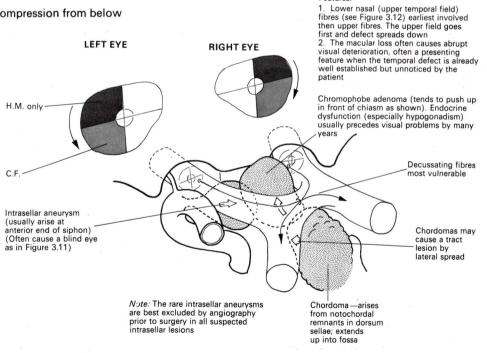

Features:
1. Lower nasal (upper temporal field) fibres (see Figure 3.12) earliest involved then upper fibres. The upper field goes first and defect spreads down
2. The macular loss often causes abrupt visual deterioration, often a presenting feature when the temporal defect is already well established but unnoticed by the patient

Chromophobe adenoma (tends to push up in front of chiasm as shown). Endocrine dysfunction (especially hypogonadism) usually precedes visual problems by many years

Decussating fibres most vulnerable

Chordomas may cause a tract lesion by lateral spread

Note: The rare intrasellar aneurysms are best excluded by angiography prior to surgery in all suspected intrasellar lesions

Chordoma—arises from notochordal remnants in dorsum sellae; extends up into fossa

Craniopharyngiomas which press on the chiasm from above and behind cause three distinct syndromes in addition to the visual problem, which consists of a bitemporal hemianopia spreading up from the *lower* fields into the upper fields (Figure 3.14).

These are:

a. In infancy the tumour may cause pituitary dwarfism.
b. In adulthood progressive visual failure occurs with variable pituitary dysfunction.
c. In old age a craniopharyngioma may block the third ventricle causing hydrocephalus, and producing dementia and progressive visual failure secondary to papilloedema.

c. *Lateral Chiasmal Compression* (Figure 3.15)

Lateral compression of the chiasm is relatively rare. The most frequent cause is dilatation of the intra-cavernous part of an arterio-sclerotic carotid artery. This condition occurs more frequently in females.

The defect is usually unilateral but may become bilateral if the chiasm is pushed across against the opposite carotid artery. If the onset is abrupt the visual problem is usually combined with a blood-shot eye and extra-ocular nerve palsies (Chapter 5). Another possible mechanism is dilatation of the third ventricle in association with chronic aqueductal stenosis or blockage of the fourth ventricle outflow. The chiasm is splayed laterally by the dilating third ventricle and is damaged by the pulsatile carotid arteries pressing against its lateral edges.

5. Optic Tract Lesions (Figure 3.15)

Optic tract lesions produce incongruous homonymous hemianopias, (incongruous defects are those in which the shape of the defect is different in the two half fields (see Figure 3.2). Although incongruity can usually be established on confrontation testing, minor degrees are best demonstrated by formal screen testing. The importance of demonstrating incongruity is that a tract lesion is almost invariably the cause if incongruity is marked. Pituitary tumours, craniopharyngiomas, chordomas and meningiomas may all produce tract lesions. Often the cerebral peduncle on the same side is damaged and mild pyramidal signs in the opposite limb may be detected. Multiple sclerosis can produce a tract lesion but this is quite rare.

All pre-geniculate visual pathway lesions cause variability in the density of the defect with the possibility of progression from a simple field defect to a red pin, to a defect also to a white pin, and finally to the inability to detect even hand movements as the defect becomes complete. Detecting early

defects requires considerable knowledge and some degree of skill but is extremely rewarding as early diagnosis really does have value in these situations.

When we come to consider lesions affecting the post-geniculate visual pathways, the situation is quite different. With the exception of attention hemianopias the defects are absolute and variable degrees of loss of vision are not seen. Therefore a 5 mm. white pin is all that is necessary to document the defect.

LESIONS AFFECTING THE VISUAL RADIATIONS

1. Optic Peduncle Lesions

Because the fibres emerging from the lateral geniculate body sweep over the trigone of the lateral ventricles, lying below and behind the capsular region (see also Chapter 9), field defects are *not* a feature of a simple capsular cerebral vascular accident. This region of the visual radiation is most often damaged by occlusion of one of the thalamo-geniculate arteries arising from the posterior cerebral artery. This produces a clinical picture which includes an homonymous hemianopia with hemi-sensory loss (posterior thalamic damage) and a very mild motor deficit which usually recovers, presumably due to oedema of the adjacent motor pathways in the internal capsule (see Chapter 9).

2. Temporal Lobe Lesions

The fibres carrying visual information from the upper temporal fields sweep forwards and downwards into the temporal lobe in what is known as Meyer's loop. In the anterior loop there is some splaying of the fibres so that an incongruous defect can be produced but this is usually of minimal degree and once the fibres have looped round to pass posteriorly, congruous defects are the rule. (A congruous defect is one which however bizarre the shape, the defect is identical in both eyes.) In patients suspected of harbouring a temporal lobe lesion careful evaluation of the upper visual fields is indicated.

3. Parietal Lobe Lesions

The part of the visual radiation lying in the anterior part of parietal lobe is carrying information from the lower visual fields. Therefore a lesion in the anterior parietal part of the radiation will produce a lower quadrantic hemianopia. This is an extremely rare field defect only encountered on one occasion by the writer, the patient being an eight-year-old boy with a cerebral abscess. These fibres are quickly rejoined

Figure 3.14. Chiasmal Compression from above

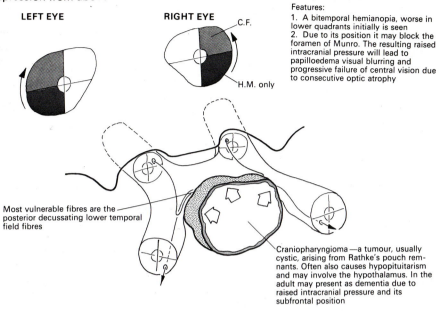

LEFT EYE

RIGHT EYE

C.F.

H.M. only

Features:
1. A bitemporal hemianopia, worse in lower quadrants initially is seen
2. Due to its position it may block the foramen of Munro. The resulting raised intracranial pressure will lead to papilloedema visual blurring and progressive failure of central vision due to consecutive optic atrophy

Most vulnerable fibres are the posterior decussating lower temporal field fibres

Craniopharyngioma—a tumour, usually cystic, arising from Rathke's pouch remnants. Often also causes hypopituitarism and may involve the hypothalamus. In the adult may present as dementia due to raised intracranial pressure and its subfrontal position

Figure 3.15. Lateral Chiasmal and Optic tract Compression

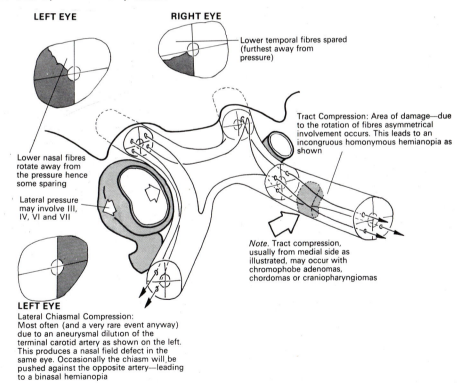

LEFT EYE

RIGHT EYE

Lower temporal fibres spared (furthest away from pressure)

Tract Compression: Area of damage—due to the rotation of fibres asymmetrical involvement occurs. This leads to an incongruous homonymous hemianopia as shown

Lower nasal fibres rotate away from the pressure hence some sparing

Lateral pressure may involve III, IV, VI and VII

Note. Tract compression, usually from medial side as illustrated, may occur with chromophobe adenomas, chordomas or craniopharyngiomas

LEFT EYE

Lateral Chiasmal Compression:
Most often (and a very rare event anyway) due to an aneurysmal dilution of the terminal carotid artery as shown on the left. This produces a nasal field defect in the same eye. Occasionally the chiasm will be pushed against the opposite artery—leading to a binasal hemianopia

by the upper field fibres sweeping up from the temporal lobe and more typically a parietal lesion damages *all* the fibres causing a complete homonymous hemianopia.

Attention hemianopias are due to peripheral parietal lesions and have been fully discussed earlier in this chapter.

4. Lesions of the Anterior Visual Cortex

The peripheral visual fields are represented in the most anterior part of the calcarine cortex. The blood supply of this area is derived from the posterior cerebral artery. Occlusion of this vessel causes infarction of this area and produces a macular sparing hemianopia. The other rare cause of this particular field defect is a meningioma of the tentorium cerebelli pressing against this area of the cortex. Vascular occlusions in this area occur quite commonly in migraine and in general a macular sparing hemianopia does not require extensive investigation. Bilateral infarction of this area leads to tunnel vision with a small ring of two to five degrees of intact vision. This is extremely disabling as patients can see only objects in the direct line of vision and cannot scan to an object in the peripheral fields, even though the visual acuity is quite normal. This may follow cerebral air or fat embolism. Non-organic tunnel vision is occasionally encountered in hysteria and is discussed below.

5. Lesions of the Macular Cortex

If the tip of one occipital pole is damaged a congruous, homonymous and extremely small hemianopia is produced. It is thought that the occipital pole has an independent blood supply from the middle cerebral artery and that this accounts for macular sparing in the posterior cerebral arterial occlusions discussed in section 4. For the same reason occasionally small hemianopic field defects may result from failure of this separate blood supply.

NON-ORGANIC VISUAL FIELD DEFECTS

The most frequently encountered field defect due to malingering or hysteria is tunnel vision or a generalised constriction of the visual field. This may vary in size during testing to the extent of producing a spiral field loss which is diagnostic of hysteria. The defect is best evaluated by using different test objects at different distances. In an organic field defect the size of the intact field increases as the distance increases. In nonorganic loss the defect remains the same size and could perhaps be more accurately called tubular vision (see Figure 3.16).

VISUAL HALLUCINATIONS

Damage to the visual pathways may cause irritative phenomena, appreciated by the patient as flashes of light or colour. More complicated visual images are usually the result of abnormal activity in visual association areas, in particular in the temporal lobes.

Retinal damage is perhaps the most familiar, as in the universal experience of "seeing stars" after a blow to the eye. Damage or ischaemia of the retina causes hallucinations confined to one eye, consisting of unformed "flashes" or "speckles" of light, like stars on a dark background. This is often the last phase of a syncopal attack before loss of consciousness and gives rise to the term "black-out". Similar disturbances of vision in one eye also occur at the onset of a migraine headache. Oedema of the retina due to central serous retinitis causes metamorphopsia (an undulating shape) and alterations in colour perception, but this is a visual aberration rather than an hallucination. Jaundice and digitalis overdose may alter colour perception so that everything appears yellow.

Optic nerve, chiasm and tract lesions do *not* cause visual hallucinations. Although complex visual hallucinations have been reported in patients with chiasmal lesions due to tumours it seems likely that these were due to simultaneous damage to the hypothalamus or medial temporal lobes caused by the same lesion.

Visual hallucinations due to occipital pole ischaemia, or due to seizures originating in this area consist of unformed blobs of colour—usually in the red-orange end of the spectrum. Undoubtedly the most common cause is ischaemia of the occipital poles occurring during or preceding a migraine attack. It is also quite possible for a patient to have repeated attacks of this sort without necessarily developing the headache and patients in this category should be kept

Figure 3.16. Diagram to illustrate Non-Organic Tunnel Vision

Note. The shaded area represents the intact visual field

1m

2m

In organic tunnel vision the size of the field at 2 metres is much larger than at 1 metre, whereas in non-organic tunnel vision the defect does not change size, as indicated under careful review. The hallucination may be hemianopic or bilateral and consist of zig-zag lines or circular lines on a dark background, like a plan of a castle, the hallucination that is also called "fortification spectra". Red and orange blobs that may alter in size and seem to explode are often described. Another variant is a sensation as if rain were running down a window pane in one half of vision. This may persist for several hours.

Formed visual images, still pictures like a tableaux, or micropsia or macropsia, where the surroundings seem to get very small or very large, are a feature of temporal lobe epileptic phenomena or occur during migrainous vascular spasm, in which there is ischaemia of the medial temporal lobe. It has been suggested that the idea for "Alice in Wonderland" was the result of macropsia during a migraine attack experienced by Lewis Carroll. One patient seen recently by the writer suffered an episode of this type as she arrived at a cross roads. The distance to the other side seemed vast and she sat in the car too frightened to move until the hallucination passed off. The static tableaux type of hallucination is known as *"déjà vu"*. These are extremely brief and consist of a feeling of familiarity with a scene that is abruptly "frozen". Typical attacks last a split second only and occur occasionally in normal people. In some patients with temporal lobe epilepsy they may occur many times a day and sometimes culminate in a seizure. More complicated and persisting visual hallucinations may occur as part of a temporal lobe attack, but occur more frequently in toxic confusional states or schizophrenia.

A feature of visual hallucinosis is that there is no detectable field defect even during the attack. However, if the hallucinations occur during the onset of ischaemic damage a defect may be detectable after the episode.

Figure 4.3. Deep Optic Cup simulating Papilloedema

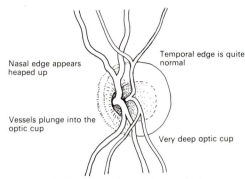

Nasal edge appears heaped up

Temporal edge is quite normal

Vessels plunge into the optic cup

Very deep optic cup

This appearance is very often mistakenly described as papilloedema. In papilloedema the cup is the first part of the disc to fill and become abnormal

Figure 4.4. Medullated Nerve Fibres

Normally nerve fibres are bare beyond the lamina cribrosa. Sometimes they are myelinated on the disc or even on to the retina as in this case

The appearance is typically flared and careful focusing will usually reveal the fibres traversing the area. This abnormality will produce a field defect as it obscures the retinal cells. The patient is unaware of the defect as it is present from birth

Papilloedema is often suspected but seldom confirmed. The early changes are very subjective, but the recent advent of fluoroscein retinal angiography has enabled the problem to be resolved in many cases. One should never rely on the absence of papilloedema as an absolute indication that intracranial pressure is not raised.

Causes of Papilloedema

Although a full discussion of the causes of papilloedema is inappropriate to the discussion of fundal appearances, a list of common causes is given in Table 2.

It should be noticed that the causes are not exclusively neurological. Raised intracranial pressure due to any mass lesion in the brain is the main cause, but conditions interfering with the circulation of the C.S.F., such as aqueductal stenosis and congenital anomalies in the posterior fossa, should always be considered.

There are a variety of other causes in many of which the mechanism of the papilloedema is obscure. In some cases a high C.S.F. protein or altered blood products block C.S.F. reabsorption by the arachnoid granulations. In some instances diffuse brain swelling is responsible and in others impaired venous drainage of the brain or of the retina itself is the cause. The common causes of central retinal vein thrombosis are therefore included in the table.

Table 2

CAUSES OF PAPILLOEDEMA:

1. Raised intracranial pressure due to mass lesions.
2. Raised intracranial pressure due to circulatory block
   —aqueductal stenosis.
   —intraventricular tumours.
   —fourth ventricle outflow block.
3. Due to cerebral oedema—post-head-injury.
   —post-cerebral anoxia.
   —benign intracranial hypertension
   —lead poisoning
   —steroid withdrawal
   —Vitamin A intoxication.
4. Due to raised C.S.F. protein or altered blood products
   —post-subarachnoid haemorrhage
   —post-meningitis
   —Guillain—Barre syndrome
   —hypertrophic polyneuritis
   —spinal cord tumours
5. The malignant phase of hypertension.
6. Metabolic disorders—hypercapnia.
   —hypocalcaemia in childhood in particular.
   —malignant thyrotoxic exopthalmos.
7. Disorders of the circulation including central retinal vein thrombosis
   —lateral sinus thrombosis.
   —jugular vein thrombosis.
   —superior vena caval obstruction.
   —polycythaemia rubra vera.
   —multiple myelomatosis.
   —macroglobulinaemia.
   —diabetes mellitus.
   —hyperlipidaemia.
   —arteriosclerotic vessels in the retina.
   —vasculitis, including temporal arteritis.

2. Secondary Optic Atrophy

If the patient survives the cause of his papilloedema, further changes may appear in the optic disc following subsidence of the papilloedema which may take six to ten weeks. Occasionally general physicians may seek neurological advice if papilloedema has not resolved within a few days of a patient receiving effective anti-hypertensive therapy. This concern is quite unnecessary: at least six weeks may elapse before significant resolution is apparent.

Even while disc swelling is still obvious, the nerve head may start to become a greyish white colour and the patient may notice decreasing visual acuity. Finally as the swelling subsides the patient is left with a flat greyish-white nerve head with very indistinct edges. This scarring process in the nerve head may lead to further serious deterioration of vision long after raised intracranial pressure has subsided. The earliest possible relief of raised pressure is therefore indicated, but no confident prognosis for vision can be given to a patient who has evidence of optic atrophy or decreased acuity when first seen. This is called consecutive or secondary optic atrophy.

3. Primary Optic Atrophy

Following any toxic insult, injury, occlusion of the central retinal artery, compressive, infiltrative or demyelinating process affecting the optic nerve, the patient may develop primary optic atrophy. The nerve head becomes extremely pale and the lamina cribosa becomes very distinct. Again, this is an extremely subjective impression and doubtful cases are often recorded as "slight pallor of discs". Many patients incorrectly suspected of suffering from multiple sclerosis have been diagnosed using this highly subjective sign as corroboratory evidence—a very unwise policy.

The normal variation in disc colour is considerable. The temporal edge of the disc is relatively avascular and always looks pale compared with the nasal half of the disc. The lamina cribrosa is often well marked and forms a very pale central area of the disc. The pallor of a normal disc may be accentuated by the rim of pigment that is often seen at the temporal edge of the disc caused by the slight retraction of the retina that occurs developmentally (Figures 4.5 and 4.6).

The visual acuity and the visual field to red are often normal and do not alone disprove the diagnosis of primary optic atrophy. The diagnosis remains an extremely subjective one although recent advances using visual evoked responses provide additional evidence of optic nerve damage.

4. Miscellaneous

1. Patients with decreasing visual acuity may have macular degeneration and a close inspection of the macular (to be

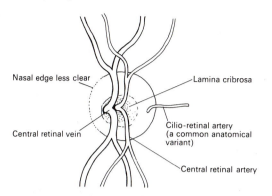

Figure 4.5. Normal Optic Disc

Nasal edge less clear

Central retinal vein

Lamina cribrosa

Cilio-retinal artery (a common anatomical variant)

Central retinal artery

Figure 4.6. Pigment Rim simulating Optic Atrophy

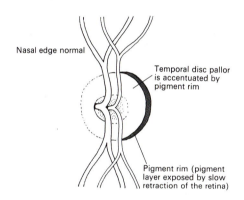

Nasal edge normal

Temporal disc pallor is accentuated by pigment rim

Pigment rim (pigment layer exposed by slow retraction of the retina)

found two disc diameters from the temporal edge of the disc) is necessary. This requires dilatation of the pupil in most instances. The normal macular is a small pale yellow spot in a slightly darker area of the retina and expert opthalmological advice is necessary for full evaluation of this region.

2. Patients with transient ischaemic attacks may have evidence of embolisation of the retinal vessels. Small highly refractile fragments of cholesterol may be seen blocking arterioles usually at the bifurcations. Distally the vessels appear pale and empty.

3. Patients with night blindness, children with epilepsy and patients with several inherited neurological disorders may have retinitis pigmentosa. This consists of spiderlike nets of pigment that are initially seen at the periphery of the retina. They may be associated with a degree of primary optic atrophy secondary to destruction of the retinal cells in these pigmented areas. Later peripheral constriction of the fields occurs with optic atrophy. Marked narrowing of the arterioles is an important diagnostic feature.

4. Rapid loss of central vision, often described by the patient as if a red or orange ball were present in front of the eye with persistent after images, metamorphopsia or micropsia, are features of a disease known as central serous retinopathy. In this condition there is marked oedema and heaping up of the retina, causing the distortion of vision. The condition occurs mainly in young males and responds to steroids. Very brief attacks of metamorphopsia are usually due to temporal lobe disorders.

Ophthalmoscopy requires a certain amount of skill. Once the skill is acquired a considerable degree of familiarity with normal fundal appearances is necessary to detect minor but possibly significant abnormalities. In many instances the interpretation of appearances is highly subjective and it is wrong to place too much reliance on disputed appearances unless corroboratory evidence using flouroscein angiography or visual evoked potentials confirms the suspected abnormality.

Chapter 5

THE THIRD, FOURTH AND SIXTH CRANIAL NERVES

These three cranial nerves control the upper eyelid, eye movements and pupils and have long intracranial courses. Due to the latter feature they are subject to damage by a wide range of disease processes at various sites. A careful history and clinical examination usually provides all the information necessary for accurate diagnosis. Difficulty in remembering the actions of the various extraocular muscles and their nerve supply is a universal problem and therefore these features are covered extensively in this chapter.

THE EXTRA-OCULAR MUSCLES

The names, positions and actions of the extra-ocular muscles are illustrated and discussed in Figures 5.1–5.4.

The main points to note are:

1. The medial rectus muscle of one eye and the lateral rectus muscle of the other work as a pair to produce lateral eye movements. The central mechanism responsible for synchronising these actions is fully discussed in Chapter 7.
2. The vertically acting rectus muscles are most effective when the eye is abducted (i.e. looking outwards) as in this position the line of pull of the muscles is along the vertical axis of the eye.

3. In the same way the oblique muscles are maximally effective when the eye is adducted (i.e. looking inwards) as their line of pull is then along the vertical axis of the eye.

These are the only important points to remember when evaluating eye movements from a neurological standpoint. All the muscles have secondary actions and some have torsional effects. It is probably because these other movements are given such emphasis in anatomical textbooks that so few can understand or remember the simple facts needed for an adequate neurological examination!

DIPLOPIA

The single symptom that indicates damage to one or other of the three nerves under discussion is diplopia. This should not be taken to imply that diplopia is *always* due to a nerve lesion. A discussion of other causes of diplopia will be found at the end of this chapter.

Explanation of Diplopia

The eyes are normally positioned so that the image falls on exactly the same spot on the retina of each eye. The slightest displacement of either eye causes diplopia as the image is

Figure 5.1. The Actions of the Extraocular Muscles

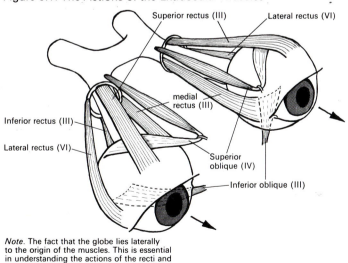

Note. The fact that the globe lies laterally to the origin of the muscles. This is essential in understanding the actions of the recti and obliques

Figure 5.2. The Actions of the Medial and Lateral Recti (lateral gaze to R side)

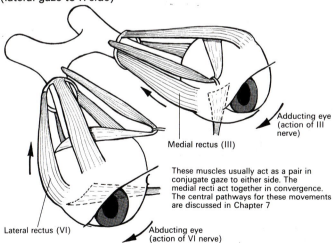

These muscles usually act as a pair in conjugate gaze to either side. The medial recti act together in convergence. The central pathways for these movements are discussed in Chapter 7

Figure 5.3

When the eye is adducted by the medial rectus the line of pull of the superior oblique becomes ideal to pull the globe up and over from behind. It is the main depressor of the adducted eye

In the primary position if the superior oblique could act alone, INTORSION would be produced. In actual fact this is only visible when a total III nerve paralysis leaves the eye free to rotate in this way

With eye abducted the inferior rectus is a strong depressor as above

Figure 5.4

With the eye adducted the inferior oblique pulls the eye from below and behind and rotates it upwards. It is the main elevator of the adducted eye

Superior rectus (III)

In the primary position if the eye were free to rotate the inferior oblique would produce EXTORSION
This movement has no useful clinical application as a lesion purely affecting this muscle is very unusual (the involvement of the other III nerve innervated muscles dominating the signs)

The superior rectus is now in the ideal position to elevate the eye upwards and outwards (i.e. directly along the axis of the muscle). It is therefore the main elevator of the abducted eye

Figure 5.5. Diagram to show the Mechanism of Diplopia
(a L VI nerve palsy is illustrated)

On looking to the L. the L. eye remains static. As the object moves the image falls on the retina to the nasal side and is projected further and further into the temporal half field, away from the macula

On gazing to the R. both eyes move sufficiently to keep the object on the macula of each eye

Straight ahead gaze—eyes hold object on the macula

The rules are:
The false image is always the outer one
The false image always comes from the affected eye

shifted to a different position on the retina of the displaced eye (confirm this by displacing one eye by gently pressing it through the eyelid).

In the case of nerve lesions the weak muscle or muscles can usually be detected by direct observation of the eye movements. Occasionally, mild lesions or other diseases may cause diplopia in which the degree of weakness is too slight to be observed. In these situations the *cover test* is useful. This test is based on the fact that the separation of the two images becomes greatest as the eyes attempt to look in the direction of the weak muscle, because the disparity in eye movements is then maximal. The false image falls progressively further away from the macula of the lagging eye and the false image is therefore *always* the *outer* image of the two. If the examiner asks the patient to follow a stick until double vision is maximal and then determines which eye he must cover to obliterate the outer image, the affected eye is identified. From the direction of the gaze the weak muscle can be determined (see Figure 5.5).

1. Third Nerve Palsy (Figure 5.6)

A complete third nerve lesion causes total paralysis of the eyelid, and diplopia *only* when the lid is held up. Severe diplopia then occurs in all directions *except* on lateral gaze to the side of the third nerve lesion (because the lateral rectus muscle is intact).

When the lid is lifted the eye will be found deviated outwards (lateral rectus action) and downwards (secondary depressant action of the superior oblique muscle). The integrity of these muscles and hence their nerve supply should be carefully evaluated to be certain that the third nerve is the only nerve affected.

To do this the examiner should test lateral gaze in the affected eye and note the disappearance of diplopia in that direction. The normal downward movement produced by the superior oblique muscle *cannot* be tested because the paralysed medial rectus does not allow the eye to adduct. Instead the secondary action of the muscle is observed. The depression of the eye is usually already apparent. If the patient makes a further effort to look downwards the eye will rotate inwards (intorsion) as the superior oblique muscle pulls sideways across the eye when it is in this position. Observation of this movement is the best evidence of an intact superior oblique muscle and hence the integrity of the IVth nerve.

The pupil may be normal or dilated and fixed to light. This important feature is fully discussed later.

2. Fourth Nerve Palsy (Figure 5.7)

A fourth nerve lesion causes weakness of the superior oblique muscle with very subtle diplopia. The weakness of the muscle in the primary position (looking straight ahead) allows the eye to rotate slightly outwards (extorsion). The very slight slant of the image will make the patient tilt his head slightly away from the side of the affected eye to line up the image from the normal eye. In children this head tilt may be misdiagnosed as torticollis. Frank diplopia occurs when the patient looks down and away from the side of the affected eye. This often leads to trouble going downstairs as two treads are seen when the patient looks downwards and sideways, as one normally does while descending stairs. Similarly, diplopia may occur while reading a newspaper or a book.

Figure 5.6. To show ptosis in complete III nerve palsy
(The eyelid sags passively—the eye can be shut tightly via the VII nerve)

Figure 5.7. To show the compensatory head tilt in a patient with a superior oblique paralysis of the right eye

To show the position of the eye when the lid is lifted
The eye is abducted (intact VI) and slightly depressed (intact IV). The pupil is dilated

To confirm intact IV nerve; note the inward rotation (intorsion) of the eye when the patient attempts to look down. This is the rotary action of the superior oblique that occurs when the eye cannot be abducted ADDUCTED

The patient has tilted his head to the L. to line up the image from the good eye with the outwardly rotated R. eye

Normally the superior oblique, by pulling across the top of the eye, slightly rotates it inwards
If paralysed the eye will rotate slightly outwards causing a slightly oblique image

Figure 5.8. To show voluntary eye closure to obliterate double vision with a VI nerve palsy of the left eye

(The lid is not ptosed—the eye is tightly shut)

To show the position of the eye when open
The affected eye is deviated towards the nose.
To prevent diplopia the patient may turn the head until the right eye is sufficiently abducted to give a single image

3. Sixth Nerve Palsy (Figure 5.8)

A sixth nerve palsy causes the greatest problem as there is no ptosis to obliterate the false image. Occasionally patients will deliberately shut the affected eye to prevent the diplopia and this can be misinterpreted as ptosis. If the examiner closes the normal eyelid, the lid on the side of the "pseudo-ptosis" will revert to a normal position. At rest the affected eye is pulled medially by the unopposed action of the medial rectus muscle. The patient may compensate by turning his head towards the weak muscle.

INTRACRANIAL ANATOMY OF THE THIRD, FOURTH AND SIXTH CRANIAL NERVES
(Figure 5.9)

Note: The nerves run a generally converging course towards the apex of the orbit from widely separate origins in the brain stem.

1. The Third Nerve (Occulomotor Nerve)

The two third nerves emerge together between the cerebral peduncles. They then splay out as they pass anteriorly lying between the posterior cerebral arteries and the superior cerebellar arteries, and then run parallel to the posterior communicating arteries until they enter the cavernous sinus. They then lie between the two layers of dura that form the lateral wall of the sinus. The nerve enters the orbit through the superior orbital fissure and divides into two main branches. The upper branch supplies the eyelid and superior rectus muscle. The lower branch supplies all the other muscles and the pupil.

2. The Fourth Nerve (Trochlear Nerve)

This nerve has several unique features. Its nucleus lies in the dorsum of the brain stem and the fibres decussate (cross over) in the substance of the superior medullary velum so that the right nerve originates in the left trochlear nucleus and vice versa. The nerve runs a very long course leaving the posterior fossa and encircling the brain stem to enter the cavernous sinus. It enters the roof of the orbit and actually crosses the third nerve in order to do so. It derives its name from the fact that the muscle it supplies (the superior oblique) passes round a trochlea (pulley) in the anterior orbital roof.

3. The Sixth Nerve (Abducens Nerve)

This nerve emerges from the front of the brain stem at the ponto-medullary junction, deep in the posterior fossa. It ascends on the front of the brain stem and then angles sharply forwards over the tip of the petrous bone to enter the back of the cavernous sinus. It lies free in the sinus, enters the orbit through the superior orbital fissure, and passes laterally to reach the lateral rectus muscle.

CAUSES OF EXTRA-OCULAR NERVE LESIONS

There are five main sites of potential damage to these nerves as indicated in Figure 5.10.

1. Nuclear and Fascicular Lesions

These will be considered in detail in the chapter on brain stem lesions (Chapter 11). There are usually other evidences of brain stem damage to confirm that this is the site of the lesion and several named syndromes involving these nerves have been described. Causes include brain stem vascular disease, multiple sclerosis, pontine gliomas, poliomyelitis, Wernicke's encephalopathy and congenital maldevelopment of the cranial nerve nuclei.

2. Lesions in the Basilar Area

All three nerves are subject to damage by basal meningeal disease processes. These include tuberculous, fungal and bacterial meningitis, carcinomatous meningitis, direct neoplastic invasion from the sinuses and nasopharynx, meningovascular syphilis, sarcoid, Guillain—Barré syndrome and Herpes Zoster. In many of these conditions there are multiple or bilateral nerve lesions to indicate a diffuse pathological process.

Aneurysmal dilation of the upper basilar artery may also cause multiple nerve palsies and in particular bilateral third nerve lesions.

Figure 5.9. The Intracranial Course and Relations of Cranial Nerves III, IV, V, VI (semi-diagrammatic)

Lateral rectus muscle (abducens nerve VI)

Superior oblique (trochlear nerve IV)

Anterior cerebral arteries

Anterior communicating artery

Optic chiasm

Dorsum sellae

Posterior cerebral artery

Edges of tentorium cerebelli joining behind the upper midbrain, forming the "ridge" of the tent

Superior orbital fissure

Ciliary ganglion (arises from inferior branch of III and joined by naso-ciliary branch of V)

V1
V2
V3

IV
VI
III

V

Carotid artery entering via the carotid canal

Posterior communicating arteries.

Free edge of tentorium cerebelli (note origin from anterior clinoid, the dura arising from the dorsum and diaphragma sella being pierced by the third nerve as it passes laterally—forming the roof of the cavernous sinus)

Figure 5.10. The Anatomical Basis of the various Lesions
Lesions as defined by sites in the text

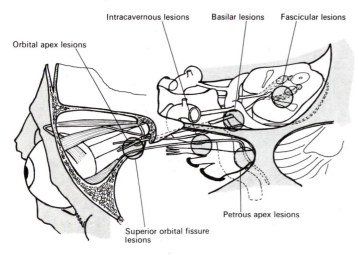

Orbital apex lesions

Intracavernous lesions   Basilar lesions   Fascicular lesions

Petrous apex lesions

Superior orbital fissure lesions

Specific involvement of the third nerve in this area occur in two ways:

1. Direct compression by a posterior communicating artery aneurysm. The onset is usually acute with severe pain and the pupil is almost always affected, and is dilated and fixed to light (Figure 5.11).

2. The nerve may be progressively damaged by the prolapsing temporal lobe, when the hemisphere is displaced by a mass. This is called a tentorial pressure cone.

Figure 5.11. Posterior communicating artery aneurysms

Aneurysms at either end (they typically occur at these sites) are likely to damage III nerve as the artery is immediately adjacent to it

The patient becomes drowsy and the pupil on the affected side becomes dilated, ptosis develops and finally a complete third nerve palsy ensues. (Figure 5.12). A third nerve palsy in this situation is very rarely false-localising (discussed fully in Chapter 23), and urgent surgical intervention is indicated.

The sixth nerve may also be affected in the basal area by increased intracranial pressure but by a different mechanism. This is a situation usually encountered in children and is often false-localising. A tumour in the posterior fossa causes hydrocephalus (dilatation of the ventricles) and the *whole* brain tries to squeeze down through the tentorium. This pushes the brain stem downwards and the sixth nerve becomes stretched over the petrous tip. One or both nerves may be affected in this way by a lesion quite remote from the nerve itself (see Figure 5.12).

Figure 5.12. Diagram to show the different mechanisms underlying III and IV nerve palsies in patients with raised intracranial pressure (seen from front)

III nerve palsy (usually unilateral)

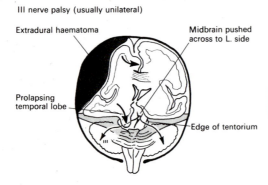

Extradural haematoma

Midbrain pushed across to L. side

Prolapsing temporal lobe

Edge of tentorium

A large extradural haematoma pushes the hemisphere sideways under the falx and downwards through the tentorium. This stretches the third nerve over the edge of the tentorium. This is a very *reliable* localising sign

VI nerve palsy (unilateral or bilateral)

Mass in third ventricle

Petrous tip

Brain stem pushed downwards

A mass in the third ventricle has caused symmetrical dilatation of both lateral ventricles. The entire brain stem is pushed downwards—pulling the VI nerve where it angulates over the petrous tip to enter the cavernous sinus. This is a very *unreliable* sign

3. Lesions at the Petrous Tip

The sixth nerve is clearly the only vulnerable nerve in this area and there are four main causes of damage.

1. Mastoiditis or middle ear infection may cause diffuse inflammation of the petrous bone and thrombosis of the overlying petrosal sinuses. This causes severe ear pain and a combination of sixth, seventh, eighth and occasionally fifth nerve lesions and is known as Gradenigo's syndrome. This must be differentiated from Ramsay-Hunt's syndrome (Geniculate Herpes Zoster) in which there is a vesicular eruption in the ear and a seventh nerve palsy and occasionally other cranial nerve lesions (see also Chapter 6).

2. Lateral sinus thrombosis secondary to mastoiditis may lead to rapidly rising intracranial pressure due to impaired cerebral venous drainage. This may cause a direct or indirect sixth nerve palsy as discussed above. To differentiate this situation from a posterior fossa abscess can be very difficult.

3. Carcinomas of the naso-pharynx or the para-nasal sinuses tend to infiltrate through the fissures of the skull base and a sudden painless sixth nerve palsy may be the first evidence of malignant disease in these tissues.

4. Benign transient sixth nerve palsies may occur in children following mild infections. This diagnosis is difficult to make and only really confirmed by the subsequent recovery, which may take several weeks.

4. Lesions in the Region of the Cavernous Sinus

1. Cavernous sinus thrombosis remains a very serious condition usually occurring as a complication of sepsis of the skin over the upper face or in the paranasal sinuses. As the sixth nerve lies free in the sinus it is the most vulnerable nerve. The sixth nerve palsy is coupled with severe pain, exophthalmus and oedema of the eyelids and later this involves the opposite eyelid as an extension of the thrombosis to the opposite cavernous sinus is almost inevitable.

2. Intrasellar tumours such as chromophobe adenomas may extend laterally into the sinus and then usually damage the third nerve (Figure 5.13).

3. Aneurysmal dilatation of the intracavernous portion of the carotid artery usually occurs in elderly hypertensive females. If the swelling of the artery is at the anterior end of the sinus, oedema of the eyelid, exophthalmos, blindness and a third nerve lesion may occur simultaneously heralded by quite severe pain. If the dilatation is at the posterior end of the sinus, the first division of the fifth nerve may be irritated with severe pain over the fifth nerve distribution (ophthalmic division) and a sixth nerve palsy. Again the eye becomes suffused and proptosed (Figures 5.14, 5.15). If the vessel actually ruptures into the sinus it is rarely fatal as the

Figure 5.13. Intrasellar mass spreading laterally

Optic chiasm compressed. Carotid siphon and nerves displaced laterally— III nerve especially vulnerable

Figure 5.14. Intracavernous aneurysm (anterior type)

Optic nerve compressed (blind eye)

III and IV most likely to be damaged

Venous pressure raised—bloodshot eye

Figure 5.15. Intracavernous aneurysm (posterior type)

VI nerve palsy and pain from V₁ irritation

Venous pressure raised—bloodshot eye

cavernous sinus will contain the haemorrhage, but a severe unilateral and later bilateral pulsatile exophthalmos occurs. This is called a carotico-cavernous fistula and may also follow a head injury if a basal fracture tears the carotid artery at its point of entry into the sinus.

5. Lesions at the Superior Orbital Fissure and Orbital Apex

There are numerous neoplasms that may arise in the posterior orbit and a fairly well-defined syndrome results. These are listed in Table 3. Because all the nerves are relatively close together palsies of the third, fourth and sixth nerves in various combinations may occur. Involvement of the fifth nerve may cause pain and later numbness in the distribution of the first division of the fifth nerve, with depression of the corneal response.

Table 3

TUMOURS ARISING IN THE ORBIT AND OPTIC FORAMINA	
Meningiomas	40%
Haemangiomas	10%
Gliomas	5%
Pseudo-tumour of the orbit	5%
Carcinoma of the lacrimal duct	
Neurofibroma	
Fibrous dysplasia of bone	
Sarcoma	
Epidermoid	
Melanoma	40%
Lipoma	
Hand–Schuller–Christian Disease	
Tolosa–Hunt Syndrome	
Arterio-venous malformations	

Some generalisations are possible:

1. Malignant infiltration of the orbit (by direct spread of carcinoma of the nasopharynx or remote spread from carcinomas in other sites) produces rapidly evolving extra-ocular nerve palsies and exophthalmos.

2. Benign tumours in the orbit may cause very slowly progressive but quite marked exophthalmos with remarkably little visual loss or nerve palsies until quite late in the course of the disease. The diplopia is often purely the result of mechanical displacement of the globe.

3. Lesions in the superior orbital fissure or intracranial lesions just behind the fissure cause nerve palsies with little or no exophthalmos.

4. Lesions in the orbit tend to cause exophthalmos as an early sign. If, in addition, there is considerable pain and redness of the eye the condition known as "pseudo-tumour of the orbit" must be considered. This is usually associated with a high E.S.R. and responds to steroids. It may well be a mild variant of the rare Tolosa–Hunt syndrome in which a mass of granulomatous tissue is found behind the eye and in the orbital fissure. The possiblity of unilateral exophthalmos with superior rectus muscle weakness being due to endocrine disease must always be excluded. Even in the absence of frank thyrotoxicosis, hyperthyroidism is the most common cause of unilateral exophthalmos.

5. Vascular tumours and arterio-venous malformations in the orbit may only cause proptosis when the patient is lying, bending forwards or performing the valsava manoeuvre.

Miscellaneous Disease Processes Causing Extra-ocular Nerve Lesions

1. There are three medical diseases that may cause acute extra-ocular nerve palsies. These are diabetes mellitus, meningo-vascular syphilis and arteriosclerosis. With the exception of diabetes the onset is usually painless (and in the writer's experience many diabetic palsies are also painless). The presumed pathology is infarction of the nerve trunk and hence in third nerve lesions due to these causes the pupil is usually spared. The prognosis in all instances is for complete recovery of function over some four to eight weeks. If recovery does not occur the diagnosis must be reconsidered. Compare this with an extra-ocular palsy due to a surgical cause which is usually painful, and in the case of a third nerve lesion *does* affect the pupillary response. Another rare "vascular" cause of extra-ocular nerve palsy is temporal arteritis; a condition confined to the elderly (over sixty years of age) (see also Chapter 20).

2. During the course of acute migraine headaches transient extra-ocular nerve palsies or a Horner's syndrome may occur. An incomplete third nerve palsy is the usual finding but less typically a sixth nerve palsy may be seen. The transience of the palsy, repeated identical attacks and the characteristics of the headache should suggest the diagnosis. The first episode may require angiographic exclusion of an aneurysm. A long history of repeated attacks may allow a confident diagnosis to be made without further investigations.

3. Third and sixth nerve lesions may occur during acute Herpes Zoster Ophthalmicus. The diagnosis is usually very obvious with an extensive vesicular eruption over the forehead preceded by severe pain. The prognosis for recovery is good.

4. Fourth nerve lesions in isolation are quite rare. Diabetes is probably the most frequent medical cause. In children

tumours infiltrating the superior medullary velum may produce bilateral fourth nerve palsies, and a similar picture occasionally follows severe head trauma, possibly due to haemorrhage into the same area. Unilateral weakness of the superior oblique commonly follows damage to the trochlear itself by injuries to the upper orbital margin.

Other Conditions Simulating Nerve Lesions

In general extra-ocular nerve palsies are "all or none"; partial palsies are relatively rare and usually *all* muscles supplied by the nerve show some degree of weakness. In the case of a fourth or sixth nerve palsy only one muscle can be affected, therefore if *two* muscles are affected the following conditions should be considered.

1. *Thyrotoxicosis*

Weakness of the superior rectus muscle and/or the lateral rectus muscle commonly causes diplopia in thyrotoxicosis irrespective of the presence of exophthalmos. The pathological changes in the muscles suggest that an inflammatory myopathic process is responsible.

2. *Myasthenia Gravis*

Diplopia and ptosis of the eyelid are the most common presenting symptoms of myasthenia gravis, and varying eye signs or fatigueability of eye movements should always raise this possibility. Many patients have had ophthalmological operations for squints later proven to be due to myasthenia gravis!

3. *Latent Strabismus*

Diplopia under conditions of fatigue, drowsiness or following impairment of vision in either eye is often due to the breaking down of a lifelong squint. A history of a childhood squint or previous orthoptic exercises usually establishes the cause. If there is no history the cover test may be useful. The examiner covers one of the patient's eyes and asks him to fix his gaze on a finger held about 18 inches away. When the other eye is uncovered it will be seen deviated inwards or outwards and will quickly pull back to line up with the other eye. This unmasks a latent deviation requiring positive muscle action to keep it compensated. Fatigue allows the eye to drift, resulting in diplopia usually in the evenings while watching TV!

4. *Progressive Ocular Myopathy*

This is a relatively rare form of muscular dystrophy in which the main muscle weakness occurs in the extra-ocular muscles and eyelids causing ptosis and diplopia. Careful examination usually discloses weakness of the facial and limb girdle muscles (also see Chapter 19). Familial ptosis is probably a mild variant of this condition that usually starts in late adulthood and may be associated with impaired upward gaze. Ptosis props fitted to the spectacle frames may be required to push the lid up off the pupil.

5. *Internuclear Ophthalmoplegia*

Multiple sclerosis may present as an extra-ocular nerve palsy, usually a sixth nerve lesion. More often diplopia occurs without weakness of any individual eye movement. This is due to disruption of the conjugate eye movement mechanism and is fully discussed in Chapter 8.

General Approach to Diplopia

Whenever a patient presents with the symptom of diplopia the following sequence of questions will usually establish the site of the lesion and provide a strong clue to the cause.

1. *Was the Onset Acute or Gradual?*

Clearly one either has or has not got diplopia, but a relentless worsening suggests infiltration of the nerves or a mechanical displacement of the globe.

2. *Is there any Variability or Remission?*

Extra-ocular nerve lesions of any cause are usually "all or none". If the symptom varies from time to time a latent strabismus or myasthenia gravis must be considered.

3. *Is there any Associated Ptosis of the Eyelid?*

An acute third nerve palsy invariably includes complete ptosis of the eyelid. Lesser degrees of ptosis or variable ptosis should suggest myasthenia gravis or a progressive ocular myopathy. Occasionally, patients with allergic swelling of the eyelid are incorrectly diagnosed as suffering from recurrent partial third nerve lesions; oedema of the eyelid during an attack establishes the diagnosis.

4. *Was there any Pain?*

A painful onset usually indicates aneurysmal dilatation of a blood vessel, either a berry aneurysm causing a third nerve palsy or an aneurysmal dilatation of the intracavernous part of carotid artery causing a third or sixth nerve palsy. Incomplete loss of eye movements and severe congestion of the eye should also raise the possibility of a granulomatous lesion in the orbit, i.e. pseudo-tumour of the orbit or Tolosa–Hunt syndrome. Herpes Zoster Opthalmicus with a nerve palsy should also be considered as the vesicular rash may take several days to appear during which time there is severe pain in the distribution of the first division of the fifth nerve.

Migraine headache may occasionally be complicated by an extra-ocular nerve palsy. A full personal and family history of headaches usually provides a clue to this possibility.

5. Is there any Exophthalmos or Proptosis?

Protrusion of the globe suggests the presence of either an aneurysm in the cavernous sinus, thrombosis of the cavernous sinus with vascular congestion or a tumour in the orbit.

The rapidity of onset and presence of pain usually enables the distinction to be made but the inflammatory conditions of the orbit which respond to steroids should also be considered. the fact that thyrotoxicosis is the commonest cause of exophthalmos should always be remembered.

Chapter 6

THE CEREBELLO-PONTINE ANGLE AND JUGULAR FORAMEN

The second major grouping of cranial nerves is found in the region known as the cerebello-pontine angle. This consists of a shallow triangle lying between the cerebellum, the lateral pons, and the inner third of the petrous ridge (see Figure 6.1). The vertical extent of the angle is from the fifth

Figure 6.1. The Skull Base

Crista galli

Dorsum sellae

Anterior cranial fossa

Petrous temporal bone

Middle cranial fossa

Pons

Internal auditory canal

The cerebello pontine angle

Posterior cranial fossa

Fourth ventricle

Cerebellar hemispheres

nerve above, on its course from the pons to the petrous apex, and the ninth nerve below, passing from the lateral medulla to the jugular foramen. The abducens nerve runs upwards and forwards on the medial edge of the area and the seventh and eighth cranial nerves traverse the angle to enter the internal auditory canal (Figure 6.5).

The hallmark of a lesion in this region is clinical evidence of damage to the seventh and eighth cranial nerves, so that a wide range of vestibular, auditory and motor abnormalities may occur. Several simple and benign conditions such as Bell's palsy enter into the differential diagnosis of more serious conditions such as acoustic nerve tumours.

It is essential to be able to evaluate the nerves in the area at the bedside, and have at least an understanding of the methods and aims of eighth nerve tests, such as auditory

function tests and the caloric test. These are described and discussed at the end of this chapter.

CLINICAL EVALUATION OF THE AFFECTED CRANIAL NERVES

1. The Trigeminal Nerve (V)

The trigeminal nerve conveys sensation from the face and provides the motor supply to the muscles of mastication, The cutaneous distribution is of great clinical importance.

Figure 6.2. The Cutaneous Distribution of the V Nerve

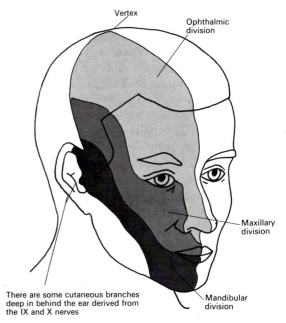

Vertex

Ophthalmic division

Maxillary division

There are some cutaneous branches deep in behind the ear derived from the IX and X nerves

Mandibular division

The sensory supply of the face is shown in Figure 6.2. Notice that the area supplied by the first division extends back to the vertex; not to the hairline and includes the nose and part of the upper lip (embryologically this is the nerve supply of the fronto-nasal process). The third division has a relatively small area of supply and it is important to remember that there is a large area over the angle of the jaw supplied by nerve roots C2 and C3. Patients with non-organic sensory

Figure 6.7. Figure to show the Position of the Semicircular Canals in the normal position

The lateral canal is tilted upwards at 30° in the rest position

Figure to show the Position of the Semicircular Canals during *The Caloric Test*

When the subject is leaning backwards at 60° the lateral canal lies vertically

and is in continuity with the subarachnoid space. A highly specialised fluid with a high protein content, known as endolymph fills the semicircular canals and the scala media of the cochlear.

The Vestibular Apparatus (Figure 6.7 and 6.8)

1. *The Semi-Circular Canals*

The semi-circular canals are three fine tubes arranged as shown in Figure 6.7. Note that the lateral canal is tilted up 30° at the front; it is *not* horizontal. The six canals work as three matched pairs in three planes as indicated in the figure. At the end of the canal that joins the utricle is a swelling called the ampulla. This contains the cupola and the hair cells. The cells are polarised to respond to movement in one direction only by the position of the single kinocilium on each cell. In the lateral canal movement towards the utricle stimulates the cupola. The vertical canals are stimulated by movement *away* from the utricle.

Activity in the canals is transmitted to the vestibular nucleus on the same side of the brain stem and then to the eye muscle nuclei as discussed in Chapter 7. The desired end result is that whatever the position of the head the eyes look straight ahead.

2. *The Otolith Organs*

The Utricular Mechanism

The otolith organ in the utricle senses tilting of the head. It is shaped like a flat plate tilted up at the anterior end. It is covered with hairs polarised towards the bend. Head tilt is sensed by the variation in pressure of the calcium carbonate crystals on the hairs produced by gravity.

The Saccular Mechanism

The organ in the saccule senses angular acceleration of the head. It is shaped like a shield with a central ridge facing forwards. Forward movement forces the crystals to attempt to slide down the slope on either side proportional to the speed and angle of the movement.

Vestibular Function Tests

1. *Gait and Stance*

Patients with a unilateral disorder of vestibular function tend to veer or fall to that side. The same is true of cerebellar disease so that any distinction between the two has to be made on other grounds. The Romberg test is *not* a specific test of vestibular function.

2. *Nystagmus*

Nystagmus is discussed in detail in Chapter 8.

3. *The Caloric Test*

This is the most useful test of vestibular function. Ideally a standardised test using thermostatically controlled water temperature should be used. The test is based on the fact that the cupola can be deflected by convection currents set up in the semi-circular canals if they are heated or cooled. The lateral canals can be easily stimulated by hot or cold fluid running through the external auditory canal. A further advantage is that the patient's head can be held still so that the resulting nystagmus is easily observed.

a. The patient sits on a couch with his head back at 60° to bring the lateral canals to the vertical position. This is because it is easier to produce convection currents in a vertical column of fluid. The test should not be performed if the ear drum is perforated.

b. Water at 30°C and 44°C is run into each ear in turn. A thermostat is used to keep the temperature steady and 250 mls. of water are allowed to flow over 40 seconds in the standardised test.

Figure 6.8. Schematic Diagram of Right Vestibular Apparatus

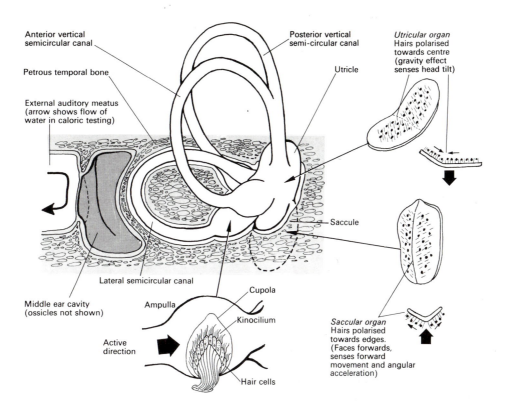

c. While the water is running the patient looks at a point straight ahead. This produces vertigo and easily observed nystagmus as the canals are stimulated or inhibited and the eyes are pushed or pulled to either side. The duration of the nystagmus is timed. The normal duration is 2 minutes ±15 seconds.

Explanation of results (Figure 6.9)

a. Cold water cools the apex of the canal and fluid flows towards the cool area *away* from the utricle. The cupola is inhibited.

b. Hot water heats the apex of the canal setting up a convection current towards the utricle. This stimulates the cupola.

c. With the knowledge that an active semicircular canal moves the eyes to the opposite side it follows that cold water upsets the balance and the normal canal pushes the eyes towards the cold stimulus. Conversely, the hot water activates the canal and pushes the eyes away from the stimulated ear.

The two abnormalities that may be detected are called canal paresis and directional preponderance.

Canal Paresis

If the semicircular canals or the VIIIth nerve are damaged an incomplete or defective response to both hot or cold water in the *affected* ear will be found.

Directional Preponderance

The central connections of the vestibular nerve are such that cold water in one ear has the same effect as hot water in the other. If it is found that nystagmus cannot be induced to one side it indicates that the vestibular nucleus of the appropriate side is defective. This is known as directional preponderance.

There are some situations in which both canal paresis and directional preponderance may be combined. This is often encountered when an acoustic nerve tumour or other posterior fossa lesion is displacing the brain stem.

4. Positional Nystagmus

When a patient's main symptom is vertigo occurring only when the head is in a certain position, positional testing is essential.

Figure 6.9. Diagram to Illustrate the Mechanism of the Caloric Test

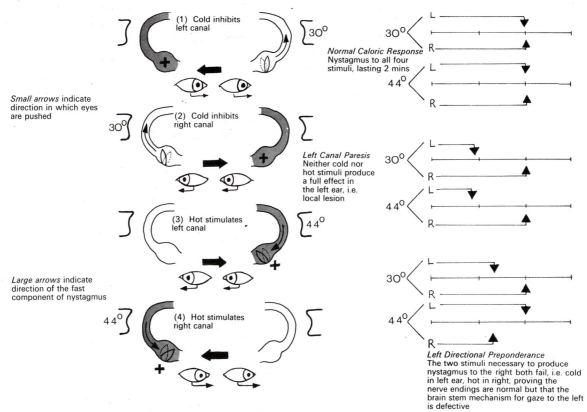

(1) Cold inhibits left canal

30°

L

R

30°

44°

Normal Caloric Response Nystagmus to all four stimuli, lasting 2 mins

Small arrows indicate direction in which eyes are pushed

30°

(2) Cold inhibits right canal

Left Canal Paresis Neither cold nor hot stimuli produce a full effect in the left ear, i.e. local lesion

30°

L

R

44°

L

R

(3) Hot stimulates left canal

44°

Large arrows indicate direction of the fast component of nystagmus

30°

L

R

L

R

44°

44°

(4) Hot stimulates right canal

Left Directional Preponderance The two stimuli necessary to produce nystagmus to the right both fail, i.e. cold in left ear, hot in right, proving the nerve endings are normal but that the brain stem mechanism for gaze to the left is defective

The patient's head is held by the examiner with the patient sitting with his back towards the end of a couch. The patient is then quickly lowered with his head turned to the right or left until the head is off the end of the couch and below the horizontal position. Acute vertigo with brisk nystagmus occurs when the affected vestibular apparatus is in the underneath position. There are two types of response.

a. Nystagmus starts after a ten to fifteen second delay, lasts some fifty seconds and is directed towards the underneath ear. If the test is repeated the response is less dramatic or absent. This is the benign type.

b. If the nystagmus comes on immediately, persists as long as the position is maintained or is in the opposite direction, it is of the central type. Repeated testing will produce repeated responses. There is a high likelihood that the patient has a tumour in the posterior fossa.

More complex vestibular tests including electronystagmography will not be discussed in detail. Their main advantage lies in the fact, that using electrical recording with the eyes closed, the optic fixation reflexes are abolished. These reflexes are strong enough to suppress peripheral vestibular nystagmus but have no effect on nystagmus due to central pathway, cerebellar nystagmus. This allows a distinction to be made that may be impossible on clinical examination.

The Auditory Apparatus (Figure 6.10)

The organ of Corti has a similar basic structure and consists of receptor hair cells arranged in a spiral tube. The cavity of the tube is divided into three compartments by two membranes stretched across its centre, a roof membrane (of Reissner) and a tightly stretched basilar membrane. The closed cavity between them is filled with endolymph and the cavities on either side with perilymph. The receptor cells lie on supporting tissue arising from the basilar membrane. The hair processes are embedded in a thin membrane that bridges across the organ of Corti, known as the tectorial membrane. When the basilar membrane vibrates in response to a sound wave the tectorial membrane has a shearing effect on the hairs. At the apex of the cochlear the membrane has a diameter of 0·5 mm. and at the base 0·04 mm., responding to low tones and high tones respectively. The pressure wave is transmitted through the perilymph by the pump-like effect of

Figure 6.10. Section of part of the Cochlear Spiral

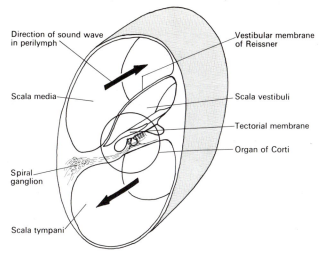

The Anatomy of the Organ of Corti

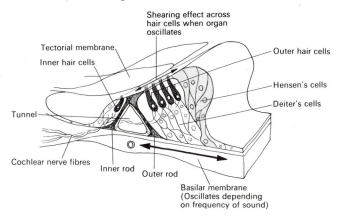

the stapes in the oval window and the shock wave passes to the round window where the energy is dissipated.

Hearing can be tested at the bedside in the following ways.

a. A simple test can be performed with a watch and quantitated by measuring the distance from the ear at which the watch can still just be heard.

b. If a watch cannot be heard at all a whispered voice at about eighteen inches should be tried, gradually raising the voice until it becomes audible. It is essential to occlude the opposite ear with a finger while performing this test.

c. The tuning fork tests help distinguish between hearing loss due to middle ear disease (conductive deafness) and that due to eighth nerve damage (perceptive deafness).

The Rinne Test

A 512 cycle tuning fork is held on the mastoid until it is no longer audible. If it is then held by the external auditory canal it will still be audible to the normal ear. This is documented as AC > BC. In perceptive deafness this situation persists, but in conductive deafness BC > AC as air conducted sound depends on intact auditory ossicles for its transmission.

The Weber Test

If the tuning fork is then placed on the vertex it should be heard equally in both ears if hearing is normal. In perceptive deafness the fork will not be heard in the affected ear. In conductive deafness, the fork will be heard equally well in both ears as the auditory ossicles are circumvented.

Electrophysiological Tests of Hearing

Classical audiometric testing includes pure tone audiometry, speech audiometry and the measurement of tone decay. These tests require considerable expertise and patient co-operation and are not easily used in young children. This is a subject in itself and can only really be appreciated by seeing the tests performed. Basically pure sounds of known frequency and intensity or a series of words are presented to the patient via earphones. The positive or correct response is plotted on standard graphs and the distinction between conductive and perceptive deafness can be made.

Recent advances in electrophysiological testing allow not only hearing to be tested but also neural activity in the cochlear, auditory nerve and brain stem pathways can be studied.

Acoustic or stapedius reflex testing is performed using an airtight probe in the external auditory meatus. The probe injects the sound, permits the pressure in the canal to be controlled and detects movement of the tympanic membrane. The stiffening of the membrane when a noise is presented to the ear is detected, requiring no co-operation from the patient.

Electrocochleography (ECog) is performed by inserting a long needle electrode through the tympanic membrane. Small potentials generated in the cochlear itself and in the auditory nerve and brain stem can be detected and studied using averaging techniques. Of special interest to neurologists, is the recording of a stream of potentials in the brain stem set up by an auditory stimulus. A series of five potentials are detected by an electrode over the mastoid process and information about brain stem function can be obtained. This promises to be of value in diseases affecting the brain stem, such as multiple sclerosis.

CLINICAL DISORDERS OF THE EIGHTH NERVE AND ITS CONNECTIONS

The insidious development of deafness and the late symptom of vertigo in cerebello-pontine angle lesions has been stressed. Only acute disorders of the eighth nerve produce dramatic symptoms such as tinnitus, acute deafness or vertigo. The most frequent cause of tinnitus is probably the rushing noise, synchronous with the pulse, that occurs in elderly arteriopathic patients and occasionally drives them to suicide. Vertigo, however, is a very frequent and distressing symptom. The most important point is to establish that the patient really has vertigo. Patients invariably use the expressions "dizzy" or "giddy" and too often these terms are uncritically accepted as vertigo. Closer questioning may reveal that the patient feels "lightheaded", "woozy" or "faint" but does *not* have the characteristic spinning sensation of vertigo. Once these "non-vertiginous" patients have been excluded relatively few disorders need be considered and most have a very characteristic history. The majority of patients in the "non-vertigo" group are suffering from an anxiety state or hyperventilation syndrome; these conditions are fully discussed in Chapter 22.

History is all important in patients with vertigo and the type of sensation, the circumstances under which it occurs, the associated symptoms, duration and frequency of attacks must all be established.

The major causes of vertigo are:

1. Benign positional vertigo
2. Vestibular neuronitis
3. Ménières Disease
4. Migraine
5. Multiple sclerosis
6. Drugs, including alcohol
7. Brain stem ischaemic attacks
8. Temporal lobe epilepsy

Benign Positional Vertigo

This condition occurs mainly in middle age. It may follow upper respiratory tract infections or quite mild head trauma. In most cases no cause can be found. This history is very striking. The patient complains of sudden attacks of vertigo while putting his head back on to the pillow to go to sleep or while getting up in the morning. Attacks during the day are unusual, and once an attack has occurred and ended, usually within fifty seconds, the patient can move about without a recurrence. The condition usually remits spontaneously over a period of weeks to months. Positional testing as described previously should be carried out and a careful distinction made between the benign form and the type indicating a tumour in the posterior fossa.

Vestibular Neuronitis

This is a common disorder that occasionally occurs in epidemic form and is thought to be due to a viral infection of Scarpa's ganglion, or of the brainstem vestibular system. The onset is abrupt with very severe ataxia and vertigo, often with severe vomiting. No position is completely comfortable and preferentially the patient lies quite still on his back. The recovery period may take several weeks with decreasing but disabling vertigo persisting during this period.

Ménière's Disease

Although this diagnosis is often suspected it is quite a rare disease of the elderly. Attacks are usually of sudden onset preceded by a full or bursting sensation in the head and followed by a roaring or hissing noise in the ear, which disappears as the ear becomes deaf later in the attack. Intense vertigo is present from the onset, but the disturbance of the otoliths is the main problem and the patient may be unable to stand or may feel as though he is somersaulting over backwards. Attacks may last up to 24 hours and leave the patient exhausted. It is the associated auditory symptoms that are the key factor in this history.

Migraine

Nausea and vertigo are common components of the migraine syndrome and many patients feel these symptoms are worse than the headache! The onset of a characteristic headache (see Chapter 20) should leave little doubt as to the diagnosis. Problems may arise when the headaches are completely replaced by the vestibular symptoms. It is essential to explore fully the previous headache history of any patient with unexplained attacks of vertigo and vomiting.

Multiple Sclerosis

Although multiple sclerosis may cause an episode of acute vertigo the majority of patients also have symptoms such as diplopia, numbness of the face, weakness or ataxia of a limb or dysarthria to indicate a more widespread brainstem lesion. None of these additional symptoms can occur with a simple disorder of the vestibular apparatus. Furthermore, in multiple sclerosis the cochlear fibres entering the brainstem may also be damaged, leading to deafness in one ear. This combination of signs may lead to diagnostic errors and Meniere's Disease may be suspected. The persistence of an attack over a two to three week period—and the patient's age—usually excludes Ménière's Disease.

Drugs

Many drugs and alcohol cause vertigo as a side effect. The drugs include all anti-convulsants, many sedatives, carbamezepine (Tegretol), some antibiotics, chloroquine, methysergide maleate (Deseril), and aspirin, which may also cause tinnitus. A careful history of drug ingestion and dosage should be regarded as part of the routine questioning in any patient who complains of vertigo.

Brain stem Vascular Disease

Although vertigo is the single most common symptom of brain stem vascular disease it does not follow that vertigo in an elderly patient is invariably due to vertebral-basilar ischaemia. As in the case of multiple sclerosis, a careful enquiry for *other* symptoms of brain stem disease should be made. It is unwise to accept this diagnosis uncritically. Brain stem vascular disease is very much overdiagnosed in elderly patients who have brief attacks of vertigo on hot days, in bathrooms and when standing up suddenly.

Temporal Lobe Epilepsy

An occasional patient with temporal lobe epilepsy will report vertigo as a symptom, often as a component of the prodromal phase of the attack. Subsequent events should leave little doubt that vertigo was part of an epileptic event. Discharges from the posterior temporal lobe are usually responsible (see also Chapters 10 and 22).

JUGULAR FORAMEN SYNDROMES

The jugular foramen is an extremely difficult area to illustrate and understand. The ninth, tenth and eleventh cranial nerves enter the internal part of the foramen lying on the medial side of the sigmoid sinus. The foramen itself angles forwards and laterally under the petrous bone which is excavated by the slight ballooning of the sigmoid sinus as it bends downwards to become the jugular bulb. The three cranial nerves emerge in front of the jugular bulb lying between it and the carotid artery which enters the carotid canal just anteriorly. There are two other structures to be considered; (a) The twelfth (hyoglossal) nerve which exits through the anterior condylar canal and comes into close relationship with the three other nerves outside the skull. (b) The cervical sympathetic which ascends into the area on the carotid artery; it does not exit from the skull via the foramen. It follows that if the cervical sympathetic is involved in a jugular foramen syndrome the lesion is certain to be outside the skull (this point is amplified later). (See Figures 6.11, 6.12)

CLINICAL EVALUATION OF THE LAST FOUR CRANIAL NERVES

1. The Glosso-Pharyngeal Nerve (IX)

A frequent error is the use of the expression "ninth nerve palsy". There is no such thing. From a practical point of view the nerve is purely sensory. The only muscle supplied by the nerve is the stylo-pharyngeus, which cannot be tested clinically. The error is made because of an almost universal misconception that the ninth nerve is motor to the palate. When the gag reflex is tested the stimulus is relayed in the ninth nerve but the resulting palatal movement is mediated by the *tenth* nerve. This reflex is too gross for accurate clinical diagnosis.

Sensation should be tested by touching the palate gently with an orange stick on each side, and then with the patient saying "Aah" touching the posterior pharyngeal wall on both sides. The patient should be asked to compare these gentle stimuli.

If there is any doubt, pain sensation should be tested in the same areas using a long hat pin. It is vital to test for such sensory loss in all the clinical situations discussed in this chapter.

Taste sensation over the posterior third of the tongue has no value in clinical diagnosis.

2. The Vagus Nerve (X)

The vagus is the motor nerve to the palate and the vocal cords. Weakness of the palate may cause nasal regurgitation of food, and nasal speech. The paralysed side of the palate does not move and is pulled across to the intact side when the patient says "Aah".

Paralysis of one vocal cord will allow that cord to lie permanently and limply in the midline. This leads to hoarseness, loss of volume of the voice and an inability to cough explosively—the so called "bovine" cough.

Examination of the tenth nerve should include examination of palatal movements, the patient's voice, and the patient's ability to cough.

3. Spinal Accessory Nerve (XI)

The spinal accessory nerve is motor to the sternomastoid and the upper part of the trapezius muscle. The complex central control of this nerve is discussed in Chapter 11. From a practical point of view, damage to the nerve itself results in wasting and weakness of the sternomastoid and upper trapezius. Like so many things in neurology these signs are very easily overlooked unless one is specifically alerted to the possibility of an abnormality.

The Syndromes

1. Vernet's Syndrome (of the Jugular Foramen)

This consists of damage to the three nerves that traverse the jugular foramen itself, i.e. cranial nerves IX, X and XI. A lesion inside the skull is more likely to cause this restricted syndrome because a lesion outside the skull is likely to affect the twelfth cranial nerve and the cervical sympathetic as well.

2. Collet–Sicard Syndrome (of the Posterior Lacero-Condylar Area)

The Collet–Sicard syndrome consists of damage to the last four cranial nerves. In Figure 6.12 it will be seen that as the foramen opens from the skull it is adjacent to the foramen lacerum, just above the condyle of the occipital bone. The last four cranial nerves lie close together in this area. This syndrome could also occur with a lesion inside the head, but an intracranial lesion extensive enough to affect all four nerves (see Figure 6.11) would usually distort the brain stem and produce signs of long tract damage.

3. Villaret's Syndrome (of the Posterior Retropharyngeal Space)

Again referring to Figure 6.12 the reader will see that in the anterior part of the area lying immediately behind the naso-pharynx, the cervical sympathetic is extremely vulnerable. Villaret's syndrome consists of damage to the IX, X, XI and XII nerves *and* a Horner's syndrome.

CAUSES OF JUGULAR-FORAMEN SYNDROMES

Lesions Inside the Skull

Any of the lesions that can cause the cerebello-pontine angle syndrome can also extend down and involve the last four cranial nerves in numerical sequence. The diagnosis is easy if the fifth and seventh nerves are also affected, as there is no lesion that could occur *outside* the skull and produce such a combination.

Tumours that specifically occur inside the skull in this region are neurinomas of the ninth, tenth or twelfth nerves. They occur most often on the twelfth nerve with a marked predilection for young females and occur on the left side in a ratio of 9:1. The reason for this is unknown. Meningiomas and epidermoid tumours (cholesteatomas) may also occur in this area and tend to cause distortion of the brain stem. This produces long tract signs and symptoms such as a mild or intermittent tetraparesis.

Lateral brain stem lesions are unusual except for vascular accidents. Although these syndromes may include a Horner's syndrome, they rarely cause diagnostic confusion because of the almost invariable spinothalamic sensory loss on the opposite side of the body which leaves no doubt that the cranial nerve damage is due to intrinsic brain stem disease (see also Chapter 11).

Lesions in the Jugular Foramen or Outside the Skull

Of the lesions discussed above both meningiomas and neurofibromas may extend out through the foramen in a dumb-bell fashion—sometimes presenting as a mass at the angle of the jaw.

A Horner's syndrome is certain evidence that the lesion is outside the skull; as the cervical sympathetic ascends *into* the area and does not pass through the foramen.

Attempts should also be made to see if a palpable mass is present at the angle of the jaw, or any cervical lymphadeno-pathy. It is important to realise that a bony hard mass is normally palpable in this area—it is the tip of the transverse process of the atlas!

Other Causes

1. Poly-Neuritis Cranialis

This is a somewhat dubious entity which basically consists of multiple cranial nerve palsies for which no cause can be established and which may well recover. The writer has seen several examples in elderly patients in whom intensive investigations including multiple naso-pharyngeal biopsies failed to demonstrate a cause and who recovered completely under observation. Some of the reported cases have also suffered from diabetes or syphilis, and the nerve lesions may represent a variety of transient nerve palsies similar to those that may involve the extra-ocular nerves. An important practical point is that although the suspicion of metastatic carcinoma must be high, irradiation without tissue diagnosis is not justified, unless relentless progression of the syndrome can be established. Isolated twelfth nerve palsies with recovery after a few weeks may occur and may be due to a similar pathology to Bell's palsy. In all cases follow up should be continued until full recovery has occurred.

2. Glomus or Carotid Body Tumours

These tumours arise in the chemo-ectodermal tissue that is normally present in the carotid body and may be found ectopically in the inner ear and around the ninth and tenth nerves. Neoplastic changes in this tissue produces highly vascular erosive tumours that may destroy the petrous temporal bone and present as a vascular nodule in the external auditory canal.

Depending on the exact site of the glomus tumour a cerebello-pontine angle syndrome associated with an internal and/or an external jugular foramen syndrome may result. These tumours occur in either sex with a peak incidence in the third and fourth decades.

3. *Glosso-Pharyngeal Neuralgia*

This very rare form of neuralgia consists of attacks of severe pain in the throat when fluid or food is swallowed. The pain is excruciating and similar to that of tic douloureux. Exploration to cut the nerve often reveals aberrant vessels coursing across the nerve or unsuspected neuro-fibromas, or cholesteatomas adjacent to the nerve. It is always wise to regard the syndrome as potentially symptomatic (i.e. indicating an underlying lesion) until proved otherwise by events or surgical exploration.

Investigation of the Jugular Foramen Syndrome

Having established the combination of nerve palsies, the two most important clinical signs to be excluded are a Horner's syndrome and evidence of brain stem compression (such as a spastic paraparesis). The former indicates an extracranial lesion and the latter an intracranial lesion.

If the lesion is outside the skull routine haematological studies and chest and paranasal sinus x-rays assume significance and direct examination of the nasopharynx and larynx is a part of the routine evaluation. Skull x-rays are rarely of value although a careful skull base film should be taken.

If the lesion is intracranial air encephalography or contrast studies (myelography) are necessary. If the lesion is outside the skull a carotid angiogram may demonstrate a mass displacing the upper carotid artery.

As an example of the jugular foramen syndrome—

CASE REPORT

A 76-year-old man presented with a history of weight loss, a mass at the angle of his jaw, dysphagia and a hoarse voice. On examination the following signs were present:

1. There was a hard tender mass at the angle of his jaw.
2. The left palate was insensitive to touch and pinprick.
3. The left palate was weak and he had a bovine cough.
4. There was wasting and weakness of the left sternomastoid and trapezius muscles.
5. The left side of the tongue was slightly wasted, fasciculating and deviated to the left on protrusion.
6. He had a left Horner's syndrome.

In this case the mass and the Horner's syndrome indicated that the lesion was extracranial. Biopsy revealed a squamous carcinoma, probably metastatic from the lung.

A certain amount of easily acquired skill is necessary to detect multiple lower cranial nerve palsies. The provisional diagnosis and investigative approach depend on the accurate detection of associated signs. Jugular foramen syndromes are examples of conditions where clinical findings alone provide nearly all the information necessary to diagnose and treat the patient.

Chapter 7

CONJUGATE EYE MOVEMENTS AND NYSTAGMUS

The eyes have central connections that function like the steering linkage on a car, allowing the eyes to move together, that is, the movements are "conjugate". In the absence of these controlling mechanisms the eyes rove in an aimless way. If these mechanisms fail to develop, as in the case of someone who is blind from birth, wild roving eye movements are a very obvious feature.

Three basic control mechanisms are established in the first few months of life, provided that the child has normal vision.

1. The ability to look in any desired direction, until an object of interest is found. These movements occur as little flicks of the eyes, called "saccadic movements". They essentially supply the brain with a series of still pictures until the desired object is located. They are under voluntary control and are initiated in the frontal lobes.

2. The ability to hold the object on the same point of the retina in spite of any movement it may make. These pursuit movements of the eyes are smooth to avoid jerky vision. They are controlled by the parieto-occipital area in close liaison with the visual cortex.

3. Ideally the eyes are held in the straight ahead position most of the time. This is achieved by the continual adjustment of the eye position in relation to the position of the head in space and is maintained by vestibular activity and proprioceptive information from the neck muscles integrated at brain stem level.

PATHWAYS OF CONJUGATE GAZE CONTROLLING MECHANISMS

It must be stressed that many of the pathways to be discussed are only presumed to exist. None of the descending pathways can be followed beyond the general area of the pretectal region and the lateral pontine reticular formation. The rough position of the pathways has been deduced from clinical evidence provided by lesions in the brain stem and their effects on eye movements.

Voluntary Gaze Mechanism (Figure 7.1)

The cortical areas controlling voluntary gaze lie in the premotor strip of the frontal lobe (area 8). This area has an intimate connection with the parietal control area, which it can override at any time to change the direction of gaze. The descending pathways pass in the corona radiata through the anterior limb and genu of the internal capsule, closely associated with the corticobulbar fibres to the brain stem nuclei. From the internal capsule the fibres rotate to lie medially and dorsally in the cerebral peduncle (follow the arrows on the figure). The main pathway passes to the pons and at some point decussates to the opposite side. The exact point is not established. Here it ends in a presumptive 'pontine centre for lateral gaze', which may lie in the para-abducent nucleus, or in the vestibular nucleus itself. The adjacent sixth nerve nucleus is activated from this area and so is the opposite paired medial rectus muscle, by a very important relay, back across the midline and up to the opposite third nerve nucleus. Thus, both eyes look to the left or right simultaneously. This relay pathway is the medial longitudinal fasciculus. The fundamental importance of this tract is shown by its presence in all vertebrates, and in its being the first tract to myelinate in man. A less well-documented pathway controlling vertical gaze also exists. Clinical evidence would suggest that this pathway is mediated via the basal ganglia and the area underlying the superior colliculus.

Pursuit Eye Movement Mechanism (Figure 7.2)

The object to be followed is located by voluntary effort. The eye "locks in" on the object, and the eyes then only move in response to movements of the object, which is kept focused on the macular part of the retina. Thus a direct relay from the visual cortex, forward to area 19 controls the movement. This area projects via corticotectal and corticotegmental fibres into the midbrain and pons. There is also a large forward projection that gives the frontal eye fields information as to where to direct voluntary gaze, although it is unlikely that the parietal area actively controls frontal eye field activity.

Vestibular and Cerebellar Influences on Eye Movements

These influences are best understood if we examine what happens when one lateral semicircular canal is stimulated.

Figure 7.1. Voluntary control (frontal eye fields)
Start at circle to follow complete pathway

Area 19 parieto-occipital eye field

Pathway mediating voluntary vertical movements and convergence

? Via basal ganglia

Via anterior limb and genu of the internal capsule

III

Medial longitudinal fasciculus (relay back up to opposite III nerve)

Start here

VI

Area 8 frontal eye field

Lateral pontine gaze centre

Adducting eye (III)

Abducting eye (VI)

Figure 7.2. Pursuit eye movements (parieto-occipital eye fields)
Start at circle to follow complete pathway

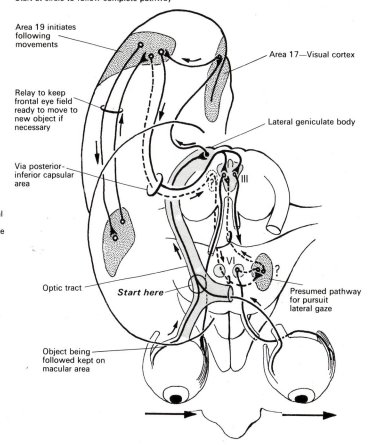

Area 19 initiates following movements

Area 17—Visual cortex

Relay to keep frontal eye field ready to move to new object if necessary

Lateral geniculate body

Via posterior-inferior capsular area

III

Optic tract

VI

Start here

?

Presumed pathway for pursuit lateral gaze

Object being followed kept on macular area

The lateral canal is only stimulated by forward movement of the endolymph within it (follow arrows on Figure 7.3 from the left labyrinth. See also Chapter 6).

If the head is rotated sharply to the left, the fluid in the left labyrinth moves forward and stimulates the cupola. For the eyes to keep looking straight ahead (the ultimate aim of the whole process) the eyes must deviate to the right side. This is performed by the activity in the medial vestibular nucleus, provoked by the canal stimulation relaying across to the opposite sixth nerve, and back up the medial longitudinal fasciculus to the third nerve nucleus on the same side. Thus both eyes simultaneously move to the right. The cerebellum plays some role through a facilitatory mechanism for the movement relayed through the fastigial nucleus of the cerebellar roof nuclei. Contributory information also comes from the proprioceptive organs of the neck muscles via the spinovestibular tract.

The role of the cerebellum is far from clear. In addition to the above, essentially vestibular reflex pathway that is facilitated by cerebellar activity, there is a prominent flocculo-oculomotor tract, the only direct cerebellar connection with the eye muscle nuclei. This pathway, by its connection with the *opposite* third nerve, and presumably by a relay down to the sixth nerve on its own side, would tend to move the eyes in the opposite direction. This pathway may help explain why nystagmus in cerebellar disease is in the opposite direction to that occurring in vestibular disease. Experimental studies on the role of the cerebellum in eye movements have produced complex results and clinical lesions and stimulation experiments often result in divergence of the eyes!

This difficulty is mentioned because whenever nystagmus is discussed, cerebellar disease is always prominent in discussion, although the nystagmus caused by cerebellar disease is the least understood and clinically the least certain cause of nystagmus that is encountered. We will refer to

Figure 7.3. Vestibular and Cerebellar Influence on Eye Movement
Start at circle to follow complete pathway

The flocculo-oculomotor tract, works in reverse to vestibular influences (?Responsible for different direction of cerebellar nystagmus)

Third nerve nucleus

Ipsilateral third nerve stimulated via relay up the medial longitudinal fasciculus

Cerebellar pathway via fastigial nucleus facilitates own side and inhibits the other

Inhibition from opposite fastigial nucleus

Contralateral abducent nucleus stimulated

Flocculo-nodular lobe

Start here

Fluid flows backwards and inhibits the lateral semi-circular canal

Fluid flows forwards and stimulates lateral semicircular canal

Medial vestibular nucleus inhibited

Medial vestibular nucleus activated

Abducent action moves eye laterally i.e. into straight-ahead position if head turned to left

Third nerve action adducting eye and completing conjugate deviation to the right side

Proprioceptive information from cervical muscles

Head has been rotated fast round to left

Direction eyes must move to maintain straight-ahead gaze

these pathways again in later discussion of the clinical features of nystagmus.

Vertical Eye Movements

Vertical eye movements do not require the participation of the sixth nerve and the controlling mechanisms lie mainly in the midbrain beneath the superior and inferior colliculi. The importance of basal ganglia pathways in these movements can be deduced from some important clinical observations to be discussed later.

The ability to converge the eyes is critical to maintaining close binocular vision. This movement utilises both medial rectus muscles simultaneously. To do this it was theorised that a midline "centre for convergence" existed, and this was long held to be in the nucleus of Perlia, lying between the third nerve nuclei. Experimental work has failed to confirm the validity of this view and divergent squints may result from damage anywhere from the thalamus to the lateral pons or cerebellar peduncles. It seems unlikely that a specific midline mechanism exists.

CLINICAL DISORDERS OF CONJUGATE GAZE MECHANISMS

In each of the controlling areas lesions that damage the pathways may cause inbalance between the two sides by either over-activity or under-activity of the damaged area.

Lesions in the Frontal Cortex and Anterior Internal Capsule

Over-activity of the Frontal Eye Field (see Figure 7.4)

Epileptic seizures arising in the appropriate area of the frontal cortex cause what are called "frontal adversive attacks". In these episodes the attack commences with the head and eyes being forcibly deviated away from the discharging frontal cortex. The side of the body to which the deviation has occurred may then be involved by focal motor activity and ultimately the attack may progress to a generalised seizure.

Under-activity of the Frontal Eye Field

Damage to the frontal eye field by a vascular occlusion may render the patient unable to look to the opposite side. This deficit is rarely seen as rapid compensation occurs and the eye movements appear to be normal within hours. However, residual evidence may be found in the patient having difficulty in maintaining gaze in that direction or in the development of some nystagmus caused by this weakness when attempting to do so. If the patient is subsequently anaesthetised or becomes comatose, the eyes will deviate towards the damaged side of the cortex, because of the unopposed activity of the intact opposite frontal lobe. The unconscious patient with a frontal lesion therefore looks away from his hemiplegic side (see Figure 7.5).

Bilateral damage to the frontal cortex or the appropriate pathways in the internal capsule may lead to total loss of voluntary control over eye movements. There are several relatively rare causes of this condition. A congenital variety exists called congenital oculomotor apraxia. The affected child moves his whole head around to find the desired object. An acquired form of oculomotor apraxia may occur

in arteriosclerotic patients who have suffered bilateral cerebral vascular accidents. If the lesions responsible are in the anterior internal capsule the loss of control of eye movements is often accompanied by other evidence of pseudo-bulbar palsy (see Chapter 9). The insidious development of the same type of damage to both pathways is seen in a condition called progressive supranuclear degeneration (Steele–Richardson–Olzewski syndrome), and may also occur as a component of Jakob–Creutzfeldt disease (see Chapter 10). Both conditions are complicated by dementia.

Lesions in the Parieto-Occipital Cortex

Over-activity of the Parieto-Occipital Cortex

Seizures originating in the parieto-occipital area cause deviation of the eyes to the opposite side, but in this situation the movement will often be accompanied by visual hallucinations. These usually consist of flashing lights and coloured blobs. A generalised convulsion may ensue but focal motor activity, other than the eye movement is not a feature of a focal seizure arising in the occipital lobe.

Under-activity of the Parieto-Occipital Cortex

Damage to the parieto-occipital cortex is often associated with other parietal lobe difficulties which may make testing impossible. Similarly, if an homonymous hemianopia coexists (as it often does if the lesion is a vascular one), the patient may be unable to follow an object because it keeps vanishing into the hemianopic field. In these cases it is essential to keep the object to be followed just inside the midline, in the intact half of the patient's vision and to move it slowly.

The nystagmus that occurs while watching passing telegraph poles from a moving train is dependent on the integrity of this fixation mechanism. Loss of this so-called opticokinetic nystagmus to one side is important clinical evidence of a lesion in the opposite parietal lobe. It is tested by spinning a drum marked with vertical lines, in front of the patient, and asking him to watch the lines. The drum is spun in opposite directions to provoke nystagmus to both right and left. This can be voluntarily suppressed by a few people but it is also a good test for hysterical blindness. The drum is spun in front of the suspected patient's eyes; if nystagmus occurs, in the direction of rotation, vision is intact.

Lesions Affecting Basal Ganglia

Although the anatomical pathways that link the basal ganglia with eye movements are unknown, there is adequate clinical evidence of their importance. For reasons that are not

Figure 7.7. Internuclear Ophthalmoplegias

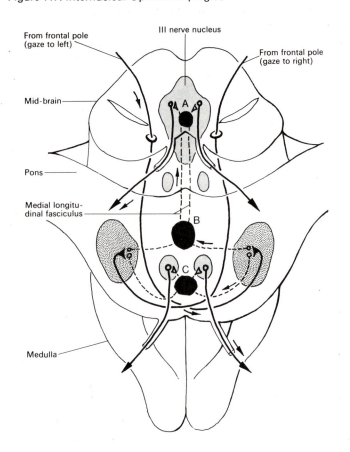

From frontal pole (gaze to left)

III nerve nucleus

From frontal pole (gaze to right)

Mid-brain

A

Pons

Medial longitudinal fasciculus

B

C

Medulla

Figure 7.7A. Lesion at A

Eyes at rest

Divergent squint due to bilateral involvement of medial recti and loss of the convergence mechanism

Figure 7.7B. Lesion at B

Classical internuclear ophthalmoplegia with ataxic nystagmus

Abduction normal— marked nystagmus

Looking to right

Adduction fails—little or no nystagmus

Adduction fails— nystagmus minimal

Looking to left

Abduction normal —marked nystagmus

Figure 7.7C. Lesion at C

Internuclear ophthalmoplegia

Abduction failure

Looking to right

Adduction full— minimal or no nystagmus

Adduction full

Looking to left

Abduction failure

and the classical variety is sometimes referred to as "internuclear ophthalmoplegia with ataxic nystagmus". The disconjugate movements plus the asymmetrical nystagmus cause frank diplopia or blurring of vision, often severe enough to prevent reading.

Neither symptom occurs in conjugate gaze palsies as the eyes maintain their relative positions at all times, but as noted previously, whenever there is weakness of conjugate movement nystagmoid movements in the direction of weak gaze are a common feature.

NYSTAGMUS

The basic pathological feature common to all causes of nystagmus is that there is weakness in maintaining the conjugate deviation of the eyes or an inbalance in the postural control of the eye movements. In either case there is

a tendency for the laterally deviated eyes to drift slowly back to the central position (this is the pathological component), and to regain the original position by a fast flick (this is the movement that is recorded as the direction of the nystagmus). One of the major problems for the student arises from the fact that nystagmus is defined in the direction of the *fast* movement which is *not* the abnormal part of the process. It is the slow drift that is pathological—*not* the more easily observed fast flick. It follows that minor degrees of nystagmus will only be manifest on full lateral gaze to the weak side. If more severe, it may appear on the slightest deviation to the weak side. If very marked, it may also be apparent at rest as fine jerky movements of the eye from side to side. Qualitatively, it may be defined as fine or coarse (based on the amplitude of movement), horizontal, vertical or rotatory. The other quality, usually described as pendular, is a specific feature of ocular nystagmus and is discussed separately below. Although at first sight the quick movement would appear to be a deliberate attempt by the occipito-parietal motor area to restore fixation, the movement persists even following transcollicular section of the brain stem. The activity is therefore thought to be generated in the pons. However, the occipito-parietal motor area does have significance in the physiological phenomenon of opticokinetic nystagmus mentioned before. It is *absence* of opticokinetic nystagmus that is pathological, and this finding points to a lesion in the pursuit gaze pathway or the opposite parieto-occipito-temporal cortex. Conversely, in cerebellar nystagmus the optic fixation reflexes may be strong enough to inhibit the slow drift and prevent nystagmus from occurring. Thus cerebellar nystagmus may only be manifest in the dark or with the eyes closed. This can be shown by electronystagmography, which is performed in the dark with the eyes closed and the eye movements are recorded electrically from electrodes placed over the eyelids.

Varieties of Nystagmus

Nystagmoid Jerks

Coarse jerking movements of the eyes occur if the patient is made to follow a moving object too far or too fast. The examiner should aim to take the edge of the iris of the adducting eye to the caruncle and no further. Similarly, if the examiner holds the object closer than two feet from the patient's eye it will cause convergence and this in turn will provoke nystagmoid jerking on minimal lateral eye movements. Nystagmoid jerks have no pathological significance; they do not represent minimal nystagmus.

Congenital Nystagmus

This condition, which is often familial, occasionally causes unnecessary concern, as it produces very dramatic nystagmus. It is present from birth. The movements are non-stop and pendular, i.e. there is no fast and slow phase, just a steady "wobble" of the eyes. The head may nod in the opposite direction, which serves to stabilise the retinal image. The movements become even more dramatic when the patient directs his gaze in any direction, but invariably the eyes oscillate from side to side—the movements do not become vertical on upward gaze. One of the features that indicates that nystagmus is of the congenital variety is that in spite of the very gross jerking the patient has no sensation of the movement of his eyes and no subjective nausea or vertigo. Recently acquired nystagmus of this severity is usually associated with nausea and vertigo on attempted lateral gaze.

An important differential diagnosis of congenital nystagmus in the first few years of life is the condition known as spasmus nutans. In this situation the child develops fast, fine but variable movements of the eyes. The head also nods, but not in a compensatory direction, usually up and down, and often the head nodding precedes the onset of the eye movements. The condition is benign but may last weeks to months. It is essential to exclude any ocular abnormality as similar eye movements occur in children with impaired vision (but not total blindness) caused by congenital macular disease, congenital cataracts, total colour blindness and albinism.

Nystagmus Caused by Vestibular Disease

Any lesion affecting the semicircular canals, the eighth nerve or the vestibular nuclei will seriously upset the push-pull effect of the vestibular control of eye movements. Let us assume that the left-sided vestibular elements have been damaged in Figure 7.3. Activity in this pathway normally pushes the eyes to the right, therefore reduced activity will lead to weakness of eye movements to the right side. On attempting gaze to this side the intact vestibular mechanism on the right, coupled with the weakness of the damaged left side will force the eyes to drift back to the midline. The quick jerk to restore the gaze will be to the right side, i.e. the nystagmus is away from the side of the vestibular lesion.

There are several distinguishing features in lesions affecting the different parts of the vestibular pathway. With destruction of the labyrinth by Ménière's Disease, nystagmus does not occur, because of central compensation for the absence of any input. A similar situation exists after acute labyrinthine destruction when the initial imbalance settles. Similarly in slowly occurring damage to the eighth nerve (an acoustic nerve tumour) compensation often prevents development of nystagmus. When it does occur in this situation it often reflects brain stem or cerebellar damage from the extension of the tumour into the cerebello-pontine angle. With central lesions of the vestibular apparatus (multiple sclerosis, cerebral vascular accidents, gliomas, syringomyelia) compensation cannot occur and the nystagmus and associated symptoms of vestibular damage tend to persist. Although nystagmus from a peripheral lesion is horizontal or rotatory, that arising from a central lesion may also be vertical. The eyes move up and down, usually doing so on attempted upward gaze. Horizontal nystagmus on looking upward is *not* vertical nystagmus. Although widely held to be pathognomonic of intrinisc brain stem disease, vertical nystagmus can result from distortion of the brain stem by an extrinsic lesion, and is quite often seen in patients with drug toxicity, especially that caused by diphenylhydantoin (Epanutin) and other anticonvulsants.

The most clearcut examples of vestibular nuclear nystagmus are seen in vascular lesions of the brain stem which are usually strictly unilateral. In multiple sclerosis, bilateral damage, and involvement of other pathways produces very complex nystagmus, such as that found in association with internuclear ophthalmoplegia as discussed above.

Nystagmus Caused by Cerebellar Lesions (see also Chapter 12)

As already mentioned the exact mechanism of cerebellar nystagmus is not known. Although nystagmus is a feature of unilateral cerebellar disease, in some cerebellar degenerations and midline cerebellar disease, nystagmus may be absent even though the patient may be so ataxic as to be unable to sit without support. Many hold that cerebellar disease only causes nystagmus when vestibular pathways are damaged, and yet this view has to explain why when nystagmus is found it is in the reverse direction to vestibular disease affecting the same side. If we consider the flocculo-occulomotor pathway in Figure 7.3, which normally tends to move the eyes *towards* the active side of the cerebellum, weakness of this activity could lead to difficulty in looking at the damaged half of the cerebellum, and the fast jerk to restore gaze would be *towards* the damaged cerebellar hemisphere. This explanation certainly fits the clinical situation as nystagmus in cerebellar disease is maximal towards the side of the lesion.

Other Causes

There are a multitude of rare varieties of nystagmus beyond the scope of this text. However, there are several common causes of nystagmus that cannot be based on anatomical features. All sedative drugs, especially barbiturates and glutethimide, and anticonvulsants, especially diphenylhydantoin (Epanutin), primidone (Mysoline) and carbamezepine (Tegretol) can cause severe vertigo and dramatic nystagmus following deliberate or accidental intoxication. Alcohol and one of its complications—Wernicke's encephalopathy—are also associated with nystagmus. Following head injuries with loss of consciousness, transient nystagmus following recovery of consciousness is quite common and does not seem to carry any serious prognostic significance. Persistent nystagmus may occur in the event of a fracture though the petrous bone damaging the labyrinth or eighth nerve (see Chapter 23).

A comprehensive list of causes of nystagmus without an understanding of the underlying pathophysiology is of little use.

The importance of testing for nystagmus correctly, and recording in detail the quality, direction and other features is not sufficiently appreciated. The almost universal finding recorded in the neurological examination of patients—"a few nystagmoid jerks" does not indicate great clinical acumen. On the contrary it demonstrates poor clinical technique and a failure to recognise that this is not a physical sign.

DISEASES AFFECTING THE CEREBRAL HEMISPHERES

There are three basic ways in which cerebral hemisphere functioning can be compromised:

1. Infiltrative or compressive neoplasms either primary or secondary.
2. Vascular lesions including vascular occlusions, haemorrhages, emboli, subdural and extradural blood clots.
3. Diffuse neuronal dysfunction either due to degenerative processes or metabolic disorders.

Neoplastic lesions tend to occur in the lobes of the brain whereas vascular lesions occur in specific vascular territories which fortunately for the diagnostician are not anatomically the same as the lobes of the brain. Finally, extremely diffuse damage to the hemispheres is usually readily recognisable although the cause can rarely be established.

Chapter 8

THE CEREBRAL HEMISPHERES: 1. THE LOBES OF THE BRAIN

GENERAL FEATURES OF DISEASE IN THE CEREBRAL HEMISPHERES

Intellectual and Behavioural Disorders

For the highest levels of intellectual functioning the entire brain must be intact. Yet quite extensive lesions in some areas may produce little or no identifiable deficit, whereas a small lesion in the dominant hemisphere may have a devastating effect on speech function and comprehension. In the presence of a cerebral neoplasm additional features such as raised intra-cranial pressure, cerebral oedema and brain displacement may add non-specific generalised intellectual or behavioural changes to the focal signs of the underlying lesion. For this reason any statement by a patient's relative to the effect that a recent intellectual decline or change in personality has occurred should be taken very seriously, even if no definite abnormality is detectable on simple testing. So often the patient himself is unaware of, or denies such a change and it is always vital to get reports from employers and workmates to supplement the history given by the patient and his family.

Memory impairment, loss of concentration, irritability, loss of motor skills or inappropriate behaviour may all mark the onset of symptoms of a cerebral lesion. As examples the following cases may be cited:

CASE REPORT

A middle-aged industrial chemist, always an extrovert, became more expansive in his behaviour and one day while driving with his wife suggested that she should drive for a while. As soon as she stepped from the car to go round to the driving seat, he drove off and left her stranded. He had no explanation for this behaviour. The only physical sign was a right Babinski response. Investigation demonstrated a large meningioma over-lying the left parietal area. No satisfactory explanation can be advanced for the behavioural upset but his behaviour was normal following the removal of the meningioma.

CASE REPORT

The doorman at a large London hotel started greeting eminent guests at the door in a familiar manner. By lunchtime numerous complaints had been received by the manager who found the doorman entertaining the occupants of the entrance hall to a selection of army songs. On examination he had bilateral extensor plantars and mild papilloedema. His behaviour until that day had been exemplary. A chest x-ray revealed a large carcinoma of the lung and subsequently multiple cerebral metastases were demonstrated by a cerebral scan.

More specific disabilities may provide clues as to the localisation of the underlying lesions.

1. Frontal lobe lesions cause striking memory impairment to the point of dementia, often coupled with marked physical inertia (see later explanation). A frequently associated feature is a deterioration in the social behaviour especially in respect of micturition. This is probably related to the location of the cortical centre for micturition in the second frontal gyrus. Urinary incontinence occurring in the early stages of the history in a patient with intellectual decline should always be regarded as indicating a frontal lesion until proven otherwise. The unusual use of bad language in inappropriate circumstances is another feature.

2. Temporal lobe disorders may also cause personality changes with memory impairment. The slow deterioration may be punctuated by episodic bizarre personality change with sudden onset and cessation. These often turn out to be complex psychomotor seizures and may last for days at a time with residual confusion between the more obvious attacks. The possibility of a temporal lobe disorder should be considered in any patient with sudden attacks of altered behaviour.

3. Parietal lobe lesions produce manifestations that vary depending on the patient's cerebral dominance. The majority of patients (including the majority of left-handed patients) are left hemisphere dominant.

Dominant hemisphere parietal lesions produce dysphasia with either inability to understand commands, inability to speak or a combination of both.

The evaluation of patients who are unable to communicate requires some degree of skill and time. A very common error and dangerous assumption is that poor communication is synonymous with confusion.

CASE REPORT

A middle-aged alcoholic female became irrational and "confused". This was attributed to an amnestic syndrome and she was transferred to a mental hospital where it was discovered that she was "dysphasic". Subsequent investigation and operation disclosed a glioma in the temporal lobe of the dominant hemisphere.

CASE REPORT

An elderly coloured male was taken to hospital and left by his relatives, who departed before giving any history. He was "confused" and could give no account of himself. The neurological service was asked to see him at their leisure with a diagnosis of "chronic brain syndrome". Examination revealed both receptive and motor dysphasia, a mild right hemiparesis and a slightly dilated left pupil in an extremely drowsy man. Immediate investigation revealed a massive subdural haematoma which was successfully evacuated.

The methods available for screening patients for dysphasia will be detailed later, but the main point must be reiterated; speech difficulties can easily be mistaken for confusion by the unwary examiner.

Lesions affecting the non-dominant parietal lobe do not affect speech function but cause unusual deficits in acquired skills such as cutting up food, dressing, getting out of the bath, and geographic orientation. The complete preservation of speech function which allows the patient to discuss, while not understanding these disabilities is a feature of the condition which is known dyspraxia.

CASE REPORT

A man came home to find his 70-year-old wife sitting in an empty bath making repeated but ineffectual efforts to get out. She could not understand why she was having such difficulty and may have been stuck in the bath for four hours. After her husband had helped her from the bath she needed help to dress. There was evidence of a right hemisphere lesion on physical examination, which proved to be due to a cerebro-vascular accident.

CASE REPORT

A 56-year-old man suffered a series of attacks of paraesthesiae in the left arm during an influenzal illness. There were no definite sequelae. On the day he returned to work he took two and a half hours to travel the half mile to work and was seen wandering in the wrong direction by neighbours. When he arrived at work he was unable to find his way to his bench. He was sent home and his wife found that he had great difficulty putting on his pyjamas. No abnormality was found on angiography but a vascular lesion of the non-dominant parietal lobe was probably the cause.

Combinations of peculiar behaviour, wearing clothes back to front, inability to dress, getting lost around the house or in the street, or sudden inability to perform skilled tasks such as carpentry are all suggestive of a lesion in the non-dominant parietal lobe.

Bedside Evaluation of Intellectual Function

An assessment of the patient's mental state, intelligence and specific evaluation for dysphasia should be made. Consider-able information in all these spheres can be obtained while passing the time of day with the patient and during the actual history taking.

His mood, attitude towards his disability, attitude towards the examiner and third parties are readily detectable without specific testing.

1. Mental State

Formal testing of the mental state is often confined to asking the patient the date and day of the week. Anyone who has spent more than a few days in a hospital bed will know how difficult this becomes! The monotony of routine, the irrelevance of the date, and the isolation from the outside world readily produces some degree of confusion about time and date in the most alert patient. General questions on the content of the day's newspaper, or the news on the radio, are usually much more useful although they are at first sight less specific than the date. Nursing reports of the patient's behaviour and manner are also extremely useful in making this general evaluation. An assessment of the patient's memory for remote, recent and immediate events should be made and wherever possible checked with a relative.

2. Intellectual Function

Testing can be performed at the bedside but subtle alterations are very unlikely to be detected by the occasional examiner. Formal psychometric testing is essential especially where no immediately obvious abnormalities are apparent. For clinical notes the "100 minus 7" test is traditionally used although for full interpretation both accuracy and the time taken are important. This is so badly affected by anxiety and fright that to base the whole assessment on this test would be entirely inappropriate. The ability to learn a lengthy sentence, such as the typical Babcock sentence, is useful however. A perseveration of errors as well as the time taken to complete the sentence gives useful information. The test sentence (which the examiner must also know by heart!) is, "There is one thing that a nation must have to be rich and great, and that is a large, secure supply of wood". Most patients can learn this sentence accurately in three to five attempts. However, the test is subject to all the problems of anxiety, speech difficulty and memory disturbance. The results are not specific for any condition. Another test of memory and concentration consists of asking the patient to learn a series of numbers forwards and backwards. Normally patients can learn seven numbers forwards and five backwards. Explaining the meaning of proverbs and general knowledge tests, the names of public figures, capitals of countries etc. can be very difficult as the general interests of the patient will influence their performance.

One dysphasic patient unable to name any simple objects or describe the meaning of simple words such as brunette was asked the meaning of "piscatorial", his face lit up and he answered in a flash "appertaining to a fish". Needless to say he was a keen fisherman. The writer experienced considerable difficulty while working in the U.S.A. when attempting dysphasia and intelligence testing as he had little common ground with the patients in public affairs or sport.

Finally, the patient's ability to repeat, paraphrase or explain a simple story can be tested. Many patients who are slightly confused regard the examiner with incredulity when the story is related and it requires a certain amount of self-control and preliminary explanations to perform this test without calling your own sanity into question.

Cowboy Story:

A cowboy went to San Francisco with his dog, which he left at a friend's house while he went to buy a new suit of clothes. Dressed in his grand new suit he came back to the dog, whistled at it, called it by name and patted it. The dog would have nothing to do with him in his new coat and hat and gave a mournful howl. Coaxing the dog was of no avail, so the cowboy went away and put his old suit on again and the dog immediately showed its wild joy on seeing its master as it thought he ought to look.

3. *Dysphasia and Dyspraxia*

Dysphasia testing is best left until one has a clear idea as to how confused or disorientated a patient is, yet as already mentioned it is important to be certain that the patient has full comprehension of the spoken word and is capable of making a well-informed, appropriate answer to a question before taking the case history. It is essential that the patient is not distressed by testing and it is best not to pursue any difficulty for too long.

a. Establish that the patient can understand the spoken word by his ability to close his eyes, stick out his tongue and show either his right or his left hand to command. A severely confused demented or dysphasic patient may stick out his tongue at the first command and may continue to stick it out on every subsequent command. This may represent perseveration or may be the only motor act that the patient can be persuaded to perform.

b. If the patient cannot understand spoken commands he may be able to read them. The same simple responses should be asked for in writing, i.e. "put out your tongue" etc. showing the command to the patient on a card.

c. The patient's spoken answers, if any, should be recorded. In patients with nominal aphasia (difficulty in naming objects) a remarkably good command of language is possible but the sentences may lack nouns. To avoid the problem he may use an alternative to the noun. A patient who was asked to name his wedding ring, pointed to his wife and said, "I've been with her a long time."

d. The patient may be able to express himself better in writing and should be asked to write his name and address and write a simple sentence to dictation.

e. Object-naming is a very simple test and is perhaps the most useful at the bedside. It can also be most distressing for the patients and casual bystanders should not be allowed to listen to or laugh at the patient's disabilities. Naming simple objects such as a pen and its nib, or a watch and its hands will usually detect nominal aphasia.

f. The patient should read and discuss a passage from a book or newspaper to test his ability to both read *and understand* what he is reading.

Abnormalities in the performance of these tests indicates impairment of understanding the written or spoken word and imply dysphasia and therefore damage to the dominant parietal lobe. Once one dysphasic difficulty has been detected the site of damage is localised and no further localising information can be added by more exhaustive testing.

Dyspraxia is the equivalent of "dysphasia" in the non-dominant parietal lobe. The presenting history usually includes examples of lost skills such as difficulty in feeding or getting out of the bath. Simple tasks such as removing the dressing gown, lighting a cigarette or folding a piece of paper are readily observed. Allowances for any motor deficits or ataxia should obviously be made but in many cases these functions are normal, making the considerable difficulty that the patient has with apparently simple tasks even more dramatic. Constructional tests using either matches to copy simple figures and shapes or drawing things from memory fall into the same category. As with dysphasia the demonstration of difficulty in one sphere of activity provides sufficient localising information. At a higher level of testing the patient's ability to draw a plan of the ward or of an area of his home can be tested. A taxi driver performed well on all tests until asked to sketch a plan of Trafalgar Square—explaining his main complaint of difficulty in doing his job!

In summary patients may appear to be confused because of general depression of intellectual function which may vary with the conscious level, or because of dysphasic difficulties causing them difficulty in both understanding and communicating verbally, or they may have problems in the performance of simple tasks due to dyspraxia. Distinction between these possibilities is vital. Dysphasia or dyspraxia indicate a focal abnormality in the dominant and non-dominant hemispheres respectively, whereas confusion may indicate an altered level of consciousness or a metabolic disorder affecting the whole brain. This would require an entirely different approach to further investigation and treatment.

Motor Disorders in Hemisphere Disease

For normal motor function the patient must have intact sensory feedback and cerebellar control of his limbs. Patients often say that they are "unsteady" or "numb" when they mean "weak". If these descriptive terms are taken at face value an entirely incorrect view of their disability will be obtained. It is essential to ask the patient to elaborate on these terms in the same way as he should be asked to elaborate on the term "blackout". In a severe parietal lobe lesion the limbs on the opposite side may lie useless and completely ignored by the patient although they may not be weak. At a less severe level the outstretched arm, held out normally when the eyes are open, may fall away when the eyes are closed; this is not due to weakness but due to deficient appreciation of its position. In cerebellar disease the outstretched arm may show wild oscillations and even rise when the eyes are shut. This outstretched arms test is a very useful one for screening a patient and should be evaluated systematically.

1. Observe the outstretched hands. Are there any abnormalities of the hands themselves, such as finger clubbing? Do they shake? Does one arm have difficulty in maintaining its position?

2. Can the patient play the piano in mid air quickly and rhythmically? If not, the less efficient hand may be affected by a mild pyramidal lesion (in a right-handed patient the movements are often normally slightly better performed with the right hand).

3. When the eyes are closed, do the hands remain level? Does one rise up or oscillate (indicates cerebellar disease)? Does one fall away (indicates defective sensation or weakness)?

If the patient is drowsy or will not move his limbs to command because of dysphasia, the spontaneous movements of the suspect limb should be observed. If the examiner pinches the skin of the patient's anterior chest wall, the patient will invariably use his best arm to pull the examiner's hand away. If the good arm is then held down while the test is repeated the affected limb will move if it is able to do so. The legs may be tested by painful stimuli to each leg in turn, and at the same time the gross sensory function of the two sides can be assessed.

Full Evaluation of Motor Function in the Presence of a Hemisphere Lesion

We have considered gross defects of motor function in the semi-conscious patient above. In many instances one is looking for a very subtle deficit and the secret of evaluation lies in knowing how to look for minor motor disability.

1. *The Face*

We have previously mentioned the problem of the asymmetrical face and the frequent assertion that this represents a mild upper motor neurone lesion. We can now elaborate on upper motor neurone facial weakness as encountered in patients with hemisphere lesions.

There are two types of facial movement, voluntary facial grimacing and smiling, and involuntary grimacing and smiling as a true emotional response. The former function is probably mediated through classical motor pathways from the motor strip and the emotional responses through supplementary motor areas lying deep in the insula and temporal lobes. Therefore, the facial movements should be carefully observed during history taking and spontaneous smiles provoked and carefully observed. Then a forced smile should be tested and the patient's ability to show the teeth (with the almost inevitable patient response "they are false").

Quite obvious facial weakness on one test may be coupled with normality on the other. The type of weakness may have localising significance, emotional weakness usually indicating a lesion affecting the temporal lobe.

2. *The Limbs*

When testing the limbs we are looking for pyramidal weakness. This concept is vital to accurate diagnosis and yet is surprisingly neglected in most textbooks and teaching, as indicated by the number of doctors who test limb power by assessing the hand grips and the strength of the quadriceps muscles. These are the two movements *least* likely to be affected in cerebral disease!

The distribution of weakness is best remembered by recalling the typical posture and gait of a patient recovering from a stroke. The arm is flexed (the flexor group of muscles being strong), and the leg extended (the extensors being strong). Functionally this is ideal; if the situation were reversed few patients would ever regain the ability to walk after a stroke.

In the arm the weak groups are those controlling shoulder abduction elbow extension, wrist extension and finger abduction. The intact spastic groups adduct the arm to the side of the body, and flex the arm at the elbow and wrist.

In the leg, the weak groups are the hip flexors, the hamstrings and the dorsiflexors of the foot. The strong spastic muscles are the glutei and quadriceps which hold the hip and knee stiff and the plantar flexors which keep the foot slightly flexed—causing it to scrape along the ground as the patient walks.

This pattern of weakness indicates damage to pyramidal pathways and is typical of a deep hemisphere lesion, or damage to the main motor pathways (the cortico-spinal tracts in the brainstem or spinal cord).

If the whole area of cortex supplying a limb is damaged the extra-pyramidal pathways are unable to take over and *global, flaccid* weakness of the limb occurs associated with brisk reflexes and an extensor plantar response. This also explains how a patient with a small infarction in the internal capsule has a good prognosis for recovery whereas if the left middle cerebral artery is occluded the prognosis for recovery is poor and the patient has the added problem of dysphasia due to the damage to the speech cortex. This is discussed further in the next chapter.

Motor Evaluation Should Answer the Following Questions

1. Is there any facial weakness, either voluntary or emotional?
2. Is there any fall away of the outstretched hands?
3. Is there any disparity between piano-playing movements of the hands or toe wiggling (the equivalent test in the feet)?
4. Is there any tone increase on the affected side?
5. Is there any reflex asymmetry (brisker on the affected side) or an extensor plantar response?
6. Is there weakness in the pyramidal distribution, bearing in mind that proximal movements (shoulder abduction and hip flexion) may be demonstrably weak when the only peripheral signs are impaired fine movements?

SENSORY DISORDERS IN HEMISPHERE DISEASE

The main symptom of damage to the sensory cortex is sensory epilepsy. This usually consists of episodes of tingling parasthesiae progressing to numbness. It is very unusual for focal pain to be produced although it can happen. Due to considerable motor representation in the sensory cortical area the sensory symptoms are often associated with some twitching of the same limb or limbs. The sensory symptoms are usually strictly unilateral.

CASE REPORT

A 70-year-old man complained of severe low back pain and pain radiating down the entire right leg. On examination an orthopaedic surgeon found brisk reflexes and an extensory plantar response. When seen the next day he was densely hemiplegic and semiconscious. A large metastatic deposit in the leg area of the sensory strip was found. It is thought that his early symptoms were a form of sensory epilepsy.

CASE REPORT

A 42-year-old engineer had suffered from attacks of tingling and numbness of the left hand, extending to the left side of the chest and head since the age of nineteen. As these episodes often occurred at meal times they had long been ascribed to "indigestion"! Three weeks before admission he suffered two major epileptic fits each beginning with these sensory symptoms but progressing to focal jerking of the arm and face and then loss of consciousness.

A loud bruit was heard over the entire right side of the head and angiography revealed an angioma occupying the bulk of the right hemisphere.

The sensory loss caused by a superficial lesion is rarely complete. In fact, *total* loss of *all* sensory modalities on one side is extremely unusual, and should raise doubts as to the organicity of the findings. Due to bilateral cortical projections and some sensory appreciation of poorly localised touch, pain and vibration at thalamic level these sensations may be relatively spared. The modalities that are specifically affected by a cortical lesion are accurate localisation of touch, two point discrimination, joint position sense and temperature appreciation. Other "popular" modalities such as the recognition of numbers scratched on the skin and stereognosis (recognition of an object placed in the hand) are really composite sensory functions requiring all modalities to be intact, and are not specific forms of sensation. They do depend on the sensations particularly appreciated at cortical level and will therefore often be very severely impaired by a cortical lesion. Asking the patient to compare the textures of bed coverings is a useful screening test, but is subject to the same objection of relative non-specificity. Abnormalities in these tests suggest diffuse damage to the sensory cortex.

To detect very minimal dysfunction the test for sensory extinction is used. The theoretical basis of the test is probably the same as that for extinction hemianopia, illustrated in figure 3.3. The patient is lightly touched on either limb and occasionally simultaneously on both limbs. The ability to recognise a light touch on one limb, but failure to detect the same touch when both limbs are touched at the same moment is called sensory extinction and has the same significance as cortical sensory loss.

If the lesion lies deep in the hemisphere at thalamic level or in the subthalmic area more dramatic sensory loss will be found. In the early stages of a progressive lesion, or in the

CASE REPORT

A 60-year-old woman had been behaving somewhat peculiarly for nearly five years. The earliest symptom was apparent while driving when passengers noticed that she always drove in and out of bus bays to the alarm of the people waiting at the bus stop. Her business acumen declined and she was unable to cope with the introduction of V.A.T. Finally, her air letters to her son in Canada arrived written only in the margins so that when the letter was opened the message was destroyed. She was extremely peculiar in affect and slightly hypomanic but there were no definite neurological signs. Investigation demonstrated a large right subfrontal meningioma.

The particular type of micturition disturbance associated with a frontal lobe lesion is an abrupt awareness that the bladder is full coupled with the inability to prevent the bladder from emptying immediately. The patient loses the ability to inhibit the micturition reflex. As personality changes ensue, this causes less and less concern (to the patient)!

CASE REPORT

A 56-year-old female became increasingly disinterested in her household duties and incontinent of urine. However, it was not until she voided on her husband's prize roses that he sought advice on her account. An enormous parasaggital meningioma was removed with full recovery.

Epileptiform attacks are a frequent feature of frontal lobe lesions. There are three types of seizure that point to a frontal lobe disturbance.

1. *Adversive Fits*

Due to the presence of the frontal eye fields in area 8, a discharge in this region often causes the head and eyes to turn away from the discharging cortex. these are called "adversive seizures" and are typical of a frontal lesion.

2. *Focal Motor Epilepsy*

Focal Jacksonian fits and unilateral motor convulsions are usually due to a lesion in or near the main motor cortex in the precentral gyrus of the frontal lobe. However, surprisingly frequently the lesion is actually found in the parietal area. The discharge in these cases probably arises in the motor cells in the sensory strip. The simultaneous onset of tingling parasthesiae with the focal fit should indicate this possibility.

3. *Status Epilepticus*

It has recently been recognised that as many as fifty per cent of patients who suffer an attack of status epilepticus *early* in the course of their illness are eventually shown to have a frontal tumour.

Patients with lesions in the orbital part of the frontal lobe or subfrontal lesions such as olfactory groove or sphenoidal ridge meningiomas may develop intellectual deficits due to frontal lobe damage. These lesions may also cause blindness in one eye or loss of sense of smell in one or other nostril, and these problems may not be noticed by the dementing patient. For this reason it is essential to examine vision and sense of smell extremely carefully in demented patients.

Because the motor strip is so far back, compared with the size of the frontal lobe, intellectual deterioration, micturition disturbance or focal epileptic attacks are often the earliest symptoms of a frontal lobe tumour, long before definite physical signs appear. The possibility of a frontal tumour should always be pursued as far as possible on suspicion alone, even if there are no physical signs.

CASE HISTORY

A 64-year-old bus driver complained of a variety of unexplained symptoms and was eventually dismissed on medical grounds. About a year later he began to become morose and uncommunicative and complained of headaches. He rapidly deteriorated and memory difficulties were noted. The picture was thought to be due to a severe retarded depression and he was admitted to a mental hospital for electroconvulsive therapy. After three treatments he became drowsy and developed a mild left hemiparesis. Neurological examination revealed gross papilloedema and a mild left hemiparesis. A very large oedematous Grade 3 astrocytoma was resected from the right frontal lobe. Following surgery the patient had no motor deficit and no recollection of events for several weeks prior to his admission.

Physical Signs of Frontal Lobe Lesions

As indicated above, physical signs may be a late feature of a frontal lobe lesion. The need to look for optic atrophy, check for normal vision in both eyes and careful testing of the sense of smell has already been mentioned.

One of the most useful tests is the grasp reflex. It is also difficult to elicit. In the fully conscious patient stroking the palm is liable to serious misinterpretation! It is easier if the examiner holds the patient's hand with two or three fingers in the palm while gently rotating and flexing the arm as tone is assessed. Then as he lets go gentle pressure is exerted against the base of the patient's fingers. An involuntary increase in the grasp which traps the examiner's fingers is a positive response. In the unconscious or drowsy patient the test is useful and performed by gently pulling against the patient's fingers. A bilateral grasp response has no localising value but a unilateral grasp reflex provides strong evidence of a disturbance in the opposite frontal lobe.

If the lesion is situated posteriorly in the lobe damage to the motor strip may cause increased reflexes and a Babinski response on the opposite side of the body. If the dominant hemisphere is affected the patient may also have motor aphasia (inability to speak but with full understanding of instructions). This is almost invariably coupled with detectable weakness of the right face and right arm.

Parasaggital lesions are particularly likely to cause micturition disturbances and intellectual upset. As the area of cortex supplying the leg lies either side of the midline at this point, increased reflexes in both legs and *bilateral* extensor plantar responses may be found. Direct disruption of frontal lobe influences over the basal ganglia and cerebellum may cause "pseudo-Parkinsonism" or "pseudo-cerebellar" signs in addition to the apathy due to dementia. It is easy in such a case to make the mistaken diagnosis of arteriosclerotic dementia and Parkinsonism. For this reason the majority of neurologists insist on full investigation before a patient is allowed to be labelled as demented with the hopeless prognosis that this diagnosis carries.

2. The Parietal Lobes (Figure 8.3)

The parietal lobes are quite small extending from the Rolandic fissure anteriorly to the parieto-occipital fissure posteriorly and the temporal lobe below. The functional overlap between parietal, occipital and temporal lobe function in this area, and the physical continuity of the lobes makes anatomical boundaries of little practical significance.

The sensory cortex is organised in the same way as the motor strip with a large representation for information from the face and arm on the lateral surface and the trunk and leg areas on the top and in the parasaggital area.

Speech function is concentrated in the supramarginal and angular gyri, and in the upper part of the adjacent temporal lobe. The visual association areas (Area 19) are adjacent to the occipital lobe (see extinction hemianopia, Chapter 3). The same region is also responsible for the phenomenon of optico-kinetic nystagmus discussed in Chapter 7.

Clinical Features of Parietal Lobe Damage

The clinical features of dominant and non-dominant parietal lobe dysfunction have been discussed earlier in this chapter. To summarise, the following physical signs should be sought in patients with a suspected parietal lobe disorder.

1. Evidence of cortical sensory loss or sensory inattention.
2. Evidence of dysphasia if a dominant hemisphere lesion is suspected.
3. Evidence of dyspraxia if a non-dominant hemisphere lesion is suspected.

Figure 8.3. Parietal and Occipital Lobes (from behind and above)

SYMPTOMS:
Parietal lobe:
Sensory seizures
Dysphasia (dominant hemisphere)
Dressing apraxia   \ (non-dominant
Geographical confusion / hemisphere)
Occipital lobe:
Seizures with flashing light aura
Visual field defects
Dyslexia and visual agnosia (if area
    19 and forward involved)

SIGNS:
Parietal lobe:
Cortical sensory loss
Sensory inattention
Attention hemianopia
Dysphasia/dyspraxia
Optico-kinetic nystagmus lost
Occipital lobe:
Homonymous field defects
Dyslexia or alexia

4. Evidence of an attention hemianopia or a frank hemianopia if a parieto-temporal lesion is present.
5. Loss of optico-kinetic nystagmus (Chapter 8).
6. "Soft" motor signs such as increased reflexes, mild facial weakness, and an extensor plantar response on the side opposite the suspected lesion.

3. The Occipital Lobes (Figure 8.3)

The occipital cortex has already been described in Chapter 3. Tumours in the occipital pole have epileptic potential but are relatively rare. Seizures preceded by visual hallucinations, consisting of unformed flashes of light and colours should be regarded as arising in the occipital lobe. Any field defect that is produced by a tumour in the lobe will not spare the macular cortex (a feature of vascular lesions, see next chapter and Chapter 3). Damage to areas 18, 19 and 37 in the adjacent parietal lobe responsible for visual association may cause varying degrees of psychic blindness such as visual agnosia (inability to recognise objects) or alexia (inability to read).

CASE REPORT

A middle-aged architect suffered from attacks of flashing lights in the right field of vision for ten years. Following one attack, vision did not recover and the hemianopia did not spare the macular. He also had great difficulty reading, writing and spelling indicating damage to the adjacent parietal area. This was not consistent with a simple vascular lesion and further investigation and operation revealed an occipito-parietal astrocytoma.

4. The Temporal Lobes (Figures 8.4, 8.5)

The anatomy of the temporal lobe is extremely difficult to grasp due to the way the lobe is folded in on itself under the overhanging frontal and parietal lobes and the extensive and important areas that are rolled in under the hemisphere. Furthermore, the connections of the lobe to the hippocampal area, the cingulate gyrus and the insula make the "functional" temporal lobe much more extensive than its physical boundaries. The "limbic system" which includes many of these functions is discussed in Chapter 12.

One can only summarise some of the many functions of the temporal lobe that find expression in clinical disorders. These include:

1. The central representation of auditory and vestibular information.
2. Memory function in the hippocampal gyrus.
3. Visual association areas.
4. Central representation of taste and smell.
5. The upper homonymous visual field pathways (Chapter 3).

Figure 8.4. The Temporal Lobe

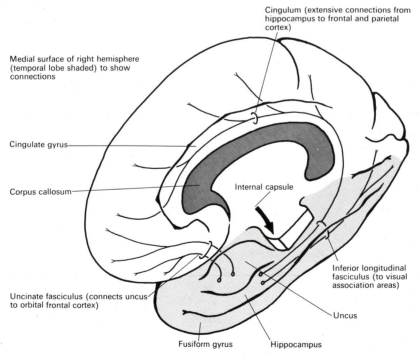

Cingulum (extensive connections from hippocampus to frontal and parietal cortex)

Medial surface of right hemisphere (temporal lobe shaded) to show connections

Cingulate gyrus

Corpus callosum

Internal capsule

Inferior longitudinal fasciculus (to visual association areas)

Uncinate fasciculus (connects uncus to orbital frontal cortex)

Uncus

Fusiform gyrus

Hippocampus

Figure 8.5. Lateral Surface of Left Temporal Lobe (anterior part shown cut off, Sylvian fissure pulled open)

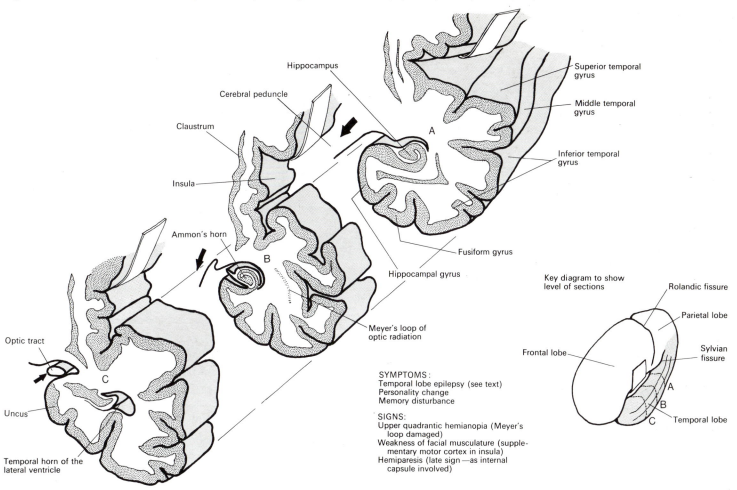

SYMPTOMS:
Temporal lobe epilepsy (see text)
Personality change
Memory disturbance

SIGNS:
Upper quadrantic hemianopia (Meyer's loop damaged)
Weakness of facial musculature (supplementary motor cortex in insula)
Hemiparesis (late sign —as internal capsule involved)

6. The entire visual radiation at the parieto-occipital-temporal junction.
7. Supplementary motor areas concerned with facial expression, eating, emotional responses to pain and pleasure.
8. Many aspects of behaviour via frontal lobe connections.
9. Central control of visceral motility, sexual and respiratory function.

Clinical Features of Temporal Lobe Disease

The clinical symptoms of temporal lobe disease can be of bewildering complexity. Fortunately the great frequency with which the disordered function is ''epileptic'' in nature makes recognition of the lesion possible. The important clinical pointer is that however bizarre and whatever the nature of the upset, the sudden onset and offset of the disturbance points to a paroxysmal disturbance in the temporal lobe, generally known as a ''psychomotor'' seizure. This term emphasises the behavioural upset that is a feature of such attacks, which is unlike any other form of epilepsy. Consciousness is not necessarily lost and motor dexterity is often maintained. These disorders are discussed in greater detail in Chapters 12 and 22.

Patients may relate a variety of typical prodromal events closely related to temporal lobe functions. They may describe vertigo, auditory or visual hallucinations, smell or taste hallucinations, unpleasant visceral symptoms, *déjà-vu* sensations, uncontrollable deep breathing, sexual fantasies or just a peculiar feeling ''as if something awful was going to happen''.

Motor accompaniments vary and peculiar grimacing, chewing, sucking or kissing mouth movements, repeated fiddling with clothing and sometimes removal of clothing may occur. Patients may drive many miles during an attack and become lost.

Focal motor seizures affecting the face and arm in particular (by activation of supplementary motor areas in the insula) may occur and the seizure may progress to loss of consciousness and a major convulsion.

Following a temporal lobe attack the patient is often very confused and in this state may physically attack over-helpful bystanders. Contrary to popular opinion, aggressive behaviour *during* the attack is very unusual.

Physical Signs of Temporal Lobe Lesions

Lesions in the temporal lobe almost invariably cause temporal lobe epilepsy unless they are extremely acute lesions such as haematomas or highly malignant gliomas. It is important to remember that only ten per cent of patients with temporal lobe seizures are harbouring a tumour, so that exclusory investigation is not indicated *unless* there are other reasons to suspect a neoplasm. The main reasons are physical signs and these are as follows.

Subtle personality change may occur. These are less dramatic than in frontal lobe lesions and may mimic depressive or psychotic disorders more often than dementia. There is a high incidence of impotence in males with temporal lobe tumours so that this symptom combined with personality change should arouse suspicion. Unilateral lesions rarely cause significant memory impairment.

A careful search for an upper quadrantic homonymous hemianopia is very important. This would provide evidence of damage to Meyer's loop (Chapter 3). If a complete hemianopia is present the lesion has spread into the adjacent parietal lobe, and appropriate parietal lobe problems may be found including dysphasia.

As the face area of the motor cortex is that most likely to be affected by a temporal lobe mass, a mild facial weakness should also be sought. Otherwise physical signs occur extremely late in the course of the disease and the picture then becomes one of a rapidly developing hemiparesis with confusion, headache, dysphasia (if on the dominant side) and personality change indicating a rapidly expanding lesion.

THE DIAGNOSIS AND INVESTIGATION OF CEREBRAL TUMOURS

The cardinal symptoms and signs of a cerebral tumour are said to be headache, vomiting and papilloedema. In fact these are very rarely the presenting symptoms unless the tumour is in the posterior fossa or has blocked the flow of C.S.F. This means that the majority of tumours produce more subtle symptoms and signs as already described in this chapter.

Headaches are discussed in detail in Chapter 20. In relation to cerebral tumours the following features are worth considering:

a. Headache is *not* an inevitable symptom of a cerebral tumour and is often so mild that the patient only mentions it in response to a direct question.
b. Less than one per cent of patients referred to hospital with headaches have a cerebral tumour.
c. Tumour headache is *not* particularly severe, it has a dull relentless quality. An association with vomiting certainly increases the chances of finding a serious cause but as a broad generalisation the more severe the headache the *less* likely it is to be due to a tumour.

Epileptic seizures in relation to tumours at different sites have already been discussed. As in the case of headache it is essential to have a sense of proportion about epilepsy and cerebral tumours:

a. In patients under twenty years of age the incidence of cerebral tumours causing epilepsy is 0·02 per cent.
b. Even in patients in the age group 45–55, the decade with the highest incidence of cerebral tumours, only ten per cent of patients with recent-onset epilepsy prove to have a cerebral tumour.
c. Epileptic seizures are more likely to occur when the underlying tumour is an infiltrating glioma than a surface lesion such as a meningioma. As gliomas occur twice as frequently as meningiomas the patient who has a fit due to a tumour usually proves to have a malignant glioma or astrocytoma.

From this it follows that a first seizure occurring in a patient aged twenty-one or more does *not* automatically mean that the patient has a cerebral tumour. Extensive investigation is only indicated if there are features discussed earlier in this chapter. In patients who have physical signs the tumour incidence rises to fifty per cent. In all patients with epilepsy a long-term follow-up is essential and the onset of physical signs should prompt investigation. A complete set of negative investigations early in the course of the illness does *not* exclude a neoplasm. Occasionally five to ten years elapse before other evidence of a slow growing tumour becomes apparent. Epilepsy due to a tumour is *not* particularly difficult to control and difficulty in controlling epilepsy is not evidence of an underlying tumour. However, if the epilepsy *starts* as an episode of status epilepticus there is a fifty per cent risk that the patient has a frontal tumour and full investigation *is* indicated in this instance.

In childhood the majority of cerebral tumours occur in the cerebellum (medulloblastomas or cystic astrocytomas), the pons and the optic nerve or chiasm. Supratentorial tumours are rare. Therefore early headache, vomiting ataxia or visual disturbance *are* common features of a tumour in the child and conversely epilepsy is very unusual. (Clinical details of posterior fossa tumours in childhood are to be found in Chapters 3, 6, 1.1 and 12.)

In the adult supratentorial tumours account for ninety per cent of cerebral neoplasms increasing the likelihood of an epileptic presentation and decreasing the incidence of headache as there is more space available for tumour expansion. Only cerebellar tumours (in the adult haemangioblastomas and metastases) and tumours that block C.S.F. flow (pinealomas, ependymomas of the fourth ventricle and intraventricular tumours) cause headache and vomiting as early features.

Pathological Features and Clinical Management

Childhood

In childhood cerebellar tumours are the main problem and pre-operative pathological diagnosis is difficult. Half the tumours consist of a small astrocytoma associated with a large cystic cavity. Complete removal with a low risk of recurrence is often possible. The other half consist of highly malignant medulloblastomas; tumours of disputed tissue origin usually arising in the vermis and extending down the superior medullary velum or peduncles into the brainstem with less possibility of complete resection. They also tend to seed the C.S.F. and secondary deposits in the lumbar theca are found. They are usually radiosensitive and combined surgery and radiotherapy (including the whole spinal canal) may achieve impressive cure rates. Pontine gliomas are discussed in Chapter 11 and optic nerve gliomas in Chapter 3. Neither are really resectable but often are moderately radiosensitive and significant symptomatic improvement and survival can be achieved. In the adult these particular gliomas occur with greatest frequency in patients with neurofibromatosis.

Adulthood

In the adult the first difference is the twenty to thirty per cent chance that *any* cerebral tumour is a metastasis. In the male carcinoma of the bronchus is the usual cause and in the female carcinoma of the breast. Therefore a chest x-ray and careful breast examination are the first and most important investigations in any patient of the appropriate sex with a cerebral tumour. Almost any other tumour may metastasise to the brain but renal carcinoma, large bowel tumours and malignant melanomas are those most likely to do so. Large bowel tumours show a particular tendency to metastasise to the cerebellum, and in general metastases occur more frequently in both the parietal lobe and cerebellum than would be anticipated if spread were on a random basis.

Primary cerebral tumours occur in the lobes in a frequency roughly proportional to the size of the lobe, i.e. frontal/temporal/parietal and occipital. The primary cerebellar tumour that specifically occurs in the adult is the haemangioblastoma. This consists of a small highly vascular nodule of tumour often in association with a large haemorrhagic cyst. Complete resection is often possible and the prognosis is probably the best for any cerebral tumour. Occasionally these tumours produce erythropoeitin and cause polycythaemia. They may also be associated with vascular tumours in the retina (Hippel—von Lindau disease).

In the cerebral hemispheres half the tumours are malignant gliomas or astrocytomas with four grades of malignancy, I–IV, in order of increasing malignancy. An important subvariant is the oligodendroglioma, which occurs mainly in the frontal lobe and shows the greatest tendency to calcify. Many patients survive fifteen to twenty-five years with this type of tumour due to its exceedingly slow growth. The general prognosis of gliomas and astrocytomas is related to both the site and histological grading. Seventy-five per cent of patients with Grade IV tumours are dead within nine months, and even with Grade I and II tumours seventy-five per cent of patients are dead within three years.

There is little to be gained by early diagnosis of these infiltrating malignant tumours for the following reasons. Those tumours arising in silent areas (i.e. in regions not associated with specific symptoms or signs) tend to remain asymptomatic until very large and even then may carry a good prognosis because they are accessible and resectable by virtue of their site. Whereas tumours arising in vital areas cause early symptoms and signs but are often inoperable because the deficit produced by surgery would be unacceptable. The chance of operation depends on the site of the tumour and survival on the histological grading. Paradoxically it is better to have a highly malignant glioma in the frontal pole than a low grade glioma in the parieto-temporal region!

The relative incidence of tumours in different sites are indicated in Figure 8.6.

Tumours outside the substance of the brain include meningiomas, intraventricular lesions, pinealomas and neurofibromas. They produce either local signs if strategically sited or non-specific signs and raised intracranial pressure if they interfere with the circulation of the C.S.F. (Figure 8.7).

year previously. Prior to admission an attack left her with permanent weakness of the left face and arm and a peculiar affect. Right carotid angiography revealed an avascular mass in the right frontal lobe. At craniotomy for glioma pus was encountered and a β-haemolytic streptococcus was cultured. She made a full recovery following surgery.

This history is typical of the sub-acute "space-occupying lesion" type of presentation, in a clinical setting in which the original source of infection is not certain.

Other infective diseases causing cerebral masses are relatively rare in Great Britain. The syphilitic intracerebral gumma has become a museum disease and intracranial tuberculoma has become an extremely rare disease although in India tuberculosis accounts for twenty per cent of all intracranial masses. Hydatid cysts are rare in Europe but account for thirty per cent of intracranial tumours in several South American countries. Clearly these disorders must be considered in immigrants and those who have served overseas in these areas.

(Other infectious diseases of the nervous system are discussed in Chapter 26.)

INVESTIGATION OF A SUSPECTED CEREBRAL MASS

Details of special investigations and interpretation are to be found in Chapter 25. Only details directly applicable to the diagnosis of cerebral tumours will be considered in this section.

1. The history and physical examination should be reviewed for any evidence to suggest an underlying primary neoplasm. Negative chest x-rays and a normal breast examination will exclude the majority of primary neoplasms. All previous surgical procedures should be reviewed. Very often patients have not been told or have forgotten the removal of a malignant tumour many years previously.

2. Plain skull films are almost always normal. Gross sella erosion is usually found only in the presence of obvious raised intracranial pressure and pineal shift usually parallels very obvious clinical evidence of a large mass in one hemisphere. Abnormal intracranial clacification may occasionally provide a diagnostic clue and the x-rays are usually abnormal in patients with a pituitary tumour. It is unusual for x-rays to do anything other than confirm clinical findings. Apparently abnormal skull films in the absence of symptoms and signs should always be interpreted with caution. This often happens when skull films are taken after a minor head injury and some unrelated abnormality is suspected.

3. An E.E.G. is more likely to be abnormal with an intrinsic tumour although it may be misleadingly normal in some cases. However, as a general rule an E.E.G. is more likely to raise false diagnostic possibilities, and when grossly abnormal often does no more than confirm very obvious physical signs. Interpretation by the clinician in charge of the case is more likely to avoid unnecessary investigation of dubious abnormalities.

4. Ultrasound investigation although finding its place at first in cerebral disease diagnosis no longer holds a significant place in investigation. The problem of reflection of sound waves from the skull have not yet been overcome and usually the shift of the midline is only certain when the clinical situation is already obvious.

The investigations discussed so far, although often showing abnormalities usually do so only when the situation is already clinically obvious. They do *not* advance the diagnosis but merely add supportive evidence and can occasionally be misleadingly normal in the most difficult clinical situations.

5. Radioisotope scanning is the first of the investigations providing accurate and occasionally pathologically useful information. The highest accuracy is achieved in meningiomas, cerebral abscesses and metastases (provided the latter are over 2 cm. in diameter). This is probably due to the combination of increased vascularity and oedema in these lesions. The diagnostic accuracy rapidly falls off in the case of gliomas and astrocytomas. Even in the most malignant tumours a false negative rate of thirty to forty per cent is possible and in low grade tumours the success rate is as low as twenty per cent. A negative scan may practically exclude meningiomas, abscesses and metastases but does *not* exclude other tumours. Furthermore acute vascular accidents cause positive scans and cannot be distinguished from a tumour unless the scan uptake decreases with time. Unfortunately the clinical situation may not allow the luxury of waiting and repeating the scan six weeks later.

6. The recent advent of computerised axial tomography (EMI scanning)—a form of computerised x-ray densitometry holds great promise for the future and although enormous advantages are already apparent the technique is still under evaluation and only available in a few centres in Great Britain.

7. Angiography was introduced in 1936 and remains an indispensable aid to tumour diagnosis. (Its role in vascular disease is discussed in the next chapter.) However, even angiography may fail to detect tumours in certain areas where shift of known vessels is not produced or lesions that do not develop a pathological circulation. However if the patient is suspected of having a tumour on one side a

carotid angiogram on the appropriate side is the investigation of choice, and the investigation most likely to indicate the site, and often the nature of the lesion.

8. Lumbar air encephalography is contraindicated in patients with suspected cerebral tumours as is lumbar puncture. There are occasional exceptions to this rule but only under close neurosurgical supervision (the whole problem is amplified in Chapter 25). In patients with tumours and particularly those with obstruction of C.S.F. pathways ventriculography is the procedure of choice unless angiography has already indicated the site and nature of the lesion. Air or sodium iophendylate (myodil) is put into the lateral ventricle via a burr hole and allowed to pass through the foramen of Munro into the third ventricle and down the aqueduct to the 4th ventricle until the site of the obstruction is seen. The shape and direction of the obstructive deformity often indicates the probable diagnosis.

The diagnosis of cerebral tumours is in the first instance based on the history and physical signs. Subsequent investigation is based on a sequence of investigations as seems appropriate to the clinical diagnosis. At all stages a continual review of the situation and the evidence provided by the tests already performed is evaluated and the need to continue the investigations considered. It is quite possible to fail to demonstrate a tumour at the first attempt and it should always be remembered that there is no absolutely exclusory test.

The need to continue to follow patients once suspected of having a tumour is evident. The expense, and risk of unnecessary investigation on the mere "suspicion" of a tumour should be apparent. Full tumour exclusion should only be considered when the clinical suspicion backed up by signs and screening investigation indicate a *real* possibility of detecting a tumour.

Chapter 9

THE CEREBRAL HEMISPHERES: 2. VASCULAR DISEASES

In the previous chapter the anatomy of the hemispheres was described and this knowledge applied to the detection of dysfunction in various areas. This has special application in the detection of cerebral tumours.

When we consider the blood supply of the cerebral hemisphere the single most important point to remember is that each lobe does not have an individual blood supply so that vascular disease usually produces an entirely different set of syndromes although on occasions some overlap with lobe disease can occur.

At the simplest level a hemiparesis means no more and no less than that there is an abnormality in the opposite hemisphere. A very common error is to assume that "hemiparesis" is synonymous with a "stroke", an assumption that may have disastrous consequences.

To make the differentiation between a neoplastic or other space occupying lesion and a stroke one must rely very substantially on the history and yet the abruptness of onset that characterises a vascular lesion *may* occur with a cerebral tumour, and conversely but much less frequently a stroke may have a sub-acute onset that mimics a tumour. Therefore, a very accurately plotted anatomical extent of the lesion can be critical in making the differential diagnosis and distinguishing those patients who should be considered for further investigation.

THE ARTERIAL BLOOD SUPPLY OF THE CEREBRAL HEMISPHERES

The hemispheres are supplied by the terminal branches of the carotid and basilar arteries. There are anastomoses between the various branches over the cortex and the efficiency of these is often critical in determining the final outcome of major vessel occlusions (Figure 9.1).

1. The Anterior Cerebral Artery (Figure 9.2)

The anterior cerebral artery sweeps forward and over the genu of the corpus callosum and then backwards as two vessels, the pericallosal and callosomarginal arteries, supplying the parasaggital cortex including the entire motor and sensory cortex controlling the leg.

Shortly after its origin the anterior cerebral artery gives off an inconstant branch known as the recurrent artery of Huebner. If present, this vessel contributes to the blood supply of the nerve fibres in the internal capsule destined to supply the cranial nerve nuclei and the arm on the opposite side.

The two anterior cerebral arteries are joined by a short anterior communicating artery which allows collateral flow to the opposite hemisphere if the carotid artery is occluded on either side. Whenever carotid ligation is contemplated in the treatment of an aneurysm the patency of this vessel has to be demonstrated angiographically before ligation is performed.

2. The Middle Cerebral Artery (Figure 9.4)

This artery originates at the bifurcation of the internal carotid artery just above the cavernous sinus. The vessel then passes laterally between the upper surface of the temporal lobe and the inferior surface of the frontal lobe to reach a position deep in the Sylvian fissure. Here it divides into three main vessels which pass upwards and backwards in the fissure giving off branches that exit along the length of the fissure to supply the surface of the hemisphere. These are the precentral, central, posterior parietal and posterior temporal arteries.

As the middle cerebral artery passes laterally it gives off a series of six to twelve long thin penetrating vessels that enter the anterior perforated substance to supply the basal ganglia and part of the internal capsule. These are the Lenticulostriate arteries. Terminal branches of the main vessel reach the occipital pole (see below) and probably provide an independent blood supply to the macular cortex at the tip of the lobe.

3. The Posterior Cerebral Artery

The posterior cerebral arteries are formed by the bifurcation of the basilar artery in the interpeduncular space (Figure 9.2 and Figure 9.4). Each vessel passes round the cerebral peduncles lying between the medial surface of the temporal lobe and the upper brain stem. Along its length each gives off vessels supplying the inferior medial surface and hippocampal area of the temporal lobe. A series of

Figure 9.1. Diagram to Show the Course of the Carotid and Vertebral Arteries in the Thorax and Neck

A, B, C are common atheroma sites
Lesions at A & B produce transient hemiparetic ischaemic attacks
Lesions at C produce brainstem ischaemic episodes
Lesions at D produce the "subclavian steal syndrome"—blood passes up the left carotid artery and back down the left vertebral artery to supply the left sub-clavian artery

Anterior cerebral arteries

Posterior cerebral arteries

Middle cerebral artery

Carotid siphon (in cavernous sinus)

Basilar artery

Carotid canal (in petrous bone)

Foramen magnum

C1

Vertebral artery

C2

Internal carotid artery

External carotid artery

C3

A

C4

C5

Common carotid artery

C6

Right sub-clavian artery

C7

Left sub-clavian artery

D1

C

D

B

Aortic arch

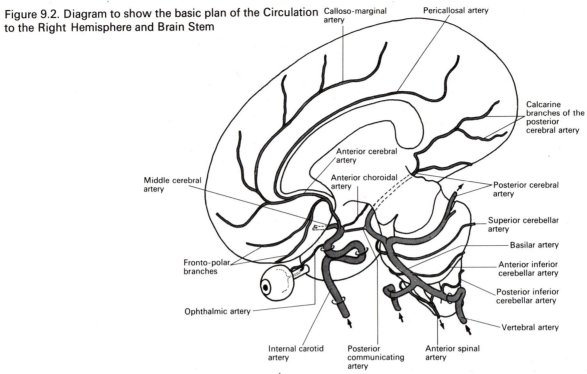

Figure 9.2. Diagram to show the basic plan of the Circulation to the Right Hemisphere and Brain Stem

Calloso-marginal artery

Pericallosal artery

Calcarine branches of the posterior cerebral artery

Anterior cerebral artery

Anterior choroidal artery

Middle cerebral artery

Posterior cerebral artery

Superior cerebellar artery

Basilar artery

Anterior inferior cerebellar artery

Posterior inferior cerebellar artery

Fronto-polar branches

Ophthalmic artery

Vertebral artery

Internal carotid artery

Posterior communicating artery

Anterior spinal artery

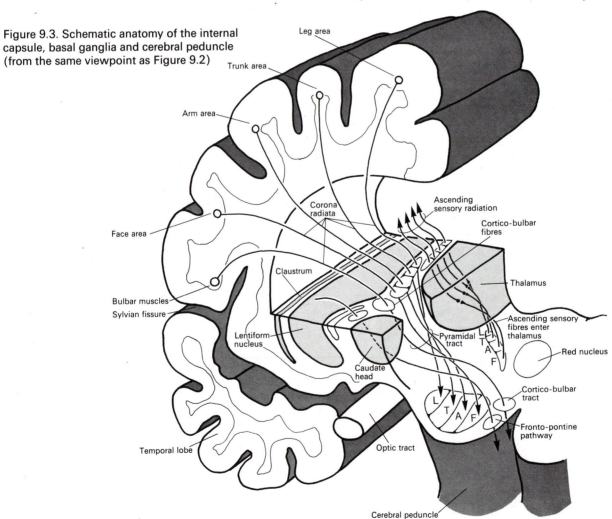

Figure 9.3. Schematic anatomy of the internal capsule, basal ganglia and cerebral peduncle (from the same viewpoint as Figure 9.2)

Leg area

Trunk area

Arm area

Ascending sensory radiation

Cortico-bulbar fibres

Corona radiata

Face area

Thalamus

Claustrum

Bulbar muscles

Ascending sensory fibres enter thalamus

Sylvian fissure

Red nucleus

Lentiform nucleus

Pyramidal tract

Caudate head

Cortico-bulbar tract

Fronto-pontine pathway

Temporal lobe

Optic tract

Cerebral peduncle

Figure 9.4. The Blood Supply of the Deep Structures of the Hemisphere

Callosomarginal Pericallosal } Arteries (Branches of the anterior cerebral artery)

Superficial branches of the middle cerebral artery

Deep branches of the middle cerebral, supply visual radiation

Vessels that tend to rupture

Thalamo-geniculate arteries

Posterior cerebral artery

Short and long penetrating arteries to the peduncle and midbrain

Trifurcation of the middle cerebral artery

6–8 lenticulo-striate arteries. Branches of the middle cerebral artery

Anterior choroidal artery

Internal carotid artery

Posterior communicating artery

Branches of posterior cerebral artery to the infero-mesial surface of the temporal lobe

Forward sweep of the anterior cerebral artery

Basilar artery

penetrating vessels supply the dorsolateral brain stem, the thalamus, posterior internal capsule and sublenticular and retrolenticular visual radiations. These are the thalamogeni-culate and thalamo-perforating arteries.

The main vessel terminates as the calcarine artery, supply-ing the visual cortex with the exception of the macular cortex at the tip of the pole. This has a dual or independent blood supply from the middle cerebral artery (see macular sparing hemianopia, Chapter 3).

THE CLINICAL PICTURES PRODUCED BY CEREBRAL BLOOD VESSEL OCCLUSIONS

The term occlusion is used reservedly. Following a C.V.A. it is unusual to find a vessel actually occluded. This is because most occlusions are probably due to embolic blockage with rapid subsequent recanalisation. However, a few minutes obstruction of flow in any vessel leads to irreversible damage to the territory supplied.

There are three main patterns of damage that can occur:

1. Occlusion of the main trunk of the parent vessel.
2. Occlusion of one of the important penetrating arteries.
3. Occlusion of one of the terminal branches.

We will consider these three possibilities for each vessel in turn.

Figure 9.5. Anterior Cerebral Artery Occlusion

Anterior Cerebral Artery Occlusion (Figure 9.5)

1. *Main Trunk Occlusions*

Anterior cerebral artery occlusions are quite rare. The picture depends to some extent on whether the recurrent artery of Heubner is present.

 a. If there is *no* recurrent artery the face and arm will not be affected, but the entire leg area of the cortex is destroyed. This causes flaccid paralysis of the leg, with cortical sensory loss.

 b. If there *is* a recurrent artery and the block occurs proximal to its origin, the anterior internal capsule will also be infarcted giving rise to a typical upper motor neurone facial weakness and a spastic arm with considerable potential for recovery (because the overlying arm cortex is intact) but a useless flaccid leg (because all cortical control of the limb is lost).

Because the paracentral lobules are also damaged, voluntary control of micturition is often impaired. Incontinence of urine is the almost invariable consequence. In some instances this combination of incontinence and flaccid weakness of the leg may lead to an ineffectual search for a cauda equina lesion. The clinical evidence against this is that in spite of the flaccidity of the leg the reflexes rapidly return and become *brisk* and the plantar response is *extensor*. These findings would be very unusual with a cauda equina lesion which usually cause areflexia and absent plantar responses (see Chapter 15).

Furthermore considerable intellectual deficit and memory disturbance may occur due to damage to fronto-parietal and fronto-temporal fibres in the cingulate gyrus.

In all cases if there is any evidence that the other leg is also affected (i.e. the lesion is not strictly unilateral) a para-saggital tumour must be excluded. Vascular occlusions affecting the hemisphere should *not* produce *bilateral* signs.

2. *Perforating Artery Occlusion*

If the recurrent artery of Heubner is present and is occluded, weakness of the face and arm will occur; this will be of pyramidal type. Even if the dominant hemisphere is involved dysphasia does not occur because the cortex is unaffected. This is a very rare syndrome.

3. *Terminal Branch Occlusion*

The terminal vessels primarily supply the cortex controlling the leg and infarction affects both motor and sensory function. Flaccid weakness of the leg with brisk reflexes and an extensor plantar response is found. The sensory loss affects accurate touch perception and joint position sense, i.e. is of the cortical type. This makes it almost impossible to mobilise the patient as even with splints to stiffen the leg the patient has lost awareness of its position. With distal lesions intellectual disturbances and bladder dysfunction may be less severe than that caused by a main trunk occlusion.

Middle Cerebral Artery Occlusions

1. *Main Trunk Occlusions* (Figure 9.6)

Middle cerebral occlusion causes massive infarction of the bulk of the hemisphere. There is often considerable cerebral oedema which may cause coma. There are also important differences between the hemispheres with global dysphasia if the dominant hemisphere is affected, and severe dyspraxia or even denial of the existence of the whole left side if the non-dominant hemisphere is affected.

From a motor point of view the lesion destroys both pyramidal and extrapyramidal mechanisms, hence a flaccid type of weakness of the face and arm, with little or no potential for recovery is found. The leg cortex is spared but is so extensively "undercut" by the lesion that even the leg rarely improves significantly.

This is quite the most devastating type of C.V.A. with very minimal improvement to be anticipated and a real chance

Figure 9.6. Distal Middle Cerebral Artery Occlusion

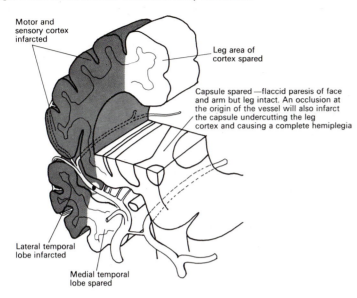

Motor and sensory cortex infarcted

Leg area of cortex spared

Capsule spared —flaccid paresis of face and arm but leg intact. An occlusion at the origin of the vessel will also infarct the capsule undercutting the leg cortex and causing a complete hemiplegia

Lateral temporal lobe infarcted

Medial temporal lobe spared

that the patient may die from the acute swelling of the infarcted hemisphere. Hemianaesthesia and a complete hemianopia are usually associated with the hemiparesis. The clinical picture can be identical with that produced by total occlusion of the carotid artery in the neck, with cross circulation via the anterior communicating artery keeping the anterior cerebral area perfused and the posterior cerebral circulation functioning normally. These anastomoses may be so efficient that patients are sometimes seen who have complete carotid artery occlusion and no neurological deficit.

2. *Perforating Artery Occlusions* (Capsular C.V.A.) (Figure 9.7)

A cerebral vascular accident due to occlusion of one of the lenticulostriate vessels is both the most frequent and the most favourable that occurs. Several of these vessels may be occluded without demonstrable effect. The evidence for this statement takes two forms. First, extrapyramidal syndromes are extremely rare in vascular disease of the brain and yet a substantial part of the basal ganglia is supplied by these vessels. Secondly, there is the evidence provided by "pseudo-bulbar palsy". The explanation of this condition is rarely understood by physicians. The mechanism is as follows; a vessel supplying the cortico-bulbar fibres to the brain stem nuclei becomes occluded. Because most of these nuclei have 50:50 innervation from each hemisphere, little or no deficit occurs and the episode may pass unnoticed. If some time later, the cortico-bulbar fibres on the *other* side are damaged the cranial nerve nuclei are abruptly deprived of

all control. Speech, chewing and swallowing become impossible. Significant recovery is unusual. The syndrome is most often seen in diabetic or hypertensive patients, as both groups are prone to develop widespread small vessel disease.

When the vessel supplying the main motor pathways of the capsule is occluded, a typical "capsular C.V.A." occurs. The only evidence of cortico-bulbar fibre damage is a mild upper motor neurone facial weakness. Both limbs on the opposite side are affected, resulting in a flaccid hemiparesis. In the acute stage no reflexes or plantar responses can be elicited. Within hours, tone starts to return, the reflexes become brisk and an extensor plantar response will be found. As the tone increases power returns in a pyramidal distribution. The flexor groups in the arm and the extensor groups in the leg become strong. The functional importance of this distribution of power results in the majority of patients leaving hospital with the typical hemiplegic gait. Physiotherapy capitalises on this functional distribution and helps the patient to learn to use the compromised limbs, but recovery would have occurred in any case.

There is rarely any sensory deficit or field defect, as both these pathways lie in the vascular territory of the posterior cerebral artery. A combination of hemiplegia, hemianaesthesia and hemianopia is not typical of capsular infarction and the prognosis in such cases is poor. These patients have either had a middle cerebral artery occlusion

Figure 9.7. Capsular Infarction (lenticulo-striate artery occlusion)

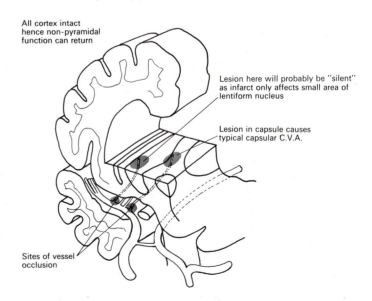

All cortex intact hence non-pyramidal function can return

Lesion here will probably be "silent" as infarct only affects small area of lentiform nucleus

Lesion in capsule causes typical capsular C.V.A.

Sites of vessel occlusion

(see above), an anterior choroidal artery occlusion (see later), or a haemorrhage into the internal capsule.

A capsular lesion is not accompanied by dysphasia because the parietal cortex is unaffected.

A distinction must be made between dysphasia and dysarthria. Dysarthria refers to poor phonation. With a capsular lesion in the acute stages, severe weakness of the face may lead to slurring of speech but the patient understands the spoken word, and uses words correctly. There is really no reason at all for there to be any confusion about the use of these terms.

3. Terminal Branch Occlusions

There are four major peripheral branches on each side.

a. The Dominant Hemisphere

The precentral artery supplies the motor areas for the face and arm and Broca's speech area. Occlusion of this vessel causes flaccid paralysis of the face and arm and total inability to speak, but with full comprehension. As the patient is also unable to write his anguish and frustration is considerable. Recovery is minimal although speech therapy may occasionally have a modest success in helping these patients to say a few key words.

If the central artery is occluded weakness of the face and arm occurs with mild dysphasic difficulties.

Occlusion of the posterior parietal artery produces *complete* aphasia with loss of comprehension and loss of speech, even though the patient may well be able to phonate and even say single irrelevant words, or new words of his own making (neologisms), or incoherent sentences of otherwise normal words (word salads). There may be a mild hemiparesis and cortical sensory loss but this is usually impossible to ascertain due to the lack of communication.

Occlusion of the superior temporal artery tends to cause receptive aphasia. The patient may be able to speak but the sentences are irrelevant and inappropriate to the examiner's question.

b. The Non-dominant Hemisphere

Superficial branch occlusions in the non-dominant hemisphere produce similar findings although the dysphasic difficulties are replaced by dyspraxia. Precentral and central branch occlusions cause a flaccid monoplegia of the arm and face. Occlusions of the posterior parietal and superior temporal arteries may cause mild sensory difficulties in the left face and arm and more generalised difficulties such as dressing apraxia or geographical disorientation and difficulty with skilled tasks.

Figure 9.8. Posterior Cerebral Artery Occlusions

Infarction of posterior capsule —causing hemisensory loss and if low enough a transient homonymous hemianopia may also occur

Infarction of occipital cortex typically causes macular sparing hemianopias due to a dual blood supply

Lower peripheral visual field

Upper peripheral visual field

Calcarine artery occluded

Penetrating branch occlusion

Main vessel occluded

Area of temporal lobe also infarcted by main vessel occlusion but unless bilateral no memory deficit occurs

Posterior Cerebral Artery Occlusions

1. Main Vessel Occlusions

The effects of a complete posterior cerebral artery occlusion can be very variable as there are anastomoses between the vessel and the middle cerebral arteries. Variable degrees of confusion and memory deficit can occur but these are more suggestive of *bilateral* damage due to occlusion of the basilar artery than occlusion of a single posterior cerebral artery. There may also be some sensory deficit and a field defect due to thalamo-geniculate artery occlusion.

2. Perforating Vessel Occlusion

Occlusion of one of the thalamo-geniculate vessels produces a more readily recognisable clinical picture. The posterior limb of the internal capsule, part of the thalamus and the visual radiation, are affected, resulting in hemianaesthesia with loss of all sensory modalities, and complete hemianopia (the visual radiation is damaged in its entirety). Often a good recovery is achieved but the main risk is the subsequent development of the Dejerine—Roussy syndrome which follows this type of C.V.A. When this happens the initial numbness is replaced by paraesthesia, or a painful sensation which becomes excruciating in severity when the affected limb is touched, or even continual pain without provocation. This thalamic pain may drive the patient to suicide and is rarely responsive to drugs or surgical procedures. Occasionally control may be achieved with Diphenylhydantoin (Epanutin) or Carbamezepine (Tegretol) combined with Imipramine (Tofranil).

If the branches to the upper brain stem are affected Hemiballismus may occur. This is the *only* extra-pyramidal syndrome typically produced by vascular disease. It consists of the abrupt onset of wild flinging movements of the limbs on one side of the body. It may subside spontaneously but can usually be arrested dramatically by 50 mgms. Chlorpromazine I.M.I.

CASE REPORT

A middle-aged woman with severe aortic stenosis was an inpatient awaiting surgery. Early one morning she acutely developed severe flinging movements of the left limbs, fracturing the left humerus against the cot side. Within minutes she had severe angina and the violent movements continued; with serious effects on the damaged limb. Within minutes of giving 50 mgs. of Chloropromazine intramuscularly all movement ceased. It did not recur. A cerebral embolus into the region of the sub-thalamic mucleus was thought to be responsible (see also Chapter 12).

3. *Terminal Branch Occlusion*

Occlusion of the calcarine artery causes a macular sparing hemianopia (see Chapter 3). This quite frequently occurs in otherwise fit young persons during the course of a migraine attack. There is no need to embark on full investigation of a patient who presents with a macular sparing hemianopia unless other physical signs are present. Incomplete lesions can cause a variety of incomplete hemianopias but in all cases the deficit will be absolutely congruous and will spare the macula, making identification easy.

Anterior Choroidal Artery Occlusions

The anterior choroidal artery arises directly from the carotid artery and runs backwards along the optic tract to the area under the internal capsule and eventually supplies the choroid plexus of the lateral ventricle. It has a variable distribution that includes the optic tract, and the basal ganglia. At one stage surgical ligation was attempted as a possible treatment for parkinsonism, but this occasionally produced devastating disabilities including hemiparesis, and was quickly abandoned.

It seems likely that some patients who develop hemiparesis, hemisensory loss and hemianopia and who clearly have not had a middle cerebral artery occlusion (i.e. no flaccidity, no drowsiness, no dysphasia or dyspraxia), have suffered an occlusion of the anterior choroidal artery and have infarcted the subcapsular area and the optic tract.

THE DEVELOPMENT OF SYMPTOMS AND SIGNS OF A VASCULAR ACCIDENT

The various clinical pictures produced by infarction of various areas of the central nervous system have been outlined. If the damage is clearly in one of these territories, the chance that the lesion is a vascular one is high. However, the majority of diagnoses of "stroke" are based on historical features. We will examine some of these features critically to show how valuable an accurate topographical diagnosis can be in substantiating a clinical impression.

The Abrupt Onset of Symptoms

The term a "stroke" emphasises the single characteristic feature of a vascular accident—the very abrupt onset. Yet so often the patient, often elderly and living alone, is found drowsy, confused and dysphasic and the mode of onset cannot be established. In such instances it is safest to pursue other diagnostic possibilities.

Drowsiness or increasing neurological deficit over a period of hours can occur following a middle cerebral occlusion but if the onset was not very abrupt, metabolic disorders, subdural or extradural haematomas, or meningeal infection must be excluded. In the elderly patient meningitis may present as a stroke-like illness, with confusion, minimal pyrexia and little neck stiffness.

A further cause of acute hemiparesis with or without confusion that should always be considered is hypoglycaemia. There is clinical and experimental evidence that poor perfusion of one hemisphere may lead to focal symptoms such as hemiparesis when the blood sugar reaches dangerously low levels.

Conversely the extremely abrupt onset of disability can occur with a cerebral tumour.

CASE REPORT

A 28-year-old pregnant woman collapsed and became deeply unconscious while preparing a meal. She had a complete right hemiparesis and fixed dilated pupils. A skull x-ray revealed half an inch of pineal shift to the left side. She died while further investigations were being arranged. She was found to have an extensive infiltrating glioma of the left thalamus. She had been asymptomatic until she collapsed.

A Stuttering Onset of Symptoms

Whenever a neurological event has occurred it is always important to establish whether there were any premonitory symptoms. For example, however abrupt the onset of the hemiparesis, if there was a prior history of several weeks' headache, personality change or ill health the diagnosis of a stroke would clearly be in doubt.

Repeated identical brief episodes of hemiparesis with full recovery quite often occur and such episodes are called transient ischaemic attacks. These are widely regarded as a sign of an impending stroke and in general angiography is indicated in an attempt to locate an operable athero-sclerotic lesion in the appropriate carotid artery. Even this assumption is not always reliable.

CASE REPORT

A 56-year-old man gave a history of several brief attacks of left-sided weakness over a six-week period. There were no residual signs and he was extremely hypertensive. Hypotensive therapy was begun and angiography was not performed in view of the very high blood pressure. A few weeks later a similar episode occurred without recovery. An angiogram performed elsewhere revealed a glioblastoma multiforme in the right hemisphere.

This is a good example of the "vascular" presentation of a neoplasm. Occasionally the reverse may occur and this is a particular feature of carotid artery occlusion.

CASE REPORT

A 38-year-old female gave a ten-month history of intermittent sensory symptoms affecting the left side, headache, memory impairment, and some personality change. Over a period of five days she developed a moderately severe left hemiparesis. Full investigation showed no sign of cerebral tumour but there was almost complete occlusion of the right carotid artery.

CASE REPORT

A 49-year-old military contracts manager for an aeroplane manufacturer gave a three-week history of episodic tingling and numbness in the left limbs. This had been associated throughout with a dull right frontal headache. Examination revealed a left attention hemianopia, left-sided facial weakness, impairment of sensation over the entire left side but no motor signs in the limbs. A tumour was suspected but a carotid angiogram revealed complete occlusion of the right internal carotid artery.

CASE REPORT

A 58-year-old company director complained of pins and needles in his left hand for two weeks which had been treated by neck traction. This was followed by attacks of clumsiness of the left hand, weakness of the left side of his face and difficulty in articulating, each attack lasting seconds only. Over three weeks things worsened until progressive weakness of the left side was apparent and he became forgetful and drowsy but denied headache. On admission he was extremely drowsy with a left hemiparesis, and a left extensor plantar; sensory testing was impossible. A right carotid angiogram showed complete carotid occlusion. Despite attempts to control cerebral oedema he deteriorated and died several days later.

The similarities in the latter case histories are remarkable and yet when the last patient was seen only six weeks after the second, the diagnosis of carotid artery occlusion did *not* seem likely on the clinical evidence. In the author's view carotid artery occlusion mimics a cerebral tumour so closely that a tumour is almost invariably the suspected diagnosis.

A Steady Improvement of the Neurological Status

Any abrupt neurological event with rapid recovery certainly qualifies for the term "a vascular event" and in the majority of instances it will prove to be due to a vascular accident. Unfortunately, in some instances, as already discussed, recovery is not the rule, and in the case of a middle cerebral artery occlusion the subsequent oedema may lead to deterioration, coma and even death. An intra-cerebral haemorrhage may produce a similar picture. This is discussed later.

Immediate loss of consciousness or an epileptic fit are extremely unusual events in an uncomplicated cerebral vascular accident. A major embolus from a fibrillating heart, an intra-cerebral haemorrhage or a sub-arachnoid haemorrhage should be suspected if either of these events occurs. Loss of consciousness or an epileptic fit should *never* be dismissed as due to a "small stroke". They are so unusual in major strokes that the likelihood of their occurring during an otherwise sub-clinical stroke seems remote.

Headache

Although severe headache of abrupt onset associated with neurological signs is most likely to occur during some form of cerebral haemorrhage, headache of moderate severity is by no means unusual in an uncomplicated occlusive cerebral vascular accident. Occasionally patients with migraine are unfortunate enough to suffer an occlusion during an attack of migraine. This is almost invariably an occlusion of the posterior cerebral artery or its terminal branches.

These problems and illustrative case histories have been included to highlight the fact that however obvious the diagnosis of "stroke" may appear to be, the subsequent physical examination should be performed to answer the question "are these signs compatible with a C.V.A. in a certain vascular territory?" This is essential to avoid compounding an error that may have been due to a misleading history.

Other Types of Cerebral Vascular Accident
Thrombotic Lesions

Whenever an occlusive cerebral vascular accident has occurred some basic disease processes that may predispose to intra-vascular thrombosis must be excluded, especially in the young patient. Haematological disorders, including polycythemia rubra vera, thrombotic thrombocytopaenic purpura, disseminated lupus erythromatosus and the heavy protein diseases should be excluded. At any age diabetes mellitus and syphilis should be considered and in the elderly a high sedimentation rate should be regarded as due to temporal arteritis until proved otherwise. All the necessary exclusory tests can be performed quite easily, and should be a routine part of the investigation of any patient with a suspected stroke. Embolisation from auricular fibrillation may be the first evidence of thyrotoxicosis, or indicate a recent myocardial infarction; and sub-acute bacterial endocarditis frequently presents as a C.V.A.

Haemorrhagic Cerebral Vascular Accidents

There are three main types of haemorrhagic cerebral vascular accidents. It is now known that very small vascular lesions previously thought to be thrombotic are small lacunar haemorrhages. Because the blood does not burst into the ventricles or sub-arachnoid space, this type of haemorrhage cannot be distinguished from a small occlusive lesion in the internal capsule or brain stem.

1. *Intracerebral haemorrhage*

A classical intracerebral haemorrhage usually results from the rupture of one of the more peripheral lenticulo-striate arteries in the region of the external capsule. The haemorrhage rapidly strips the soft tissue under the cortex and may rupture into the sylvian fissure or into the lateral ventricle. In either event the typical clinical picture is of a sudden fulminating headache with rapidly deepening loss of consciousness and tentorial herniation. The ipsilateral pupil and then both pupils dilate and become fixed to light. In a typical case death ensues within fifteen minutes to a few hours of the onset (brain stem haemorrhage is discussed in Chapter 12).

2. *Angiomas*

A less dramatic form of cerebral haemorrhage is associated with cerebral arterio-venous malformations or angiomas. Many such lesions remain asymptomatic throughout the patient's life. In many cases focal epilepsy is the main problem. In others recurrent subarachnoid haemorrhage occurs and as a rule there is a good recovery between attacks. This is because the haemorrhage is from sinusoidal vessels under low pressure, lacking the destructive power of a jet of arterial blood from a ruptured Berry aneurysm or an artery. Finally an acute intracerebral haemorrhage with the development of signs due to a stable intracerebral haem-

atoma may be the first symptom of an angioma. In the latter case evacuation of the clot is essential but in general the prognosis for cerebral angiomas is extremely good and surgical attack is only indicated for intractable focal epilepsy or intracerebral haematoma. Recurrent subarachnoid haemorrhage may cause dementia due to hydrocephalus. This is thought to occur when the arachnoid villi become blocked by blood products, and C.S.F. resorption is impaired. A shunt procedure will often be of benefit to the patient in these cases.

CASE REPORT

A 52-year-old man had lunch and drinks with friends. A little later while walking his dog he was seen to stumble and fall down a bank. When helped to his feet he was noted to have clumsiness of the right leg. He insisted on going home and for several hours seemed to be well. However the next morning he had a series of Jacksonian fits starting in the right arm and becoming generalised. During one of these he fell and injured the occipital region and remained drowsy. He was admitted to hospital. On examination he was drowsy with a flaccid weakness of the right arm and a spastic weakness of the right leg. He had bilateral extensor plantar responses. The differential diagnostic possibilities were legion but rapid deterioration in his conscious level required urgent surgical help. He was found to have an intracerebral haematoma in the posterior frontal pole associated with two separate arterio-venous malformations. Following evacuation of the haematoma he made a good recovery.

3. *Sub-Arachnoid Haemorrhage*

Sub-arachnoid haemorrhage due to aneurysms on the vessels traversing the sub-arachnoid space represents a common and frequently lethal cause of intracranial haemorrhage. Although these aneurysms may arise at embryologically weak points on the vessel wall, they are no longer regarded as congenital. Aneurysms are only found in children in association with coarctation of the aorta or hypertension due to renal disease. At all ages the presence of an aneurysm tends to parallel the height of the blood pressure. This is most dramatically demonstrated by the sudden change in sex ratio after the age of 50. Until the age of 50 the ratio of females to males is 3:2. Over 50 it rises to 10:1. This is thought to be due to the better long-term survival of females with significant hypertension leading to the development of aneurysms in the 50–70 age group.

Less than fifteen per cent of patients have symptoms prior to rupture and these usually consist of premonitory headaches over a few days. Headache, acute nausea and vomiting and neck stiffness are the hallmarks of subarachnoid haemorrhage. Transient cardiac arythmias or glycosuria often occur in a patient who has had a subarachnoid haemorrhage for reasons that are not clear.

Figure 9.9. Schematic diagram to show the Usual Sites of Aneurysms (Figures on the illustration as a percentage of total)

Incidence: Posterior circulation 4%
Internal carotid circulation 42%
Anterior cerebral circulation 34%
Middle cerebral circulation 20%

Anterior cerebral aneurysms
Asymptomatic before rupture
Sudden confusional state
Typical S.A.H. symptoms

Middle cerebral aneurysms
Asymptomatic before rupture
Hemiparesis, seizures, hemisensory loss
Dysphasia S.A.H. symptoms
Intracerebral haematoma

Middle cerebral artery
Anterior cerebral artery
Posterior communicating artery
Anterior communicating artery
Posterior cerebral arteries
Ophthalmic artery

Posterior communicating aneurysms
Headaches/III nerve palsy before rupture
Typical S.A.H. after rupture

Basilar artery

Vertebral aneurysms
Asymptomatic until rupture. Very lethal

Cavernous sinus

Ophthalmic Aneurysms
Eye pain, headache, visual loss
IV nerve palsy before rupture
Typical S.A.H. symptoms

Carotid siphon
Internal carotid artery

Carotid aneurysms
Asymptomatic until rupture
Typical S.A.H. symptoms

Aneurysm sites and associated symptoms are fully illustrated in Figure 9.9. If there are no signs except those of subarachnoid blood (headache, photophobia, neck stiffness, vomiting, bilateral extensor plantar response) no prediction as to the site of the aneurysm can be made.

The extremely controversial subject of the correct management of subarachnoid haemorrhage is beyond the scope of the present book. Referral to a neurological centre is indicated in all cases and if focal hemisphere signs are present confirmatory lumbar puncture is best deferred. These signs may indicate an intracerebral clot and lumbar puncture may confirm the diagnosis but kill the patient.

4. *Haemorrhage into Tumours*

When a patient with a cerebral tumour develops symptoms very rapidly it is often assumed that there has been a haemorrhage into the tumour. This is a very rare event—the sudden symptoms are usually produced by necrosis and oedema in the tumour as it outgrows its blood supply. The *only* tumour that characteristically bleeds is a metastatic deposit from a malignant melanoma. Many patients with cerebral metastases from malignant melanomas present with what at first sight is a simple sub-arachnoid haemorrhage.

CASE REPORT

A 36-year-old man collapsed while cycling uphill into a head wind. He was found semi-conscious and hemiplegic. On admission he had a stiff neck and a dense left hemiplegia with sensory loss. C.S.F. examination revealed heavily blood stained fluid. Twelve years previously he had had a malignant melanoma resected from his leg. Angiography revealed an avascular mass in the right parietal lobe. Craniotomy revealed a haematoma and the remains of a melanotic deposit into which the haemorrhage had occurred.

THE INVESTIGATION AND MANAGEMENT OF SUSPECTED CEREBRAL VASCULAR DISEASE

The three considerations that should be applied to this clinical situation are:

a. Is the site and extent of the lesion typical of occlusion of an identifiable vessel?

b. Is there any underlying haematological or biochemical disorder that could have predisposed to or mimicked a C.V.A.?

c. Are there any causative factors such as hypertension, auricular fibrillation, vessel stenosis or myocardial infarction that can be identified and treated?

a. This entire chapter has been devoted to the recognition of symptoms and signs that are typical of vascular accident. Anything that casts doubt on this diagnosis should prompt immediate further investigation.

b. Underlying disorders that predispose to cerebral vascular accidents include anaemia, polycythaemia, diabetes mellitus, malignant or severe hypertension, inflammatory vascular disease and in the elderly temporal arteritis. Heavy protein diseases such as myelomatosis should also be excluded.

Careful exclusion of cardiac arrhythmia, cardiac murmurs and subacute bacterial endocarditis by clinical examination, ECG and blood cultures should always be performed. Thyrotoxicosis should be excluded if the patient has auricular fibrillation as in the elderly the clinical evidence of this disorder may be minimal or absent.

Two special conditions related to diabetes mellitus are of great importance. Hypoglycaemia may cause focal signs such as a hemiparesis persisting for twenty-four hours or more with recovery. This possibility should always be considered with an intermittent clinical picture, and it is important to realise that the patient may remain fully conscious throughout the episode. It may occur in patients on oral antidiabetic drugs or insulin and rarely as a presenting symptom of primary hypoglycaemia. The second condition is hyperosmolar non-ketotic coma. The exact relationship of this condition to diabetes is uncertain. The biochemical syndrome consists of marked hyperglycaemia (often a glucose level over 1000 mgms. per cent) with marked dehydration and gross increase in serum osmolarity. Many patients with this condition develop focal neurological signs before becoming comatose. The condition is fatal unless recognised. An important clue is marked dehydration in a patient who has only been ill for a few hours. There is no ketosis which is the main distinguishing feature from diabetic coma.

c. Once it has been established that the patient has had a simple cerebral vascular accident without evidence of underlying disease the difficult problem of further management arises. Management depends on the clinical situation:

1. *The Patient who has a Completed Infarct*

Angiography is unnecessary as the surgical restoration of circulation to the damaged hemisphere usually causes haemorrhage into the infarct. This also may occur if anti-coagulants are used. Investigation is only indicated if other possibilities such as a subdural haematoma or tumour are suspected.

2. *The Patient who has Made a Complete Recovery*

This situation constitutes a "transient ischaemic attack". Definitions of "transient" vary from full recovery in one hour to twenty-four hours, but in general it is accepted that there should be no residual physical signs.

a. Any source of emboli should be excluded as discussed above. It should be remembered that in some series as many as thirty per cent of emboli originated in the heart, often in an area of myocardial infarction. Anti-coagulants are indicated unless there are any specific contra-indications and most physicians are reluctant to anti-coagulate patients over 65 years of age. Within the last two years soluble aspirin 300 mgms. twice daily has been used as an alternative to anti-coagulants. This form of treatment can be safely used in the over 65 age group and is thought to act by reducing platelet stickiness.

b. If the blood pressure is elevated anti-coagulants are contra-indicated and there is evidence that lowering the blood pressure often prevents further attacks. Hypotensive therapy should be pursued aggressively in this situation *whatever* the patient's age. There is no evidence to support a widely held belief that lowering the blood pressure is harmful to these patients. They may well develop symptoms of postural hypotension but this does *not* cause further cerebral vascular accidents.

c. If no source of emboli is found and the patient is normotensive the question of carotid angiography must be considered. Enthusiasm for this procedure is greatly increased if the patient has a bruit over one or other carotid artery. The problem with a bruit is that sometimes it *does* indicate local narrowing of the vessel, sometimes *no* cause is found and sometimes it is due to increased blood flow in the *normal* vessel because the other carotid artery is completely occluded. Angiography therefore carries considerable risks; it may complete a partial occlusion, particularly if the needle is pushed through the narrow area, or cause further cerebral ischaemia if the vessel injected proves to be the *normal* vessel. There are many and varied statistics as to the mortality and morbidity of angiography in this group of patients and even in centres where aggressive angiography is undertaken surprisingly few patients are found who have surgically amenable lesions.

3. *The patient Who is Having a Series of Attacks with Increasing Disability*

This situation is sometimes referred to as a "stuttering hemiparesis" or a "stroke in evolution". In this group of patients a progressive thrombosis of the carotid artery is usually responsible and the risk of *completing* the thrombosis during angiography is high. In the writer's view immediate anti-coagulation by heparinisation is the correct management and even this is often unsuccessful in preventing completion of the stoke.

In the author's view each patient with cerebral vascular disease presents an entirely different set of problems and the statistics of cerebral vascular disease become meaningless perfusion in the territory of one or both posterior cerebral arteries. An extreme example of this type of transient temporal lobe dysfunction in migraine occurred in a patient recently under the author's care and is worth quoting in detail.

CASE REPORT

A 46-year-old carpenter of previously exemplary character went swimming with his daughter early one Sunday morning. On his return he completed his income tax forms and started to mow his lawn. Shortly afterwards he went indoors and told his wife his vision was "funny" and he thought he was developing a headache. He went to lie down and a few minutes later when his wife took him a cup of tea he complained that he could not see or hear. He then became drowsy and if disturbed became extremely violent. He remained in this state for forty-eight hours. C.S.F. examination to exclude a subarachnoid haemorrhage and blood sugar determination to exclude hypoglycaemia were both normal. At this stage it was discovered that both his father and brother suffered from severe migraine. A tentative diagnosis of a somnolent state with a rage reaction due to medial temporal lobe ischaemia was made. On the third day the patient sat up in bed very bewildered and completely normal mentally. He had no recollection of events after his wife came into the room. He was able to relate that the visual upset was loss of the right visual field and that this had happened on previous occasions and had been followed by a headache. There seems little doubt that these were isolated migraine headaches. Several EEGs taken during the period of confusion were within normal limits.

This case indicates the extremely narrow area between "normal" and abnormal behaviour, not dependent on a gross disturbance of cerebral function but due to quite limited areas of dysfunction, usually in the region known as the limbic system, or its cortical connections.

4. *Dementia*

Dementia is a problem common to neurology and psychiatry and is usually divided into pre-senile dementia (onset before age of 65) and senile dementia. This classification places undue emphasis on the pre-senile group, because at any age dementia is a devastating problem both for the patient and even more so for the distraught relatives. At *any* age *full* investigation to exclude any treatable cause is vital. This is so important that a later section of this chapter is devoted to the causes and investigation of dementia.

The patient is to some extent protected from the full impact of his illness by loss of insight into his condition. There are many diagnostic and management problems in dementia, two of which are worth mentioning at this stage. A previously intelligent patient may react to the onset of dementia by developing obsessional behaviour patterns to avoid embarrassment or by becoming severely depressed. In either case it is easy to overlook the underlying intellectual decline. In the later stages of dementia patients may react with paranoid suspicion, often directed at the closest relatives whose concern is regarded with suspicion by the patient who may alter his will in others' favour. Testamentary capacity in these patients is a difficult medico-legal problem as favoured relatives often become involved in the patient's delusional system.

Although dementia often indicates diffuse loss of cerebral substance occasionally exactly the same situation is produced by quite local lesions particularly in the parasagittal or subfrontal regions. Typical case histories have been quoted in Chapter 8. Symptomatic dementia of this type is often due to interference with the activity of the cingulum or the orbital surface of the frontal lobe, both areas with important connections to the limbic system.

To understand the wide range of clinical features and disturbances of mood and affect that occur in diseases affecting these regions a broad grasp of the anatomy of the interconnections of the cerebral cortex and the limbic system and hypothalamus is necessary.

THE LIMBIC SYSTEM (Figure 10.1)

There are several definitions of the limbic lobe depending on whether anatomical or physiological considerations are paramount. Most current definitions exclude much of the olfactory apparatus and its central connections. The older terms, rhinencephalon, fornicate lobe or "smell" brain are not therefore synonymous with what is known clinically as the "limbic" system.

The limbic system includes the hippocampus and hippocampal gyrus, the uncus, amygdala, cingulate gyrus, part of the insula, the septal area, the isthmus, Broca's olfactory area and the orbital surface of the frontal pole. Embryologically the inner surface of the temporal lobe rolls in on itself, forming the curved groups of cells known as Ammons Horn which lie in the floor of the lateral ventricle as the hippocampus. The hippocampal gyrus is the area overlying the hippocampus which is visible on the surface of the posterior end of the temporal lobe immediately behind the bulge overlying the amygdala. The main fibre tract from the hippocampal area is the fimbria which is joined by other fibres from adjacent areas to form a dense bundle called the fornix which sweeps posteriorly and then up and over anteriorly to distribute to all areas of the hypothalamus but particularly to the mammillary body and parts of the thalamus. Some fibres from the fimbria decussate directly to the

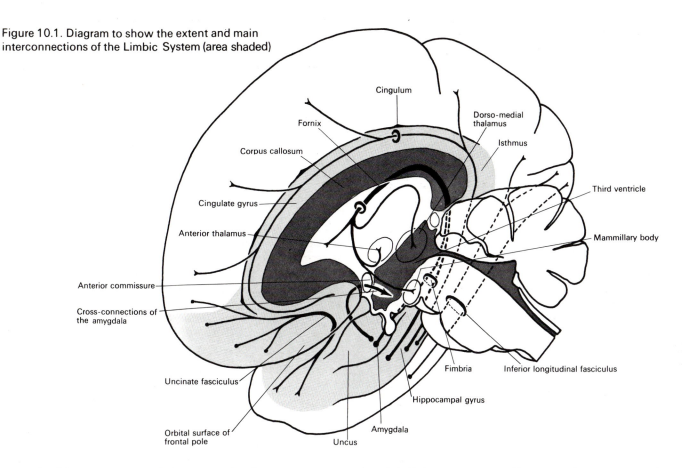

Figure 10.1. Diagram to show the extent and main interconnections of the Limbic System (area shaded)

Labels in figure:
Cingulum
Fornix
Dorso-medial thalamus
Isthmus
Corpus callosum
Cingulate gyrus
Third ventricle
Anterior thalamus
Mammillary body
Anterior commissure
Cross-connections of the amygdala
Uncinate fasciculus
Fimbria
Inferior longitudinal fasciculus
Hippocampal gyrus
Orbital surface of frontal pole
Amygdala
Uncus

opposite hippocampus and there are also important cross connections between the amygdala on each side through the anterior commissure.

Damage in the region of the amygdala is associated with rage reactions, hyperphagia (over-eating) and increased sexual activity. Lesions in the region of the uncus are associated with olfactory and gustatory hallucinations sometimes known as "uncinate fits". In fact seizures starting in any part of the temporal lobe have a unique opportunity to spread and involve other areas or both temporal lobes resulting in a wide range of physical and emotional phenomena that may occur during a "psychomotor seizure".

The cingulate gyrus lies above the corpus callosum, its connecting pathways traversing the isthmus posteriorly and extending as far forward as Broca's olfactory area. Operations directed at these pathways and the connections from the cingulate gyrus to the thalamus (see also Figure 10.2) form the basis of psycho-surgical procedures. These include frontal leucotomy and cingulotomy which may be performed in patients with phobic anxiety states and chronic pain syndromes; in the latter case producing blunting of the emotional response to pain although not abolishing the pain

itself. In recent years direct attacks on pain pathways have become more popular than psychosurgical procedures in the treatment of patients with intractable pain.

THE HYPOTHALAMUS (Figure 10.2)

Although the hypothalamus is *not* included in the limbic system from a functional point of view its exclusion is hard to understand as much of the expression of activity in the limbic system occurs via its important connections with the hypothalamus. The main afferent connections of the hypothalamus are derived from the fornix which is distributed to all the hypothalamic nuclei and terminates in the mamillary body. Olfactory information reaches the hypothalamus via the medial forebrain bundle which also receives information from other areas of the limbic system and forms the main longitudinal tract between the various hypothalamic nuclei as it lies along the lateral border of the hypothalamic area. Cortical activity reaches the hypothalamus directly and via the thalamus. From below, the hypothalamus receives visceral and gustatory sensation via both the dorsal longitudinal fasciculus and the reticular formation. Much of this

101

Figure 10.2. Diagram to show the main afferent and efferent connections of the Hypothalamus

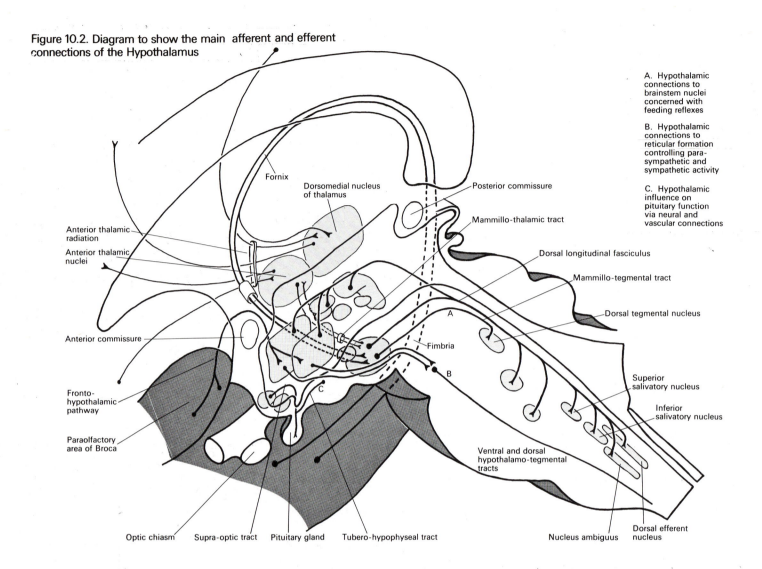

A. Hypothalamic connections to brainstem nuclei concerned with feeding reflexes

B. Hypothalamic connections to reticular formation controlling para-sympathetic and sympathetic activity

C. Hypothalamic influence on pituitary function via neural and vascular connections

visceral sensation is relayed to the cortex via the mammillo-thalamic tract and thalamus.

The efferent connections of the hypothalamus include ascending projections into the limbic system, the cortex, and thalamus and descending projections to the tegmentum, the reticular formation and the cranial nerve nuclei over the pathways already described (note: in the illustration the medial forebrain bundle and both afferent and efferent components of the main tracts are not shown to avoid over complicating the diagram).

Hypothalamic activity is mediated in three ways:

1. by control of the activity of sympathetic and para-sympathetic nervous system including the adrenal medulla.
2. extensive projections into the reticular formation.

3. through control of pituitary function by both direct neural connections (the supra-optico hypophyseal and tubero-hypophyseal tracts) and via the portal vascular system which carries the various releasing factors to the gland which liberate trophic hormones.

Functional Grouping of Hypothalamic Nuclei (Figure 10.3)

A detailed knowledge of the names and positions of the various hypothalamic nuclei is not essential for clinical purposes, but there are some rough generalisations that can be made as to the functional grouping of the nuclei.

The anterior nuclei including the supraoptic and para-ventricular nuclei are particularly concerned with fluid balance via ADH (anti-diuretic hormone) secretion and control of the thirst mechanism. The central nuclei are concerned with body temperature regulation by control over skin blood vessels and sweating mechanisms. Damage to these areas may cause diabetes insipidus, complete adipsia, hyperpyrexia, pulmonary oedema or acute gastric erosions. This part of the hypothalamus is particularly likely to be damaged by pituitary tumours, craniopharyngiomas, head injuries and intracranial surgery directed at tumours in this region.

Figure 10.3. Clinical Effects of Hypothalamic Lesions

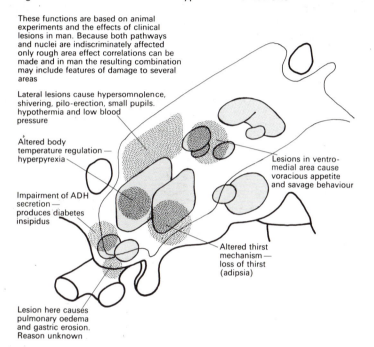

These functions are based on animal experiments and the effects of clinical lesions in man. Because both pathways and nuclei are indiscriminately affected only rough area effect correlations can be made and in man the resulting combination may include features of damage to several areas

Lateral lesions cause hypersomnolence, shivering, pilo-erection, small pupils. hypothermia and low blood pressure

Altered body temperature regulation — hyperpyrexia

Impairment of ADH secretion — produces diabetes insipidus

Lesions in ventro-medial area cause voracious appetite and savage behaviour

Altered thirst mechanism — loss of thirst (adipsia)

Lesion here causes pulmonary oedema and gastric erosion. Reason unknown

The posterior hypothalamus contains the dorsal nuclei, the posterior hypothalamic nucleus, and the supramammillary and mammillary nuclei and is mainly concerned with appetite, satiety, feeding reflexes, peristalsis and the control of the various secretions associated with eating and digestion. Lesions in this region are fortunately unusual and maybe associated with total loss of appetite leading to gross emaciation or gross overeating with obesity and altered personality often characterised by extremely bad temper and aggression.

Study of the lateral hypothalamic area is complicated by the fact that the inter-connecting pathways run through the area so that the clinical signs may indicate damage to either the nuclei or the tracts. Lesions in the lateral area are characterised by somnolence, disturbances of body temperature control and occasionally altered appetite.

The following case histories give some idea of the problems presented by hypothalamic disorders.

CASE REPORT

An 18-year-old boy became obese and somnolent and complained of visual failure. A suprasellar lesion was found which at surgery proved to be an extensive craniopharyngioma. Following surgery he was blind, and developed diabetes insipidus coupled with total loss of the thirst mechanism. Frequent episodes of drowsiness and epileptic seizures paralleled gross changes in hydration which could not be controlled by hormone replacement therapy and careful fluid balance control. He died a few weeks later.

CASE REPORT

A 32-year-old Indian lady flew to England to join her husband who had emigrated two years earlier. The husband had been informed prior to her arrival that she had been unwell with a personality disorder and had needed psychiatric treatment. He did not recognise her at the airport. Her weight had increased by 60 lb. She was apathetic and sleepy and took little interest in her surroundings. It was suspected that she had a visual disturbance of some sort. The optic discs appeared normal but formal field testing was impossible as the patient kept falling asleep. Her body temperature was low at 35°C and she woke up only long enough to eat a meal. Investigation revealed a large suprasellar mass. She died during surgical exploration. Post mortem revealed an extensive craniopharyngioma.

CLINICAL DISORDERS OF THE TEMPORAL LOBE–LIMBIC–HYPOTHALAMIC SYSTEM

Due to the anatomical extent of the limbic system and its widespread cortical connections lesions in many areas can give rise to an unusually complex range of symptoms. Due to the considerable importance of the area in special sense perception and visceral function these symptoms take unusual forms often including hallucinations. The area also has considerable importance in memory function and consciousness and several rare and unusual disorders of memory and sleep may have a basis in disordered limbic function.

1. Temporal Lobe Epilepsy

The most varied range of abnormalities undoubtedly occur in temporal lobe epilepsy and we can now consider some of these in an anatomical setting (see also Chapter 8).

1. Disturbances of hearing and balance. The cortical representation of hearing and balance are found in the upper temporal gyri just below the Sylvian fissure and discharges starting in this area typically produce auditory and vestibular symptoms.

CASE REPORT

For example, a 19-year-old shop assistant complained that for six months he had had brief attacks of a "whirring" noise in the head followed by a sensation as if he were pitching forwards which on several occasions had led to a fall. These attacks had occurred as often as six times a day and had never lasted more than thirty seconds. He had not lost consciousness. An EEG revealed seizure discharges originating in the right temporal lobe.

2. Seizures originating in the visual association areas in the parieto-temporal-occipital region may give rise to complex visual hallucinations. However *déjà-vu* phenomena, in which the patient's surroundings suddenly seem frozen and familiar, may have their origin in memory function abnormalities and are more likely to be due to hippocampal dysfunction.

3. Discharges arising in the region of the amygdala or uncus typically cause olfactory or gustatory hallucinations. These are very brief in duration and usually unpleasant in nature; often likened to "rotting cabbage" or "burning rubber". The brevity of the attack causes difficulty in identifying the odour; patients often complain that before they can take a second sniff the smell has gone. Persistent unpleasant smells are unlikely to indicate temporal lobe dysfunction. Such symptoms are often psychogenically determined or due to chronic suppurative sinus disease (sometimes known as ozena).

4. Altered awareness during the period of an attack or sometimes half-recalled events are characteristic of a temporal lobe attack and are probably related to hippocampal dysfunction, preventing complete sequential memory storage. Often bystanders cannot detect any change in the patient apart from rather deliberate movements frequently described as "zombie-like". Sometimes overtly peculiar behaviour may occur. One of the author's patients came to himself in a bus queue having completely destroyed his umbrella slowly and deliberately in front of bewildered onlookers.

5. The insula cortex deep in the Sylvian fissure is concerned with the involuntary motor activity of visceral function. Common motor accompaniments of a temporal lobe attack are lip smacking or chewing movements, which often provide an important diagnostic clue in episodes that might otherwise be mistaken for petit mal. Occasionally other visceral activity occurs and one of the author's patients frequently terminated her attacks by involuntary defecation which she was quite unable to prevent although fully conscious.

6. Another characteristic feature of temporal lobe attacks are visceral sensations. These commonly include epigastric "rising sensations", nausea, increased peristalsis and colicky pain or peculiar tingling and numbness in the perineum. These are sensations normally relayed through the reticular formation to the thalamus and hypothalamus and ultimately discharged to the temporal and frontal cortices.

7. A few patients have been reported whose attacks include heightened sexual activity, including masturbation to orgasm. The responsible discharges seem to arise in the medial temporal lobe. A central representation for sexual function in this region may be responsible for impotence in patients with temporal lobe neoplasms.

8. It is important to remember that "temporal lobe" phenomena may occur when cortical areas with close connections to the temporal lobe are damaged. These regions particularly include the orbital surface of the frontal lobe and the parasagittal region. Occasionally tumours quite remote from the temporal lobe may cause "temporal lobe epilepsy".

2. Disorders of Memory

Memory disorders usually follow damage to the medial temporal lobe and its connections to the mammillary body and upper brain stem. It follows that symmetrical lesions are usually responsible and unilateral temporal lobe lesions or surgical extirpation of one temporal lobe should *not* affect memory. Bilateral removal of the anterior temporal lobe produces the Kluver–Bucy syndrome which is characterised by psychic blindness (inability to identify friends and relatives), pathological overeating, heightened sexual activity and altered emotional responses. Some of these features may reflect the memory loss, the continued eating and sexual activity being due to incomplete recollection of previous indulgences.

Because bilateral damage is necessary for disorders of memory metabolic or infective processes are the usual cause, i.e. anoxia, hypoglycaemia and limbic encephalitis (sometimes associated with malignant disease and sometimes due to herpes simplex encephalitis). Bilateral posterior cerebral artery occlusion (due to an embolus lodged at the bifurcation of the basilar artery or sometimes occurring during a migraine attack) may cause transient or permanent memory deficit. Severe head injuries typically cause amnesia for the events of the injury and sometimes for the period immediately preceding the injury. This may be due to acute cell trauma, bilateral temporal lobe bruising, or dysfunction secondary to anoxia due to other injuries or post-traumatic cerebral swelling.

Two particularly interesting causes of amnesia are electro-convulsive therapy and Korsakoff's psychosis. In E.C.T. electric shocks sufficient to provoke an epileptic seizure are applied to one or both frontal lobes. Surprisingly this not only produces amnesia for the E.C.T. but also causes amnesia for events prior to the E.C.T. and following a large series of treatments patients may suffer permanent memory deficits. The explanation of this is unknown. Korsakoff's psychosis occurs in alcoholics usually as a permanent sequel to an attack of Wernicke's encephalopathy. The brain stem symptoms (nystagmus, extraocular nerve palsies and dysarthria) usually respond rapidly to vitamin therapy, but a permanent memory deficit with a particular tendency to upset temporal relationships occurs. This may be the cause of confabulation which is a striking but *not* diagnostic feature of the condition. There is often defective recognition of events and defective sequencing so that the patient often inaccurately relates past events as if they had happened recently. The responsible lesion is thought to be the haemorrhage and atrophy that is found in the mammillary bodies. Significant recovery from this condition is unusual.

Memory deficit is a constant feature of dementia and this problem is discussed in detail later in this chapter.

3. Disorders Affecting Sleep and Eating Habits

There are a few rare and peculiar disorders in which sleep and sometimes appetite are affected. Many have no known pathological basis and yet the association of the clinical features strongly suggests an underlying disorder of hypothalamic/limbic dysfunction.

Various encephalitic disorders cause pathological disorders of sleep including African trypanosomiasis and particularly Von Economo's encephalitis or encephalitis lethargica. In this disorder prolonged sleeping or complete reversal of the diurnal sleep pattern are the dominating features of the acute stage. Survivors later develop parkinsonian syndromes but in acutely fatal cases the bulk of the pathological changes are found in the peri-aqueductal grey matter rather than in the basal ganglia.

A peculiar disorder that usually occurs in young males is the Klein–Levin syndrome. This may follow an infective illness and is characterised by prolonged periods of sleeping coupled with peculiar behaviour and voracious appetite during the periods in which the patient is awake. Attacks lasting days to weeks may occur over several years. At the opposite extreme is the condition known as anorexia nervosa which usually occurs in females, and although a neurotic basis is suspected the combination of altered personality, complete anorexia and amenorrhea strongly suggest a hypothalamic/limbic system disturbance.

The "Pickwickian" syndrome, named after the fat boy in Dickens's novel *The Pickwick Papers* is a combination of extreme obesity, alveolar hypoventilation, carbon dioxide retention and frequent brief attacks of sleep in a setting of continual drowsiness. The sleep component may be a combination of fatigue due to sheer bulk and metabolic factors

but the whole syndrome could well start as a hypothalamic disorder. The patient quoted earlier who had a craniopharyngioma represents a minor degree of this syndrome.

Rarely cerebral tumours, particularly pinealomas and midbrain tumours, may produce pathological drowsy states in which the patient may appear to be in a coma but the eyes remain open and the patient may be able to indicate alertness by eye movement. This state is known as "akinetic mutism" and the alert but immobile condition as "coma vigil". The lesions responsible usually damage the midbrain reticular formation and include the tumours mentioned above and vascular lesions, particularly thrombosis of the upper segment of the basilar artery.

Finally we should mention narcolepsy. Although there is no known pathological basis for this disorder the combination of pathological sleepiness, hypnagogic hallucinations, paralysis and sudden collapse of posture all suggest dysfunction in the limbic-basal ganglia region. Narcolepsy should always be carefully distinguished from other causes of pathological drowsiness and full details of the condition are given in Chapter 22.

4. Dementia

In previous chapters we have referred to dementia as a presenting symptom. It is always essential to regard dementia as a symptom and not as a diagnosis. The only exception is in the very elderly in whom dementia is usually due to senile changes in the brain. Dementia should always be regarded as a symptom requiring urgent and complete investigation.

Dementia may be simply defined as failing intellectual function. There are three major components and various admixtures of the three may cause very variable clinical syndromes.

a. *Cognitive Dysfunction*

This includes memory deficit, failing judgement, difficulty in abstract thought and rumination on the past, progressing to total confusion for time and place and failure to identify even close relatives. In the very early stages perseveration of thoughts, losing the thread of conversations and even frank confabulation may occur, the latter not being a specific problem of alcoholism but occurring in any disorder in which memory is impaired.

b. *Disorders of Mood and Affect*

The patients' response to developing dementia varies widely. Some patients become extremely anxious and seek reassurance. Others react in a short-tempered way with relatives who cannot keep up with their disordered thought his speech became slurred. He thought it was the altitude and staggered outside for fresh air but found he could barely walk and his right leg was weak. He was driven down the winding mountain road with steadily increasing vertigo, slurred speech and vomiting. He made a steady recovery over the next two days and when he became mobile he noticed that he was bumping into things on his right side. When examined a week later the only residual physical sign was a right macular sparing hemianopia typical of a posterior cerebral artery occlusion.

It seems likely that this is an example of a large embolus or shower of emboli producing an on-going brain stem ischaemic episode with the final lodgement of the clot in the terminal reaches of the territory as discussed above.

Brain Stem Dysfunction Caused by Intracranial Haemorrhage

There are several ways in which intracranial haemorrhage can affect the brain stem.

An acute haemorrhage into the pons itself causes a very characteristic clinical picture. The patient becomes unconscious, and develops periodic respiration, pin-point pupils, loss of reflex eye movements and a spastic tetraplegia. Death may occur within hours, but should the patient survive for several days the body temperature steadily rises to about 106°F (42°C) before death. Haemorrhage into the cerebral hemisphere may track down the cerebral peduncle and produce a midbrain lesion. If the haematoma ruptures into the ventricular system the rapid rush of blood into the fourth ventricle may produce acute brain stem dysfunction with cardiac and respiratory arrest.

A primary haemorrhage into the cerebellum produces its lethal effect by brain stem distortion. Surgical evacuation offers a significant chance of recovery and it is vital to recognise this condition immediately. The onset is acute with occipital headache, vomiting and ataxia. Within a variable period consciousness becomes impaired with the onset of gaze palsies, bilateral pyramidal signs and periodic respiration. Death follows rapidly unless surgical evacuation of the clot is attempted.

Subarachnoid haemorrhage may produce a very similar picture. The onset is heralded by sudden headache often associated with nausea, vomiting and vertigo. These features occur so frequently that the bleeding is often mistakenly thought to come from an aneurysm in the posterior fossa. The similarity between this and the previously discussed condition should indicate that it is unwise to rush into performing a lumbar puncture in a case of suspected subarachnoid haemorrhage. An intracerebral haematoma is "space occupying" in the same way as a tumour. The risks of lumbar puncture are the same, and in the case of a cerebellar haematoma the risk is considerable. Lumbar puncture is *never* a life-saving procedure in subarachnoid haemorrhage and should not be allowed to become a life-threatening investigation. Expert neurological advice should be obtained before performing a lumbar puncture when the patient is rapidly deteriorating.

Multiple Sclerosis and the Brain Stem

Multiple sclerosis often affects the brain stem. In an established case of multiple sclerosis the diagnosis is easy. If it is the first event the diagnosis can be very difficult. Fortunately there are certain features that strongly suggest that the cause of a brain stem lesion is multiple sclerosis. The medial longitudinal bundle is extremely vulnerable and any form of internuclear ophthalmoplegia is very likely to be caused by demyelination in the brain stem. Isolated VIth nerve palsies are another common manifestation. Bilateral vestibular pathway damage with rotatory nystagmus on lateral gaze and vertical nystagmus on upward gaze is unlikely to be caused by any other disorder. The subsequent spontaneous recovery of any of these findings makes the diagnosis almost certain. The hallmark of brain stem multiple sclerosis is probably the combination of bilateral cerebellar and pyramidal signs. The patient may only complain of ataxia and slurring of speech, but examination often reveals that in addition to the anticipated cerebellar signs there are bilateral pyramidal signs. These include a brisk jaw jerk, pathologically brisk reflexes and bilateral extensor plantar responses. Although these signs strongly suggest the diagnosis of multiple sclerosis, it is always worth remembering that nothing can be regarded as absolutely pathognomonic of this condition.

Pontine Glioma

If a young child or a patient with neurofibromatosis develops brain stem signs the possibility of a brain stem glioma should be considered. In other situations or age groups this diagnosis is extremely difficult to make and multiple sclerosis is usually suspected. Any delay in diagnosis is potentially serious as many pontine gliomas are radiosensitive and early diagnosis and treatment may offer some hope of a prolonged remission. Many of these tumours start in the region of the VIth nerve nucleus and any combination of a VIth and VIIth nerve palsy should be regarded with suspicion. Minimal motor signs, brisk reflexes and extensor plantar responses are often present but hemiplegia is not an early symptom. The sensory pathways seem to be extremely resistant to infiltration by these tumours and patients often die of the disease without detectable sensory loss. Careful documentation of the signs and the recognition of new lesions in the brainstem should indicate the correct diagnosis if there is initial uncertainty. In spite of gross enlargement of the pons, blockage of the aqueduct is unusual and therefore headache is not a constant feature of the clinical picture.

Other Posterior Fossa Tumours

Cerebellar tumours in childhood produce rapidly progressive cerebellar signs and raised intracranial pressure. Medullo-blastomas may infiltrate the brain stem via the cerebellar peduncles. Ependymomas arising in the floor of the fourth ventricle produce unheralded vomiting and the presence of papilloedema usually excludes the diagnosis of a primary pontine tumour. Cystic astrocytomas do not invade the brain stem but may threaten the viability of the brain stem by mechanical distortion if the diagnosis is long delayed. Posterior fossa tumours other than metastases are relatively rare in adulthood. They also tend to be slow-growing producing a much less florid clinical picture than in child-hood and differential diagnosis may be extremely difficult. Pineal tumours produce raised intracranial pressure and evidence of upper midbrain compression such as Parinaud's syndrome. Acoustic nerve tumours usually produce signs of a cerebellopontine angle lesion. Rarely the signs of brain stem distortion dominate the clinical picture (see Chapter 6) Chordomas, cholesteatomas and meningiomas may arise in front of the brainstem. All may produce intermittent brain-stem symptoms mimicking multiple sclerosis or transient ischaemic attacks. Transient VIth nerve palsies, ataxia and pyramidal signs may be found. Even vertical nystagmus, often held to be diagnostic of an intrinsic brain stem lesion, can occur with extrinsic compression of the brain stem. Tumours in the region of the foramen magnum, usually meningiomas or neurofibromas, are notorious for producing recurrent episodes of tetraparesis and ultimately tetraplegia. A careful myelographic search in the region of the foramen magnum should always be made before ascribing such symptoms to multiple sclerosis.

Metabolic Brain Stem Dysfunction

The toxic effects of alcohol and many drugs are caused by reversible metabolic effects on the brain stem. Severe vertigo, ataxia, dysarthria, and nystagmus are common side-effects of anticonvulsant drugs. Diphenylhydantoin (Epanutin) (Dilantin U.S.P.) may even cause a reversible internuclear ophthalmoplegia. The diagnosis of deliberate or accidental overdose of Epanutin should be suspected in any patient having repeated attacks of drowsiness, ataxia, dysarthria and nystagmus. An overdose of glutethimide causes drowsiness, widely dilated pupils and brisk reflexes stimulating a brain stem lesion. Extensor plantars may occur transiently during drug overdosage and deflect attention from the desirability of obtaining blood samples for drug levels in *any* drowsy or unconscious patient.

Wernicke's encephalopathy is a serious complication of alcoholism. In addition to the characteristic mental change of gross confusion with memory loss there is a potentially fatal disturbance of brain stem function. Extra-ocular nerve palsies, usually VIth nerve palsies, conjugate gaze palsies, nystagmus and ataxia are the main features. These signs are readily reversible following parenteral therapy with Vitamin B_1. It should be remembered that this condition can also occur in patients who are malnourished for medical reasons such as malabsorption or following postoperative vomiting.

Central pontine myelinolysis is a rare lethal condition closely related to Wernicke's encephalopathy, occurring in the same clinical setting and with the same signs. The diagnosis is usually made at post mortem when the patient has failed to respond to Vitamin B_1 therapy.

Brain stem angiomas and brain stem encephalitis are ex-ceptionally rare and usually gain more prominence in differ-ential diagnostic discussions than they deserve. In the majority of cases where either diagnosis is entertained the patient is eventually found to have another condition. Encephalitis of the brain stem caused by herpes simplex virus has recently been reported and a rhomboencephalitis associated with Listeria monocytogenes meningitis also occurs.

Congenital anomalies of the foramen magnum may lead to the development of brain stem problems in later life. The syndrome of vertebrobasilar ischaemia may be caused by an anomalous odontoid peg or basilar invagination and syrin-gomyelia and syringobulbia are probably related to con-genital abnormalities of the foramen magnum. These con-ditions are fully discussed in Chapter 15.

Brain stem lesions occur quite frequently and may repre-sent an immediate threat to the patient's life or a delayed threat from complications such as aspiration pneumonia. Prompt accurate diagnosis is essential and this can best be achieved with a sound anatomical knowledge and an idea of the common causes of brain stem disease and their clinical behaviour.

The investigation of a lesion distorting the brain stem is difficult. Vertebral angiography is assuming increasing im-portance both in diagnosis and pre-operative assessment of the vascular supply of extrinsic tumours such as acoustic neuromas. Pneumo-encephalography causes little risk if the lesion *is* in the brain stem itself and often reveals characteris-tic displacement of the aqueduct and fourth ventricle. If it transpires that the lesion is in the cerebellum the risk of this procedure is so great that it is absolutely contra-indicated. In such cases ventriculography, in which the air or contrast medium is introduced through a burr hole into one or other lateral ventricle, is used. The risks of this procedure and potential complications are only acceptable when a lesion is known to be present; it cannot be regarded as a routine screening test. In most instances it is performed in theatre as a prelude to surgery. Simple isotope scanning is not very useful; if a lesion is seen it helps, but small lesions can easily escape detection. Computerised axial tomography (E.M.I. scanning) can detect lesions as small as 1 cm. in diameter and holds promise for the future for investigation of the posterior fossa but facilities are so limited at present that availability is the determining factor for performing the test. Myeloencephalography, in which myodil, introduced through the lumbar route, is allowed to run into the head, has some use particularly in extrinsic lesions such as neurofibromas, meningiomas and acoustic nerve tumours but unfortunately only indicates the site and extent of the lesion. It cannot indicate the possible pathology and carries all the risks of lumbar puncture *if* intracranial pressure is raised (Investigation techniques are discussed in greater detail in Chapter 25.)

Chapter 12

THE EXTRAPYRAMIDAL SYSTEM AND THE CEREBELLUM

There are anatomical, pathological and clinical reasons for considering disorders of the extrapyramidal system and cerebellum together.

Anatomical knowledge of the architecturally homogenous cerebellum has always been in advance of clinical knowledge. There are few physical signs of cerebellar disease and direct clinico-anatomical correlation is rarely possible. Often the resulting physical signs and symptoms are due to distortion of the brain stem and interference with the circulation of the C.S.F.

In contrast many disorders were long thought to be due to lesions in the extrapyramidal system and yet pathological findings were minimal or absent. Even now the anatomical extent of the extrapyramidal system is disputed, hence the expression "extrapyramidal system" rather than the more restrictive title "basal ganglia disease".

Since the relatively recent demonstration that many of these disorders have a neurochemical basis an entirely different concept of the functioning of the system has emerged. It is now apparent that far from the cerebellum being the "head ganglion of the proprioceptive system" with direct control over movement it merely serves as an integrating centre for postural information which it relays to the cerebral cortex and the basal ganglia. This explains the similarities of the symptoms and signs of extrapyramidal and cerebellar disease which may cause diagnostic confusion. Disease in both areas causes abnormalities of gait and unwanted additional movements either at rest or on attempted movement.

Unfortunately, such dynamic clinical disorders do not readily lend themselves to an illustrative approach. Instead an attempt has been made to provide a clear description of the various clinical signs and a disease classification based on clinical similarities and the age of the patient. The latter is particularly important in cerebellar disease in which the diagnostic possibilities are quite different in the child and adult.

ANATOMICAL CONSIDERATIONS (Figure 12.1)

Movement is initiated through the direct cortico-spinal or pyramidal system which is very highly developed in man. At the same time the continual postural adjustments that under-lie smooth and co-ordinated movement are initiated by the cortico-pallidal system which projects mainly into the putamen. To complete the volitional side of activity there are the important cortico-ponto-cerebellar projections, which enter the cerebellum through the very large brachium pontis (middle cerebellar peduncle). Therefore all three parts of the C.N.S. concerned in movement are simultaneously alerted to the onset, intended direction and aim of a movement.

It is only in disease states that the extent and importance of the non-pyramidal mechanisms become apparent.

The main sensory input to the system comes from the muscle, tendon and joint position sense nerve endings, mainly via the spino-cerebellar tracts, and from the vestibular apparatus via the vestibular nuclei. Information from both sources enters the cerebellum through the inferior cerebellar peduncle (the restiform body).

The cyto-architecture of the cerebellar cortex is uniquely arranged to allow the projection of a vast amount of information on to the extensive dendritic net of each purkinje cell and models explaining this in computer and mathematical terms have been made. The large axon from each purkinje cell projects to the central cerebellar nuclei; mainly to the dentate nucleus on the same side. This nucleus relays the information to the opposite ventral-lateral thalamus and cortex via the dentato-rubral, rubro-thalamic, dentato-thalamic and thalamo-cortical projections. These pathways leave the cerebellum in the brachium conjunctivum (superior cerebellar peduncle) and decussate through the region of, or relay in, the red nucleus. The information reaching the thalamus is then projected to the extrapyramidal cortical areas and direct to the basal ganglia particularly to the putamen, caudate and external globus pallidus. This completes a group of circuits involving cortical, basal ganglia and cerebellar components; the cortex initiating the activity and the cerebellar input providing the necessary feed-back information.

In addition to these outer circuits there is a very important inner loop which appears to have an inhibitory feed-back effect on the globus pallidus. This is a relay through the subthalamic nucleus (of Luys). Damage to this circuit literally unleashes one of the most dramatic conditions in neurology, the syndrome known as hemi-ballismus.

The other efferent pathways from the basal ganglia

Figure 12.1. Scheme of Extrapyramidal/Cerebellar System

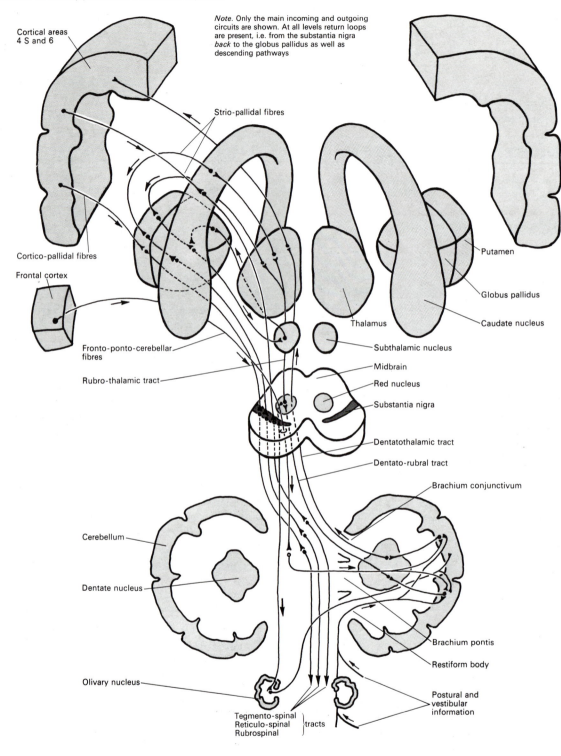

Cortical areas
4 S and 6

Note. Only the main incoming and outgoing
circuits are shown. At all levels return loops
are present, i.e. from the substantia nigra
back to the globus pallidus as well as
descending pathways

Strio-pallidal fibres

Cortico-pallidal fibres

Frontal cortex

Fronto-ponto-cerebellar
fibres

Rubro-thalamic tract

Cerebellum

Dentate nucleus

Olivary nucleus

Putamen

Globus pallidus

Caudate nucleus

Thalamus

Subthalamic nucleus

Midbrain

Red nucleus

Substantia nigra

Dentatothalamic tract

Dentato-rubral tract

Brachium conjunctivum

Brachium pontis

Restiform body

Postural and
vestibular
information

Tegmento-spinal
Reticulo-spinal ⟩ tracts
Rubrospinal

remain uncertain. Certainly an important pathway to the substantia nigra is known to exist but the exact routes of extrapyramidal activity below this level are unknown. The projections probably include tegmento-spinal, rubro-spinal, reticulo-spinal and olivo-spinal tracts. The relay through the olivary nucleus includes a circuit back into the cerebellum. Damage in this pathway has been implicated in disorders characterised by myoclonic phenomena.

The pathways described and illustrated represent only a fraction of the total neuronal circuitry involved in normal extrapyramidal function. Those included provide the best framework for clinical discussion.

PATHOLOGICAL AND BIOCHEMICAL CONSIDERATIONS

Parkinsonism was the first recognised and certainly the most studied disease of the extrapyramidal system. In spite of intensive pathological study the only constant finding was depigmentation and loss of neurones in the substantia nigra. In the period 1918–1927 a pandemic of a viral disorder known as encephalitis lethargica (Von Economo's encephalitis) occurred. This was associated with very gross disturbances of sleep, behaviour and every possible combination of abnormal movement. In patients dying of the disorder no constant pathological findings that could account for the physical signs were obtained. In recent years the severe and occasionally irreversible facial dyskinesias and dystonias caused by phenothiazine tranquillisers provided further evidence of obvious clinical disease in the absence of pathological abnormalities.

It is only in the last twenty years that histochemical studies of the brain have produced the dramatic breakthrough that indicated that these conditions are due to neurochemical disorders in the absence of neuronal damage. The normality of the underlying neural pathways has been adequately confirmed clinically by the dramatic restoration of near normal function to patients immobilised by parkinsonism for decades, by the oral administration of transmitter precursors such as L-Dopa. Acetylcholine, nor-adrenaline, dopamine and serotonin are the known transmitters but only the acetylcholine/dopamine system is understood. It would appear that it is not a simple matter of stimulatory and inhibitory transmitters in balance. There is evidence that both acetylcholine and dopamine have stimulant effects in some areas and inhibitory effects in others. However, some rough generalisations in the present state of knowledge indicate the possible relationship of the two systems:

In normal extrapyramidal function it would seem that a balance between cholinergic and dopaminergic pathways exists, whether these be inhibitory or stimulatory.

1. A decrease in activity in the cholinergic pathways or an increase in dopaminergic pathway activity causes choreiform movements. For example in Huntington's chorea severe degeneration of the caudate nucleus, in which most cholinergic neurones are concentrated, is a prominent feature. Conversely, if an excessive dose of L-Dopa is given to parkinsonian patients they develop choreiform movements.

2. An increase in cholinergic activity or a decrease in dopaminergic activity causes parkinsonism, a combination of tremor, rigidity and slowness of movement. Hence atropine-like drugs which block cholinergic neurones are of benefit in parkinsonism, and drugs that deplete or block dopaminergic neurones will worsen or cause parkinsonism. Such drugs include reserpine and the phenothiazines.

It follows from these therapeutic and biochemical considerations and the fact that depression often complicates parkinsonism and that antipsychotic drugs produce parkinsonism that there is a possibility that mental disorders are related to similar but as yet unidentified alterations in the neurotransmitters.

The complexity of these pathways which are actually closed loops with different transmitters at different synapses certainly explains the peculiarities and paucity of pathological findings. For example, histochemically and clinically it is clear that in parkinsonism the main problem lies in the dopaminergic synapses in the pallidum and yet the main pathological change is found in the synaptic area of the substantia nigra. It also explains why a lesion in one site does not necessarily indicate a specific function for that area. For example it would be incorrect to assume that because chorea occurs if the caudate is damaged that the normal function of the caudate is to prevent chorea. However, the assumption that damage to one circuit leads to an inbalance that could be corrected by deliberately destroying another circuit formed the theoretical basis for the moderately successful stereotactic operations for parkinsonism which enjoyed a vogue before the introduction of L-Dopa. There is still a place for such surgery in some conditions and this will be indicated in a later discussion.

CLINICAL FEATURES OF EXTRAPYRAMIDAL DISEASE

There are a wide range of movement disorders and physical signs associated with disease in the extrapyramidal system.

and following carbon monoxide poisoning (leaking car exhaust, unsuccessful suicide bid).

Drug-induced parkinsonism causes little tremor but considerable cogwheel rigidity and bradykinesia. A full list of drugs that may cause parkinsonism is included in Chapter 24. Oculogyric crises are the only additional feature in drug-induced disease. Very rarely parkinsonism follows a head injury. The rarity probably reflects the fact that a head injury of sufficient severity to damage the basal ganglia is likely to prove fatal.

Postencephalitic Parkinsonism

This condition occurs as an immediate and delayed complication of Von Economo's encephalitis. The peak incidence of this condition has now passed but isolated patients manifesting some of the features very typical of the post-encephalitic variety are still seen. Historically, there have been several pandemics of this disorder over several hundred years and it may well appear again.

These features are:

1. Reversed-Argyll–Robertson pupils (see Chapter 2)
2. Oculo-gyric crises (see Chapter 8).
3. Seborrhoeic dermatitis of the forehead and face.
4. Severe sialorrhoea (drooling of saliva).
5. Respiratory tics, intractable hiccoughs.
6. Behavioural disturbances.

Arteriosclerotic Parkinsonism

In the writer's opinion this is *not* parkinsonism; arteriosclerotic rigidity is a better term. The patient or relative usually gives a history of the abrupt onset of mental and physical slowing coupled with slurred speech, drooling of saliva, difficulty chewing and swallowing and immobility.

There is no tremor, the main physical findings are very marked rigidity and slowness of movement without features typical of parkinsonian bradykinesia such as the feet getting stuck. In fact the gait consists of quick short, shuffling steps known as "Marche au petits pas".

On physical examination pseudo-bulbar dysarthria, a brisk jaw jerk, brisk reflexes and bilateral extensor plantars provide evidence of diffuse cerebral damage. In idiopathic parkinsonism the reflexes are unaffected and the plantar responses are usually flexor.

This diagnosis has great practical significance. The use of anti-parkinsonian drugs in these patients almost invariably provokes severe confusion and visual hallucinations without any beneficial effect on their physical disabilities. Only diazepam seems to be of some help to these patients.

Intellectual Function and Depression in Parkinsonism

It was previously held that parkinsonism was not associated with intellectual deterioration. Since the advent of the marked physical improvement produced by L-Dopa it has become apparent that at least half the patients with parkinsonism have a moderate to severe degree of intellectual impairment. Although at first it was thought that this had been unmasked by L-Dopa there is growing concern that in some cases the therapy is in some way responsible for the sometimes abrupt dementia that may occur in patients on L-Dopa.

Depression has always been recognised as a part of the parkinsonism syndrome and lately the suspicion that it is an integral part of the disease rather than a reaction to the disease has been raised. This is discussed further in Chapter 24.

Varying degrees of parkinsonism complicate several rare disorders including Shy–Drager syndrome. In this disease a combination of parkinsonism, autonomic neuropathy and motor neurone disease occurs more or less simultaneously. It is a very rare but an exceedingly unpleasant and lethal disease. Nearly all reported patients have presented with micturition disturbances, either retention or incontinence of urine and severe constipation. Postural hypotension causes frequent syncopal attacks and careful physical examination will usually detect evidence of both parkinsonism and motor neurone disease. The normal course of the disease is death within two to four years of the onset.

CASE REPORT

A 48-year-old female was admitted to hospital with a history of unsteadiness of gait, severe constipation, urinary retention and syncopal attacks. She was discharged with the diagnosis of hysteria. When reviewed in the clinic only six months later she had obvious parkinsonism with gross bradykinesia, a postural hypotensive drop from 120/80 to 60/0 and severe sphincter disturbance. She steadily deteriorated over the next few months developing widespread muscle wasting and fasciculation. This is a classical example of the Shy–Drager syndrome.

Parkinsonism associated with dementia and motor neurone disease constitutes the syndrome known as Jakob–Creutzfeldt Disease (see Chapter 10).

The treatment of parkinsonism is detailed in Chapter 24.

Sydenham's Chorea

This condition has become a rare disease with the decreased incidence of rheumatic fever. It typically occurs within three months of an attack of rheumatic fever in patients between 5 and 20 years of age. It has an insidious onset and in half the patients is unilateral. It is frequently dominated by an emotional upset that very easily leads to a mistaken diagnosis of hysteria. The typical choreiform movements subside in three to six months. Occasionally an unusual variant of this condition in younger children produces a flaccid hemiparesis.

Chorea gravidarum probably represents a recurrence of Sydenham's chorea during a subsequent pregnancy, and has also declined in frequency. Some doubt has been thrown on this explanation by the recent recognition of typical chorea syndromes produced by the birth control pill. Furthermore one of the author's patients with chorea due to the pill developed the condition three months after the completion of a chorea-free pregnancy, making an underlying neural deficit unlikely.

Other Rare Causes of Chorea

Chorea has been reported in association with systemic lupus erythematosus, polycythaemia rubra vera, thyrotoxicosis, diphenylhydantoin (epanutin) intoxication, phenothiazine hypersensitivity and as a complication of excessive doses of L-Dopa. Some elderly patients develop choreiform movements spontaneously which may raise the possibility of Huntington's Chorea. This is usually senile chorea without genetic significance.

Huntington's Chorea

Huntington's chorea is certainly one of the most unpleasant diseases known. This is not only because it is inherited as an autosomal dominant with complete penetrance but because of the nature of the disease itself.

Rarely the disorder may manifest itself in childhood and is then somewhat atypical with considerable rigidity and even parkinsonian features rather than chorea; even epilepsy may occasionally be the first symptom. Family studies have suggested a high incidence of anti-social, alcoholic or psychopathic behaviour as a premorbid personality change in patients with this disease, but it has been argued that these phenomena merely reflect the young person's knowledge of the possibility that he will get the disease that has killed so many of his family. When one realises that the death often involves ten years of relentless generalised choreiform movements with progressive dementia this alternative explanation seems reasonable. Apart from the movement disorder and dementia which usually begins in the third decade there are no physical signs. Reflexes are usually normal, plantar responses are flexor and continence is only impaired with the onset of severe dementia. In some cases dementia may precede the movement disorder by several years or vice versa.

Perhaps the greatest hope lies in the recently devised test which may enable future sufferers to be detected before they can have children. This is based on the demonstration that low doses of L-Dopa induce choreiform movements in a certain percentage of relatives of patients with Huntington's chorea and does not do so in control patients. The predictive value of the test will have to await proof that these L-Dopa sensitive patients go on to develop the disease. Although genetically this will be a valuable advance the ethical dilemma that will result when discussing the test results with the patient is obvious.

Some symptomatic relief from the movements may be achieved with haloperidol or thiopropazate but relentless progression is the rule.

Athetoid and Dystonic Diseases

Dystonia is a feature of many rare diseases and their rarity justifies only a brief description of some of the clinical and biochemical features.

1. Kernicterus

Children who have had kernicterus (neonatal jaundice) may develop athetoid posturing of the limbs later, between the ages of 5 and 15. This problem has been greatly reduced by the treatment of Rhesus negative babies by exchange transfusion and latterly prevention in utero by immunisation procedures.

2. Wilson's Disease

This is a rare inborn error of copper metabolism in which copper is deposited in the basal ganglia and liver. A wide range of tremors, athetoid and dystonic movements develop but cirrhosis of the liver is the most serious feature. One of the diagnostic clinical features is a fine brown dust-like ring around the edge of the limbus of the cornea called a Kayser–Fleischer ring. The serum copper and caeruloplasmin levels (the copper transport protein) are greatly decreased. The disorder is now treatable with penicillamine but early recognition of the disorder is essential for complete control.

3. Hallevorden-Spatz Disease

This is a rare degenerative disease of children that causes progressive dystonia, hyperkinetic movements and retinitis pigmentosa. The aetiology is unknown; the course is one of progressive physical and mental deterioration.

4. Lesch–Nyhan Disease

Lesch–Nyhan Disease is the most recently recognised of these disorders. It is associated with severe athetoid/dystonic movements and self-mutilation. The latter is not uncommon in mentally defective children but is particularly severe in this disorder in which the children will eat their lips, tongue and fingers unless all the teeth are removed. It is associated with very high serum uric acid levels but the relationship of this finding to the movement disorder is unknown.

5. Dystonia Musculorum Deformans

This condition is inherited either as an autosomal recessive or dominant gene. The recessive variety is particularly common in Jewish families and usually produces severe disability. The dominant variety demonstrates variable penetrance with very mild disability in some affected members of the family. In the fully developed form the patient's body is pulled into grossly abnormal dystonic postures and jerked by frequent choreiform movements.

6. Paroxysmal Choreoathetosis (Reflex Epilepsy)

This is also often inherited as an autosomal dominant. In typical form sudden brief choreoathetoid postures or movements follow a sudden movement. One young male patient of the author's dreaded fielding in cricket. If he had to run for the ball his first few strides were dominated by bizarre writhing movements of his right limbs. His brother and mother had the same problems although his mother had outgrown the problem and was a first class pianist.

The commonest types of dystonia are known as the segmental torsion dystonias as opposed to the disorders discussed above which involve all or most of the body.

7. Spasmodic Torticollis

This extremely unpleasant and disabling condition affects the middle aged of either sex. The head is turned to one or other side and typically the shoulder on the same side is slightly hunched up as if to meet the chin. Initially the movement is spasmodic often occurring when the patient reaches out for something but later the spasm is continual with severe cramp-like pain in the contracting muscles and aching in the neck. In some cases the patient or preferably *someone else* can easily get the head back to the normal position by gentle pressure applied to the side of the chin. For years this was regarded as a psychological disorder but the overwhelming opinion amongst neurologists is that this is an organic syndrome related to the torsion dystonias.

8. Writer's Cramp

Writer's cramp was previously regarded as a neurotic syndrome in pre-retirement clerical workers. Current opinion now recognises that this occurs in many patients as an organic extrapyramidal syndrome and in fact many patients go on to develop parkinsonism or other dystonic syndromes.

9. Blepharoclonus and Blepharospasm

This condition occurs in an older age group and consists of frequent and prolonged episodes of forced eye closure. As in the case of writer's cramp it may be an early feature of parkinsonism.

10. Facial Dyskinesias

This group of disorders have been increasingly recognised as a complication of phenothiazine therapy but in fact these chewing, chomping movements of the face, lips and tongue often occur in elderly demented patients and in patients with mental subnormality. It is possible that the self-mutilation of the lips in the latter group and in the Lesch–Nyhan syndrome is merely a gross aberration of these movements. In addition to the facial movements repeated swallowing or tongue protrusion may occur.

11. Drug Induced Dystonias

The commonest cause of dystonic syndromes at the present time is drug hypersensitivity. The drugs responsible include all the phenothiazines, tricyclic antidepressants, benzo-diazepines and L-Dopa. In fact it is the recognition that all the syndromes described above and formerly thought to be due to neurosis, occur during drug reactions that has completely altered medical opinion to the general acceptance that these are organic disorders.

Drug-induced disorders include blepharospasm, oculogyric crisis, facial spasms, tongue protrusion, webbing of the neck due to muscle contraction, torticollis, antecollis, retrocollis, hyperextension of the back, lateral flexion of the spine, dystonic postures of the limbs and fine jerking restless movements of the limbs (sometimes called peripheral akathisia).

Although drug therapy is generally ineffective in the organic disorders, in drug-induced cases, increasing the dose of the offending drug or treatment with an alternative phenothiazine may prove as effective as withdrawing the drug. In fact on occasions the movement disorder may develop *after* the offending drug is withdrawn (tardive dyskinesia). This is particularly true of the facial movement group.

There are important differences between the different types of phenothiazine and extrapyramidal syndromes.

Piperazine side chain drugs: tri-fluo-perazine (Stelazine), fluphenazine (Modecate), perphenazine (Fentazine), prochlorperazine (Stemetil), are particularly likely to produce *acute* onset dystonia—often after a single dose in young females. It is interesting that it is the anti-emetic effect that is often the indication for the use of the drug, and that metoclopramide (Maxalon) an anti-emetic drug unrelated to the phenothiazines, may also produce acute dystonic syndromes. These are hypersensitivity reactions.

The chloro-substituted agents such as chlorpromazine are more likely to produce parkinsonian syndromes after many years of use, and are usually responsible for the tardive dyskinesias. Clearly these drugs are not producing hypersensitivity reactions but chronic alterations in transmitter substances.

Myoclonic Disorders

In Infancy and Childhood

Myoclonic jerking and myoclonic epilepsy are features of several conditions in infancy. These range from the progressive lipoidosis of Krabbe causing dementia and ultimately death to non-progressive and remitting conditions such as the myoclonic encephalopathy of infancy. In this condition brief shock-like muscle contractions follow startle or attempted movement. This condition may respond to ACTH and remit without sequelae. Infantile myoclonic spasms or "salaam" attacks are more serious and associated with a classical EEG appearance known as hypsoarrythmia. The attacks start in the first year of life and consist of a cry followed by trunk flexion or a brief "lightning jerk" of the entire body with extension of the legs and upturned eyes. Eventually, after two to three years, the attacks cease but are usually superseded by other forms of epilepsy and almost invariably the child is found to have suffered considerable cerebral damage.

In the second decade another group of disorders occur. These include simple myoclonic epilepsy with occasional grand mal attacks and myoclonic jerks complicating petit mal or idiopathic grand mal. A highly lethal variant is known as Lafora-Body disease. In this condition what starts as myoclonic epilepsy is rapidly followed by cortical blindness and increasing dementia. Lafora bodies are mucopolysaccharide cellular inclusions found in nerve cells, and in the supra-renal glands and kidneys. All patients die within six years of the onset. Another important disorder, which is usually fatal, has been recently recognised as due to an abnormal immune response to the measles virus. This is the condition known as subacute sclerosing leucoencephalopathy and occurs in the age range 5–20 years. The affected patient has usually had measles very early in life (before 2 years of age). The onset includes intellectual or behavioural problems, myoclonic jerking, spasticity, rigidity and increasing dementia leading to death over a period of one to two years. The C.S.F. globulins are markedly elevated and immunological evidence suggests that an abnormal immune response to intra-neuronal measles virus is responsible. The EEG is characterised by an extremely flat tracing with occasional bursts of high voltage spikes associated with visible myoclonic jerks. In recent years a few patients who have apparently recovered from this condition have been reported.

In the Adult

Myoclonic jerking preceding an epileptic fit occurs in some 10 per cent of epileptic patients. It is particularly likely to occur in the first hour or two after waking and often warns the patient that an attack is pending.

Myoclonic jerking occurs in some families with Friedreich's ataxia and as a specific component of Ramsay–Hunt cerebellar degeneration (dyssynergia cerebellaris myoclonica), which is discussed in detail in the next section. Some families have been reported in which parkinsonism and myoclonus appear in different members and some patients with myoclonic epilepsy may develop a parkinsonian state in later life.

A rare disorder known as Jones–Nevin syndrome (subacute spongiform encephalopathy) is also associated with myoclonus. Patients with this condition develop rapidly progressive dementia and myoclonic jerking, usually between the ages of 50 and 70. The aetiology is unknown but there is considerable overlap with Jakob–Creutzfeldt syndrome and it is thought that the two disorders may be variants of the same condition. Jakob–Creutzfeldt disease has been shown to be due to a virus infection.

There are many other disorders in which myoclonic jerking may occur of even greater rarity than those already mentioned. As a general rule in view of the possible serious implications any patient with myoclonic jerking should be referred for an expert opinion.

THE CEREBELLUM

For clinical purposes there is little to be gained by attempting to learn the complicated anatomy of the cerebellum with its confusing double nomenclature.

Basic Anatomy

The anatomy of the cerebellum and its connections is shown in Figures 12.2, 12.3 and 12.4.

There are two basic regions, the midline structures and the cerebellar hemispheres. The midline groups include the lingula anteriorly, the vermis in the middle and the flocculonodular lobe posteriorly. The lobes are divided into a small

Figure 12.2. Schematic diagram of the Cerebellum in relation to the Brain Stem

This is the same angle of view as in the brain stem illustrations in chapter 11

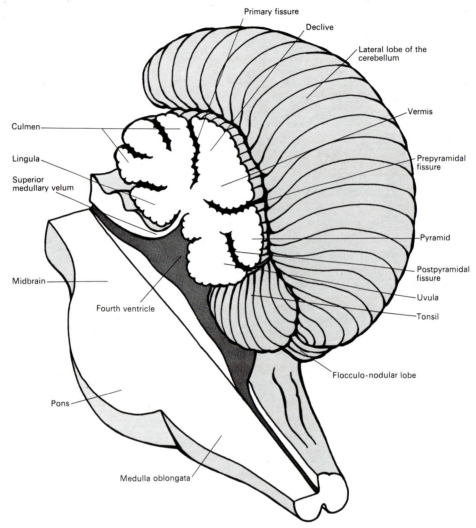

anterior lobe and a large posterior lobe. Each hemisphere contains a large main nucleus, the dentate, through which the bulk of efferent cerebellar information is discharged. There are smaller roof nuclei which are mainly concerned with vestibular reflexes and occular movements.

Clinically lesions affecting the midline group produce severe ataxia. Lesions in the lingula extend into the superior medullary velum producing fourth nerve palsies or into the superior cerebellar peduncle producing severe tremor of the arm on the same side. Lesions in the vermis cause severe ataxia; often making it impossible for the patient to sit or stand unsupported. Lesions in the flocculo-nodular region

cause ataxia, vertigo (due to damage to vestibular reflex pathways) and vomiting if they extend into the floor of the fourth ventricle. Tumours at all midline sites tend to cause early obstruction of the aqueduct or fourth ventricle resulting in headache and papilloedema.

The signs of a lesion in the lobes depend on the symmetry. A unilateral lesion produces classical cerebellar signs in the limbs on the same side (see later). Symmetrical involvement of both hemispheres, as happens in some of the cerebellar degenerations may produce quite mild symmetrical signs with moderate gait ataxia.

The most dramatic "cerebellar" signs are found in diseases

Figure 12.3. The Cerebellum—Main Afferent Connections

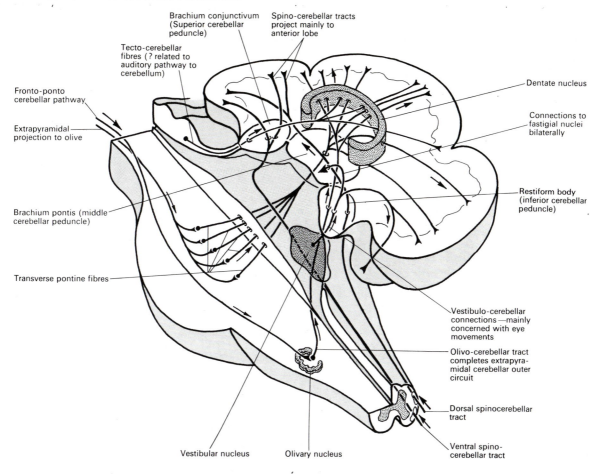

Brachium conjunctivum (Superior cerebellar peduncle)

Spino-cerebellar tracts project mainly to anterior lobe

Tecto-cerebellar fibres (? related to auditory pathway to cerebellum)

Fronto-ponto cerebellar pathway

Extrapyramidal projection to olive

Brachium pontis (middle cerebellar peduncle)

Transverse pontine fibres

Dentate nucleus

Connections to fastigial nuclei bilaterally

Restiform body (inferior cerebellar peduncle)

Vestibulo-cerebellar connections—mainly concerned with eye movements

Olivo-cerebellar tract completes extrapyramidal cerebellar outer circuit

Dorsal spinocerebellar tract

Vestibular nucleus

Olivary nucleus

Ventral spino-cerebellar tract

Figure 12.4. The Cerebellum—Main Efferent Connections

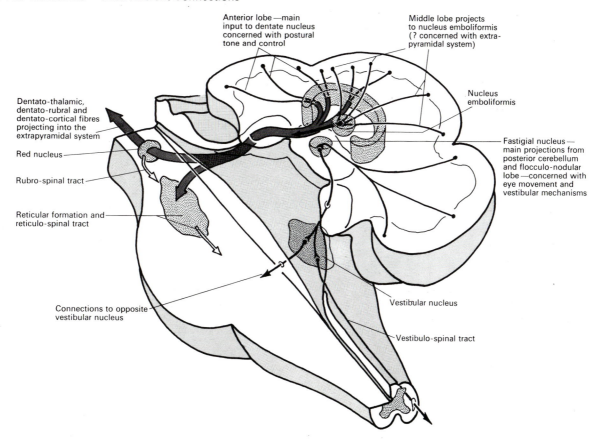

Anterior lobe—main input to dentate nucleus concerned with postural tone and control

Middle lobe projects to nucleus emboliformis (? concerned with extra-pyramidal system)

Dentato-thalamic, dentato-rubral and dentato-cortical fibres projecting into the extrapyramidal system

Red nucleus

Rubro-spinal tract

Reticular formation and reticulo-spinal tract

Nucleus emboliformis

Fastigial nucleus—main projections from posterior cerebellum and flocculo-nodular lobe—concerned with eye movement and vestibular mechanisms

Connections to opposite vestibular nucleus

Vestibular nucleus

Vestibulo-spinal tract

which damage cerebellar connections in the brain stem, either the main efferent pathways in the superior cerebellar peduncle or the inflow pathways in the inferior and middle cerebellar peduncles. One of the most difficult false-localising signs in neurology may result from a lesion affecting the fronto-ponto-cerebellar pathway.

CASE REPORT

A patient seen recently by the writer, a 50-year-old female had a known history of carcinoma of the breast. She presented with a short history of headache, vomiting and drowsiness. On examination she had marked papilloedema, left-sided cerebellar signs and bilateral extensor plantar responses. A confident clinical diagnosis of a left-sided cerebellar metastasis was made but on further investigation a right frontal metastasis was found!

CLINICAL SIGNS OF CEREBELLAR DISEASE

The most important physical sign of cerebellar disease is ataxia. This is best defined as inco-ordinated or inaccurate movement *which is not* due to paresis, alteration in tone, loss of postural sense or the intrusion of involuntary movements. For this reason the majority of neurologists do *not* test cerebellar function until they are certain that the patient has normal power, tone and sensation.

In children there are three common findings that may easily be mistaken for ataxia. These are the intrusion of choreiform movements, myoclonic jerks or minor status epilepticus (status petit mal). In the latter variety the child will sit drooling, with a blank expression on its face and all voluntary movements are performed with little pauses and sudden jolts. The EEG is diagnostic.

In the adult there are also three common clinical errors. Mild pyramidal weakness may easily produce "ataxia" on cerebellar testing unless allowances are made for the weakness. Many extrapyramidal disorders in their early stages produce "pseudo-paresis" or "pseudo-ataxia" unless the rigidity and involuntary movements are identified. Extremely anxious patients frequently perform very badly on formal cerebellar function tests due to tremulousness.

1. Gait Ataxia

A patient who has gait difficulty due to a cerebellar disorder is frightened to stand. He spreads his feet apart and will hold on to any support that is available. He will not fall but may reel from side to side even when supported and consistently to the same side if a unilateral lesion is present. Minimal degrees of gait ataxia are best detected by asking the patient to walk on a line. After one or two inaccurate steps the patient refuses to go further and reverts to a wide based stance. Although patients in this position tend to wobble even more when they close their eyes they do not fall. This is often referred to as a positive Romberg Test, but as discussed in Chapter 6 this is not strictly accurate.

An important gait abnormality also often misdiagnosed as ataxia occurs in elderly females. It has been called the 3F syndrome (Fear of Further Falling). It typically occurs after an elderly female has had an attack of vertigo, syncope or a drop attack. They will only walk in a bizarre posture, pushing one foot forward tentatively while leaning right back on the other. The arms are held at 90° to the body, slightly forward with the hands facing downward. They insist on a relative walking behind them, and insist on reaching forward to sit on a chair long before they reach it. They do *not* fall. This seems to be an entirely functional disorder that is extremely difficult to cure. Even prolonged physiotherapy seems to provide little reassurance and as soon as they attempt to walk alone they revert to the classical and ridiculous posture.

2. Truncal Ataxia

Truncal ataxia is a particular feature of midline cerebellar lesions. The patient may be unable to sit or stand without support with a tendency to fall backwards. Unless the flocculo-nodular lobe is involved there may be no other definite symptoms or signs. Limb ataxia is minimal or absent.

3. Limb Ataxia

Cerebellar function in the limbs is tested in several ways. In Chapter 9 we have discussed the value of observing the patient's outstretched hands as a screening test for disorders of pyramidal and proprioceptive function. In pure cerebellar disease the outstretched hand on the affected side tends to hyperpronate so that the palm faces outwards, and rises, often to 12" above the level of the other hand. In severe cerebellar disease some tremulous movements appear. If the examiner presses down gently on the patient's outstretched hands and suddenly releases the pressure the affected hand flies up completely out of control.

When these tests have been performed the patient's ability to touch the tip of his nose and then the examiner's index finger is tested. This is known as the finger/nose test. If postural sense has already been tested there is *no need* for the patient to attempt the test with his eyes closed. In fact, the value of the test is greatly enhanced if the examiner moves the target finger, varying both the direction *and* distance from the patient's nose. In this way quite mild inco-ordination, terminal intention tremor and dysmetria (over-shooting) can be detected.

The equivalent test in the legs is the heel/knee/shin test. The patient is asked to place the tip of the heel (not the sole of the foot) on the tibial tubercle of the other leg and run the heel down the shin. The heel is then *lifted* off and replaced on the tibial tubercle. The foot is *not* rubbed up and down the shin. If the sole of the foot is allowed to sit astride the shin the foot slides up and down with the tibia acting as a guide! Some mild inco-ordination is within normal limits for this test, particularly in the elderly with painful hips or knee joints. The test must be performed properly and over-interpretation of minor abnormalities should be avoided.

Unilateral ataxia is a reliable indication of disease affecting the cerebellar hemisphere on the same side. If severe, it could indicate disease affecting cerebellar input on the same side, the decussated dentato-rubro-thalamic pathway damage or even a lesion in the opposite frontal pole. When one adds the possibility of subtle ataxia produced by pyramidal lesions and posture sense loss the clinical difficulty occasionally experienced in diagnosing a cerebellar lesion with confidence is understandable.

4. Rapid Alternating Movements

On completion of the ataxia tests a variety of simple rapid movement tests are performed. These detect fragmentation of movement or inaccuracy of movement which is accentuated by the speed at which the movement is attempted. This is known as dysdiadochokinesia. The most useful tests are those in which the patient taps himself on the back of one hand as fast as he can or taps his foot on the floor or against the examiner's hand. This test is also subject to the proviso that there should be no pyramidal deficit. Finally, the patient is asked to make a fist and with his elbow half flexed tries to pronate and supinate the fore-arm as fast as possible. In an abnormal situation the movement is slow and irregular and the shoulder joint will start to abduct and adduct wildly as the whole arm becomes involved in the effort.

5. Other Signs

The signs already discussed, difficult as they are to elicit, are definite evidence of cerebellar dysfunction. There are a variety of other signs that are occasionally even more difficult to elicit and less certain in their interpretation.

Tone: In cerebellar disease the tone of the muscles is reduced on the side of the lesion. Reduced tone is a highly subjective phenomenon and although occasionally it is unequivocally reduced this is by no means invariably true.

Reflexes: In parallel with the decrease in tone the reflexes tend to be less brisk and rather slower in rise and fall producing what is known as a pendular jerk. Again, this is highly subjective and in the majority of patients no definite abnormality of the reflexes is found.

Nystagmus: As discussed in Chapter 8, nystagmus is not an essential feature of cerebellar disease, and if found usually reflects involvement of the flocculo-nodular lobe. If present the nystagmus is maximal towards the side of the lesion.

Dysarthria: Cerebellar disease affects the auto-regulation of breathing and particularly its integration with speech. This tends to produce spluttering staccato speech. So-called scanning dysarthria is more typical of combined pyramidal-cerebellar lesions and usually occurs in multiple sclerosis.

Writing: Writing is often affected and typically the patient enlarges his writing to make it more legible—quite the reverse of parkinsonism in which the writing becomes smaller.

Head Posture: there are three ways in which head posture may be altered by cerebellar disease. All produce a head tilt to one side. Lesions in the superior medullary velum may cause a fourth nerve palsy and lead to head tilt to compensate for diplopia. A cerebellar hemisphere lesion may unbalance postural tone, leading to a head tilt towards the side of the lesion. Lesions in the flocculo-nodular lobe causing raised intracranial pressure may directly irritate the dura in the posterior fossa, causing neck stiffness and tilting and retraction of the head to one side.

Vomiting: In view of the difficulties encountered in making a definite diagnosis of cerebellar disease on clinical evidence the considerable significance of vomiting in patients with cerebellar tumours deserves special mention. The characteristic features may be remembered as the 3 P's; postural, positional and projectile vomiting. The vomiting is typically very sudden without nausea and hence tends to be projectile. It typically occurs if the patient is in a certain position and very commonly if the patient attempts to sit up suddenly. The writer would regard the latter feature as diagnostic of a cerebellar tumour *even* in the absence of other physical signs.

CASE REPORT

A 36-year-old self-employed builder had been under a great deal of pressure and developed mild headaches and attacks of sudden vomiting. There were absolutely no physical signs but if he suddenly sat up from lying he almost invariably vomited. An E.M.I. scan revealed a cystic midline tumour, confirmed by operation. The patient and his medical advisers thought his symptoms were due to anxiety.

In summary pure cerebellar disease may produce very definite symptoms, particularly unsteadiness of gait, but remarkably subtle physical signs often dominated by a single feature, such as truncal ataxia. Patients with very florid physical signs usually have involvement of cerebellar connections in the brainstem. For the same reason extensive surgical resection of part of the cerebellum may produce remarkably little residual deficit, and even metastatic lesions may be treated surgically in anticipation of an acceptable end result.

CEREBELLAR DISEASE IN CHILDHOOD

In childhood there are five main categories of disease that may affect the cerebellum. Some of these are detailed elsewhere and will not be discussed in detail here.

Congenital Lesions

These conditions include various maldevelopments of the cerebellum, often associated with Arnold–Chiari malformation or the Dandy–Walker syndrome (see Chapter 15). Often the associated meningocoele or raised intracranial pressure are the presenting symptoms, but mild cases of Arnold–Chiari syndrome may not produce symptoms until two years of age. As in the case of extrapyramidal disorders it is worth remembering that ataxia cannot become fully manifest until the pyramidal system becomes functional. Apparently "acute" movement or gait disorders starting in the second year of life are frequently found to be due to congenital abnormalities or neonatal brain damage. One condition that genuinely causes a delayed presentation dominated by ataxia is congenital aqueduct stenosis. Some patients with this condition may present in their teens, with symptoms which include ataxia, VI nerve palsies, enlargement of the head, papilloedema with visual failure and declining intellectual function. The onset may be very insidious and the condition is easily misdiagnosed as a cerebellar tumour.

Metabolic Disorders

There are several metabolic disorders which may cause cerebellar dysfunction and ataxia. These include metachromatic leucodystrophy, Bassen–Kornzweig disease and Refsum's syndrome, which are discussed in Chapter 16. There are five additional disorders.

1. Ataxia in children may be due to drugs, especially anticonvulsants and in particular diphenylhydantoin and primidone. Occasionally acute ataxia and drowsiness may be found to be due to alcohol if the child has had access to spirits.

2. Ataxia, papilloedema and drowsiness may be due to lead poisoning and consequent cerebral swelling. This is easily misdiagnosed as a cerebellar tumour.

3. Maple Syrup urine disease. This is one of the rare disorders of amino-acid metabolism in which episodic ataxia occurs, often precipitated by infection. During attacks increased amounts of valine, leucine and isoleucine are excreted in the urine. Between attacks there is no abnormality.

4. Hartnup disease. This disease is due to impaired absorption of Tryptophan. Episodic ataxia precipitated by infection and usually associated with a dry, scaly red pellagra-like skin rash occurs. Variable amino-aciduria is found even between attacks.

5. Ataxia—Telangiectasia (Louis–Bar syndrome). The main features of this progressive disorder are telangiectasia of the conjunctivae (usually misdiagnosed as chronic conjunctivitis), progressive cerebellar degeneration and a tendency to infection in those patients who have agammaglobulinaemia which is occasionally associated with this disorder. Progressive ataxia and mental impairment, and early death from infection is the usual course of the disease.

Infectious Disorders

Acute viral infection of the cerebellum has been reported, or at least patients in whom the signs of viral encephalitis have been dominated by ataxia.

An acute ataxic syndrome may occur after *any* of the exanthemata of childhood and infectious mononucleosis. There is a specific association with chicken pox; in which severe ataxia may start within three weeks of the initial infection and almost always subsides over several months. Chicken pox "cerebellitis" usually occurs in children under two years of age and is rare in older children. In all cases of "post-infectious" ataxia in childhood it is important to exclude the metabolic disorders that can be triggered by infection (see above).

Children with Guillain–Barré syndrome may appear to be ataxic on initial examination. This is due to proximal motor weakness or sensory deficit and re-emphasises the importance of being certain that ataxia is not "pseudo-ataxia".

Degenerative Disorders

The commonest inherited form of spino-cerebellar degeneration is Friedreich's ataxia which usually causes symptoms between the ages of 5 and 10. It is fully discussed in Chapter 14. The majority of inherited cerebellar degenerations present in adulthood and are certainly the longest delayed in onset of all "inherited" disorders. Two varieties may cause symptoms in childhood. Olivo-pontocerebellar atrophy which causes dysarthria and ataxia in the adult may cause progressive spastic paralysis and death in the child. Ramsay–Hunt syndrome (dyssynergia cerebellaris myoclonica), in childhood causes a mild progressive ataxia complicated by sudden myoclonic jerking which may be sufficiently severe to throw the child to the ground in addition to falls directly due to the ataxia.

Tumours

Tumours have been considered in Chapter 8. It is pertinent to recall that the majority of cerebral tumours in childhood occur in the cerebellum and that there are two types; the highly malignant medulloblastoma which produces a "midline" picture with gross truncal ataxia and the benign cystic astrocytoma which may start in the midline but later spreads laterally as a large cystic extension into one or other hemisphere and produces a typical unilateral cerebellar syndrome.

The presenting symptom of cerebellar tumours in the child is usually ataxia, closely followed by headache, vomiting and papilloedema. The main differential diagnoses are lead poisoning and aqueductal stenosis. Pontine gliomas do *not* cause C.S.F. obstruction and are more likely to produce cranial nerve palsies (see Chapter 11).

CEREBELLAR DISEASE IN THE ADULT

In the adult the causes of cerebellar disease are quite different. Vascular disease is a rare cause of cerebellar dysfunction except that due to involvement of cerebellar pathways in a brainstem lesion. Acute intracerebellar haemorrhage has been described in Chapter 11. Several hereditary disorders typically cause their first symptoms in late adulthood. Tumours are rare if one excludes acoustic nerve tumours, and are usually metastatic, the one exception being the cerebellar haemangioblastoma. Finally, there are several "toxic" causes of cerebellar disease, alcohol being the main offender.

Inherited Cerebellar Disease

Friedreich's ataxia has already been discussed and usually causes symptoms in childhood. There are three major inherited cerebellar degenerations.

1. *Ramsay–Hunt syndrome* (dyssynergia cerebellaris progressiva or myoclonica). This consists of the insidious development of cerebellar ataxia often associated with myoclonus. It usually begins in the third decade of life and upper limb ataxia of severe degree rather than gait ataxia is the rule. This is consistent with the main pathological lesion which is in the dentate nucleus and its pathway to the thalamus.

2. *Olivo-Ponto-Cerebellar Atrophy* (of Dejerine–Thomas). This disorder is dominated by dysarthria, and for reasons that are not clear sphincter dysfunction occurs with incontinence of urine and impotence. Generalised jerking at rest rather than a pure ataxia occurs with rigidity rather than hypotonia. The pathology varies but degeneration of the olivary and pontine nuclei and loss of cerebellar Purkinje cells are the usual histological findings.

3. *Cerebellar Ataxia with Spasticity* (Marie and Sanger-Brown). This is a late onset disorder which is strongly hereditary and is dominated by ataxia. Unlike other heredofamilial degenerations, the reflexes are brisk and there is severe spasticity of the lower limbs. Optic atrophy is a frequent finding and the disorder is easily misdiagnosed as multiple sclerosis unless the progressive nature is recognised or a positive family history is obtained.

In all these disorders some decline in intellectual function is common even though the brunt of the damage falls on the cerebellum. The familial nature may be obscured by the early death of parents (before they could develop the disease) or separation from siblings by the time the disease occurs. Careful family tracing may reveal several siblings in different parts of the country with the same disease masquerading under different diagnostic labels.

"Toxic" Cerebellar Degeneration

There are a variety of possible causes of "toxic" cerebellar degeneration, characterised by loss of Purkinje cells and in some cases confined to fairly discrete areas of the cerebellum. Alcohol is the commonest cause and may produce very severe but reversible acute ataxia during intoxication, slowly worsening ataxia or severe acute irreversible ataxia during an attack of Wernicke's encephalopathy. The brunt of the damage falls on the anterior lobe and severe gait ataxia is the result.

Anticonvulsant drugs cause reversible ataxia in acute overdosage but there is no doubt that chronic and occasionally acute overdoses of diphenylhydantoin can produce irreversible cerebellar damage.

Carbon monoxide poisoning may produce acute destruction of the cerebellar cortex.

CASE REPORT

An elderly man attempted suicide in a gas oven. He was found and taken to hospital semiconscious. He was given oxygen and within twenty-four hours appeared normal. Ten days later he became acutely ataxic, dysarthric and dysphagic. He was tube fed but his condition deteriorated and he died a few days later. At post mortem the cerebellum had a jelly-like consistency and was completely destroyed.

Malignant disease usually causes metastatic cerebellar disease but cerebellar degeneration complicating carcinomas, and malignant lymphomas *without* direct metastasis does occur—but rather less often than the impression that is sometimes given in discussion. In general a patient with malignant disease who develops cerebellar signs is much more likely to have a metastasis in the cerebellum than a degenerative disorder.

Neoplastic Involvement

Metastatic malignant disease accounts for the majority of cerebellar tumours in the adult. Carcinoma of the lung and breast are usually responsible but a surprisingly high proportion are metastatic from large bowel tumours, particularly those in the descending and recto-sigmoid colon.

Primary tumours are rare although occasionally medulloblastomas may occur in the adult. Primary gliomas are also rare. The most frequent tumour is the benign haemangioblastoma—often a very small vascular nodule associated with a large cyst. The prognosis is excellent although recurrences are quite frequent. Occasionally these tumours produce erythropoietin and are associated with polycythaemia. Extrinsic compression of the cerebellum by acoustic neuromas has been considered in Chapter 6.

Multiple Sclerosis

"Cerebellar" signs in multiple sclerosis are common but in the majority of cases the lesions are in the brain stem cerebellar pathways and the cerebellar signs are almost invariably associated with internuclear ophthalmoplegia, long tract signs and evidence of bilateral pyramidal lesions.

Cerebellar disease can be difficult to diagnose, but having made the diagnosis there are a wide range of diagnostic possibilities. In the adult a very detailed family history and enquiry into drug and alcohol intake is essential. In the child urgent investigation to exclude a tumour should take priority.

DISEASES AFFECTING THE SPINAL CORD

The next three chapters cover diseases affecting the spinal cord. We will consider not only intrinsic disease of the cord, but also damage due to lesions of the spinal cord coverings, the vertebral canal and the spinal cord blood supply.

The subject is dealt with in three main sections and these should ideally be read in sequence for full understanding, as the clinical features are fully described in the first chapter and referred to in subsequent chapters to avoid repetition.

The most important anatomical feature of the spinal cord is rarely appreciated and that is the relationship of the cord to the vertebral column. The cord extends from the foramen magnum to the first lumbar vertebra. Too often, a lesion causing very high cord compression may be missed at myelography if the contrast medium is not followed up to the foramen magnum. At the opposite extreme a lesion below L1 vertebral level *cannot* compress the spinal cord and can only damage the cauda equina. Yet frequently the first investigation performed in a patient with a spastic paraparesis is an X-ray of the lumbar-sacral spine! This also explains why there is no risk of impaling the spinal cord during a lumbar puncture, provided that an interspace below L1/2 level is used. (See also Chapter 25.) These extremely important practical points will all be amplified in later sections.

detected. It is usually worth showing the patient what is required with his eyes open and then going on to do the formal test with the eyes closed or averted. Very small movements over a range of 1 mm. should be detectable at the fingers and larger movements of 3—4 mm. at the toes. With severe impairment even movements of the wrist and ankle joints may not be detected by the patient.

Finally, a note on sensory levels. As will be seen in later sections, it is important to search for a level below which cutaneous sensation is impaired. One can only do this with a good appreciation of the various physiological sensory levels that exist. These are indicated in Figure 13.5. It will be seen that these occur at the groin, the costal margin and just below the clavicle. It is very easy to mistake these physiological transitions to more sensitive areas of the body as sensory levels if one is not aware of their existence.

Chapter 14

METABOLIC, INFECTIVE AND VASCULAR DISORDERS

In many textbooks the discussion of spinal cord disease centres around conditions such as tabes dorsalis and sub-acute combined degeneration of the cord. These conditions are now so rare that to base a whole chapter on them would not be representative of either their frequency or the author's familiarity with these conditions. In this chapter we will consider cord disorders in order of clinical importance. Certainly the most frequently encountered spinal cord disease at this time is the rather poorly understood condition known as progressive cervical myelopathy, which in some instances may be associated with cervical spondylosis. Cord lesions related to fracture dislocations of the spine are covered in Chapter 23.

Progressive Cervical Myelopathy

This condition may be encountered in either sex, usually between the ages of 30 and 70. In fact, it is a negative diagnosis; it is the label attached to those patients who have a clinical picture suggestive of compression of the cervical spinal cord with negative myelographic studies and nothing in the history or cerebro-spinal fluid to enable a diagnosis of multiple sclerosis to be made. The condition may be an abortive or localised form of spinal cord demyelination occurring in an older age group and occasional patients may go on to develop other manifestations to suggest that this is a mild form of multiple sclerosis.

Typically the patient attends hospital with the symptoms of a mild to moderately severe paraparesis. In most instances there are no sensory symptoms and bladder function is unimpaired. The signs are often confined to the motor system and in general all reflexes are brisk and both plantar responses are extensor, but the weakness is confined to the legs. Weakness of the arms is a late and minor problem if the arms become involved at all. In the older patients in this group physiological loss of vibration sense to the knees may be an additional feature and the only sensory finding.

One of the main diagnostic problems is the role of cervical spondylosis. In this older age group about half the patients would be expected to have a moderate degree of cervical spondylosis and whether this is playing a role in patho-genesis is a debatable point. There is little doubt that cervical spondylosis may cause cervical cord compression and in any patient with a complete block on myelography decom-

pressive surgery is indicated, and occasionally beneficial. With lesser degrees of spondylosis operation is usually unhelpful. In these instances, rather than regarding surgery as a failure, it is probably more accurate to accept that the diagnosis was incorrect in the first instance. For the same reason there is no convincing evidence that the use of a cervical collar has any beneficial effect in these patients and in many instances the added discomfort seems to make them less able to cope with the problems presented by the paraparesis. In the author's opinion myelography should always be performed for reasons exemplified by the following two case reports.

CASE REPORT

A 53-year-old man developed a slowly progressive paraparesis over two years. There were no signs to indicate damage to the nervous system outside the spinal cord. His plain cervical spine x-rays were normal and myelography was performed with considerable reluctance. Complete spinal block at C7 was demonstrated and was due to a neuro-fibroma. Surgery cured all his symptoms.

CASE REPORT

A 58-year-old woman had been observed in the neurology clinic for nearly three years as a case of cervical spondylosis with myelopathy. On routine review it was felt that the spondylosis was relatively mild as judged from the plain x-rays and that the signs were those of a spastic tetraparesis with fine lateral nystagmus and a very brisk jaw jerk, suggestive of a very high cord compression. Myelography was therefore performed and a meningioma in the foramen magnum was demonstrated.

However skilled the clinician there are *no* clinical features that allow confident exclusion of spinal cord compression to be made on clinical grounds alone. Myelography is mandatory even if one is then left with the rather unsatisfactory diagnostic label of progressive cervical myelopathy. (Myelopathy due to cervical spondylosis is discussed in greater detail in the next chapter.)

Multiple Sclerosis (Figure 14.1)

In Europe and North America multiple sclerosis is another frequent cause of spinal cord disease. As in the case of progressive cervical myelopathy the clinical picture may be indistinguishable from spinal cord compression and often

In the majority of patients with tabes dorsalis there are also evidences of disease elsewhere. Nearly all patients have Argyll–Robertson pupils and many have optic atrophy with peripheral visual field loss. Damage to the upper motor neurone is revealed by extensor plantar responses (again the reflexes cannot become brisk because they are already abolished by the root damage). If extensor plantar responses are present it is presumed that long tract damage has occurred and the condition is then known as taboparesis. This is the third condition that may cause this combination of absent reflexes and extensor plantar responses.

Radiation Myelopathy

This is a subject of considerable and increasing importance. It is almost exclusively a complication of radiation to the thorax, particularly that directed at the bronchi or oesophagus, rather than the smaller doses used in treatment of the mediastinal lymph nodes, in Hodgkin's disease. Better techniques with rotating portals can do little to limit the dose received by the cord when the oesophagus is irradiated as it lies in the centre of the field. The critical dose may be as low as 1,800 rads. Characteristically, there is a nine- to eighteen-month delay before the onset of the cord damage. Sensory symptoms are prominent with spino-thalamic sensory loss coupled with a mild spastic paraparesis. It is difficult to distinguish from rapidly developing cord compression due to metastatic disease unless sensory symptoms dominate the early picture which is very unusual in cord compression as discussed later. This provides an important clue to the diagnosis of radiation myelopathy. The distinction is extremely important as further radiation directed at a presumed metastasis carries the serious risk of worsening the situation if radiation myelopathy is the actual diagnosis.

Finally, we must consider the important differences between the diseases listed above with intrinsic tumours of the spinal cord and spinal cord compression.

1. SPINAL CORD COMPRESSION

Spinal cord compression may be caused by lesions arising on the nerve roots, the coverings of the spinal cord, in the extra-dural fat or from lesions of the vertebral column itself. At this stage we will consider only the features of the history and the clinical signs that suggest that the patient is suffering from spinal cord compression.

The clinical feature of cord compression that must be emphasised is that the symptoms and signs are dominated by motor pathway damage. The reasons for this are not entirely clear, but may be related to the blood supply of the spinal cord and in particular to the venous drainage. This is discussed in more detail later in this chapter, but basically any impairment of venous drainage will tend to lead to oedema and poor capillary circulation in the watershed zone of the spinal cord, which includes the cortico-spinal pathways. The earliest symptoms are those of a mild spastic paraparesis. The patient may complain of slight dragging of the feet and heaviness of the legs as described in the previous chapter. These symptoms may develop over a period of months in some instances or in a matter of hours in the case of acute lesions and occasionally instantaneously. Impending irreversible cord damage is indicated by either the onset of micturition disturbance or sensory symptoms. Difficulty in initiating micturition or urinary retention may occur quite suddenly, and usually indicates that rapidly progressive deterioration is about to occur. Sensory symptoms have a similar significance and may start as a tingling sensation in the soles of the feet which then ascends. This may reach a fixed level in a matter of hours or advance slowly over several days. In either event it is unwise to delay action until the level becomes fixed.

In summary therefore, spinal cord compression is dominated in the early stages by motor symptoms and signs and the onset of sensory features heralds a phase of rapid deterioration leading to irreversible cord damage. The clinical sequence and signs at the various stages are summarised in Figure 14.6.

2. INTRINSIC TUMOURS OF THE SPINAL CORD

The clinical history and signs of an intrinsic lesion in the spinal cord are quite the reverse of cord compression. The anatomical feature that determines the sequence of events is the course of the pain and temperature pathways in the central spinal cord. These are the fibres most likely to be damaged in the early stages. Initially, a lesion in the central spinal cord (ependymoma, glioma or syringomyelic cavity) will irritate and destroy pain and temperature fibres as they cross the cord, but *only* at the level of the lesion.

No long tract damage can occur at this stage so that a narrow segment of pain and temperature loss is produced. The pain is of deep spino-thalamic type, but the sensory loss may not be detected unless pain sensation is carefully tested. Occasionally, a patient accidentally discovers the sensory loss when he drops a lighted cigarette on the skin or notices an area of impaired sensation while bathing in warm water.

Later as the lesion extends laterally the reflex arc is blocked and the reflexes disappear. This rarely produces any symptoms as far as the patient is concerned, but any patient with

Figure 14.6. Cord Compression (A lesion at D9 on left side is shown)

Note. Although sensory loss is shown developing in sequence, it must be stressed that in most cases the motor signs dominate the clinical picture

A

A neurofibroma on the left D 9. dorsal root is shown

The root is irritated causing root pain at D9

B

The cord is now seriously distorted and definite sensory loss occurs in the root zone and in the opposite spinothalamic distribution

C

The terminal stage of cord compression has been reached. Total paralysis of the legs with rapidly ascending sensory loss occurs

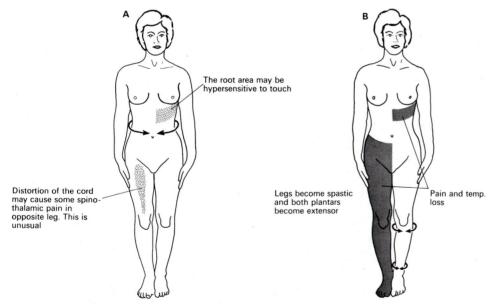

A

The root area may be hypersensitive to touch

Distortion of the cord may cause some spino-thalamic pain in opposite leg. This is unusual

Root pain may be worse on coughing
Tight band or cold bands around abdomen noticed
May be some deep pain in opposite limb
No sensory loss may be detected
Leg reflexes may be brisk
Plantar may be extensor
May be urinary urgency

B

Legs become spastic and both plantars become extensor

Pain and temp. loss

Root area now numb
Band sensations in legs occur
Opposite leg may feel "different"
Partial Brown-Séquard lesion
Radicular loss of sensation
Pain and temp. loss in opposite leg
(May be some joint position sense loss on same side)
Legs now spastic and weak
Reflexes brisk. Plantars extensor
May be marked sphincter upset

C

All modalities lost

Final stage—may be acute after long stage A and B or can go from A—C over a matter of hours
Sensory level to *all* modalities to level of lesion
Flaccid, areflexic paralysis in spinal shock phase.
Reflexes often *increased* above the level of transection

Figure 14.7. Development of a Central Cord Lesion

This picture would be seen in syringomyelia, ependymoma, and intrinsic glioma or astrocytoma. The progress of the signs relates directly to degree of involvement shown in the cord sections

A

Some local involvement of entering dural column fibres

Early pyramidal lesion

Central lesion causes spontaneous pain and band of pain loss over involved segments

Spontaneous pain

Deep nagging pain in shoulders
Sensory loss may be found by accident by patient
No signs except a thin band of pain loss

Plantars flexor

B

Lesion extending into right half of the cord damaging the sympathetic and reflex arcs

Cervical sympathetic damaged—Horner's syndrome

Reflex arc blocked

A right Horner's syndrome has developed

Pain and temperature loss

Arms and hands waste
Arm reflexes abolished on right side

Spastic paraparesis develops

Leg reflexes brisk, plantars now extensor

Pain may persist
Frequent burns and non-healing cuts on hands
Hands become thinned and weak
Definite pain/temperature loss but touch usually normal
Arm reflexes absent
Abdominals go, and leg jerks brisk
Some pyramidal leg weakness and extensor plantars. Bladder often spared

C

Lesion spreading to involve both corticospinal tracts and into the right spinothalamic tract and into right dorsal horn

Sacral fibres still intact

If spinothalamic tract itself involved sensory levels spread down

Horner's syndrome (now bilateral and very difficult to diagnose)

Spinothalamic sensory loss extends into face (See chapter 15)

If the lesion extends into the dorsal horns loss of joint position sense and light touch may be found in the hand

Spinothalamic loss starts to extend downwards as the tract is invaded

Sacral sparing

Late stages
Whole body may have lost pain as spinothalamic tracts involved from inside out—hence outer sacral fibres last (sacral sparing)
Local involvement of dorsal root zone may produce joint position sense loss in the upper limbs
Bladder involved

spino-thalamic symptoms should be carefully checked for loss of reflexes. Reflex loss applies only to lesions affecting the standard reflex arcs in the arms and the legs. In the cervical cord the sympathetic will be affected at this stage producing a unilateral or bilateral Horner's syndrome. If the lesion extends into the anterior horn cells focal wasting and weakness may appear, typically affecting the small muscles of the hand. The location of these new signs will depend on the site of the lesion. If the lesion is in the mid-thoracic cord, it is very unlikely that the patient will notice wasting and weakness of individual intercostal muscles, although this should certainly be looked for in a patient with spino-thalamic symptoms in the thoracic region. It is only when the cord becomes expanded that the long tracts become involved. This may take several years. Bilateral pyramidal signs then appear with brisk reflexes in the legs and extensor plantar responses. The inner part of the spino-thalamic tract may be damaged causing descending spino-thalamic sensory loss. In the final stages of the process only the peripheral fibres carrying sensation from the sacral area will survive and the patient develops what is known as sacral sparing, a rare but diagnostic feature of an intrinsic lesion of the spinal cord. The dorsal columns seem very resistant to infiltration by tumours and in general dorsal column signs are a late feature of intrinsic lesions. The sequence and anatomical correlation of the signs at various stages are illustrated in Figure 14.7.

THE BLOOD SUPPLY OF THE SPINAL CORD
(Figure 14.8)

The spinal cord is not supplied by segmental arteries or by a continuous vessel running down its length. There is a fairly constant territorial distribution of blood supply in the transverse plane. The central area is supplied by the sulcal arteries which are given off alternately from each side of the anterior spinal artery which lies in the ventral sulcus of the cord. The anterior spinal artery also gives off circumferential arteries which lie on the surface of the cord forming a surface plexus by anastomosing with branches of the posterior spinal arteries and supplying the periphery of the cord. The paired posterior spinal arteries form a plexus over the dorsal columns, which they supply. The posterior spinal arteries are less defined than the anterior spinal artery, although even this vessel may be incomplete and often peters out at lower dorsal cord levels and starts again below as a new vessel.

Although these small vessels are affected by disease processes such as syphilis, diabetes, arteritis and arteriosclerosis clinical disorders of the cord circulation are usually due to disease in the feeder vessels which replenish the artery at various points along its course.

The anterior spinal artery arises from the vertebral arteries in the foramen magnum as two vessels that join to become a single vessel opposite the odontoid peg. It is replenished by a fairly constant vessel which enters the canal on the C3 or C4 root and comes from the thyrocervical trunk which may be damaged in surgical procedures in the neck. This upper part of the vessel supplies the cord down to about D4.

The dorsal spinal cord segment of the artery is supplied by a variable branch from one of the intercostal arteries but the main feeder vessel is the arteria magna of Adamkewicz. This arises from the D10, D11 or D12 intercostal artery in seventy-five per cent of patients. It is easily damaged during thoracic operations, sympathectomy, nephrectomy, adrenal exploration, lumbar aortography and intercostal nerve blocks. In any of these procedures damage to the vessel may cause infarction of the entire lumbar enlargement and the thoracic cord up to mid-dorsal level.

The terminal spinal cord and the nerve roots of the cauda equina are supplied by a variable vessel entering the canal on one of the upper lumbar roots.

Vascular Syndromes

The surgical causes of vascular cord disease have been listed above.

Medical causes are dominated by atheromatous changes in the vessels and in particular disease of the vertebral arteries occluding the origin of the anterior spinal artery, which causes infarction of the central medulla (see Chapter 11).

At any cord level diabetes mellitus, syphilis, any coagulopathy, embolic phenomena (subacute bacterial endocarditis, atrial fibrillation, myocardial infarction), dissecting aneurysm of the aorta, intravascular air bubbles in decompression sickness, and sickle cell disease are notable causes of feeder vessel occlusion.

When the arteria magna is occluded by any of these processes the level of the lesion is usually found between D4 and D6. The entire anterior half of the cord is infarcted so that the picture is that of an acute flaccid paraplegia, with retention of urine, spinothalamic sensory loss to the level of the lesion but with complete preservation of joint position sense and touch. The onset is often accompanied by local pain in the back.

The lumbar feeder vessel may be involved in disc lesions in patients with congenitally narrowed lumbar canals causing the syndrome of "intermittent claudication of the cauda equina". In this condition root pain and weakness appear during exercise and rapidly pass off when the patient rests. Decompressive laminectomy usually relieves this condition.

Acute Cauda Equina Syndrome

An acute disc prolapse at the L2/3 level may cause bilateral multiple root lesions. The patient complains of severe bilateral leg pain, flaccid paralysis of both legs and retention of urine. This is a surgical emergency; and immediate exploration of the cauda equina is indicated.

One other rarity worth including is the condition known as "claudication of the cauda equina". The patient complains that while walking he develops root pain and leg weakness, usually a foot drop. This rapidly recovers on resting. This is usually due to a combination of a disc lesion and a congenitally narrowed lumbar theca which interferes with the blood supply of the spinal cord during activity. The situation is rather similar to the narrow cervical canal that predisposes to cord compression in cervical spondylosis.

CAUDA EQUINA LESIONS

A lesion in the spinal canal at any level below the D10 vertebra can cause a cauda equina syndrome. There is often a tendency to think of the cauda equina as comprising only the nerve roots lying in the sacrum. It includes the terminal spinal cord, all the spinal roots from D12 to S5 and the filum terminale—the fibrous band that extends from the tip of the cord to attach to the sacrum (see Figure 15.7).

Cauda Equina Lesions in Childhood

The embryology of the vertebral column has already been described and the variety of developmental defects that may occur in the lumbar-sacral region mentioned. It is important to remember that *disc* lesions are exceedingly rare before 15 years of age.

1. Symptoms present since birth

Spina Bifida Occulta

Many patients with spina bifida occulta remain asymptomatic throughout life but associated developmental abnormalities may cause problems. Progressive wasting and weakness affecting particularly L4, L5 and S1 are found. Absent ankle jerks and trophic changes in the feet often first manifest as recurrent chilblains may be found. The picture may remain static but close follow-up until seven years of age is necessary to exclude any progression.

Spina Bifida Cystica

Severe defects in the vertebral column are associated with variable degrees of neural abnormality. These include bulging meninges (meningocoele), a sac containing parts of the terminal cord and nerve roots (myelomeningocoele), and a lump of malformed neural tissue lying free on the surface (myelocoele). Both latter varieties are often associated with Arnold–Chiari malformation and initial surgical enthusiasm for active treatment is now being tempered by the ethical dilemma presented as the grossly disabled survivors reach adulthood. Further discussion of this tragic and emotive subject is beyond the scope of the present text.

2. Symptoms occurring in later childhood

Mild developmental abnormalities may not produce any disability at birth but the ascent of the spinal cord in the first five years of life may cause problems due to cord stretching. Occasionally symptoms or signs may not occur until adulthood. The development of any weakness, numbness, trophic change or disparity in the size or shape of the feet should prompt careful investigation. Progressive symptoms may require surgery even in the absence of myelographic abnormalities as a tethered cord may not produce myelographic signs.

Pain is an unusual feature in the developmental cauda equina syndromes of childhood. Pain should prompt an urgent search for evidence of primary malignant disease in the vertebral column or sacrum, retro-peritoneal malignancy and the possibility of seeding of the lumbar theca by a medulloblastoma should be considered.

CASE REPORT

A 16-year-old boy went camping at Easter. The weather was extremely bad and he developed a "chill". He came home early looking very pale, had a low-grade fever, severe low backache and pain in the left thigh. Over the next three weeks he lost weight and the main symptoms continued. On examination he looked very ill, but there was no hepatosplenomegaly or lymphadenopathy. The left knee jerk was absent. He was investigated for malignant disease and found to be suffering from acute lymphatic leukaemia. His symptoms remitted with appropriate chemotherapy.

Cauda Equina Lesions in the Adult

There are three main clinical pictures.

a. *The Lateral Cauda Equina Syndrome* (Figure 15.9)

The most frequent cause of the lateral cauda equina syndrome is a neurofibroma. Rarely, a high disc lesion may be responsible. The symptoms include anterior thigh pain, quadriceps wasting, weakness of inversion of the foot (L4 root lesion) and an absent knee jerk. If the lesion is very high and lies lateral to the terminal spinal cord there may even be pyramidal signs *below* the lesion, in which case the ankle jerks may be very brisk with ankle clonus and an extensor plantar response. In this situation sphincter disturbance is likely to be due to cord compression.

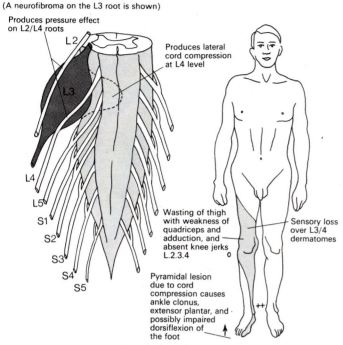

Figure 15.9. High lateral Cauda Equina lesion
(A neurofibroma on the L3 root is shown)

Produces pressure effect on L2/L4 roots

L2

L3

Produces lateral cord compression at L4 level

L4

L5

S1

S2

S3

S4

S5

Wasting of thigh with weakness of quadriceps and adduction, and absent knee jerks L.2.3.4

Sensory loss over L3/4 dermatomes

Pyramidal lesion due to cord compression causes ankle clonus, extensor plantar, and possibly impaired dorsiflexion of the foot

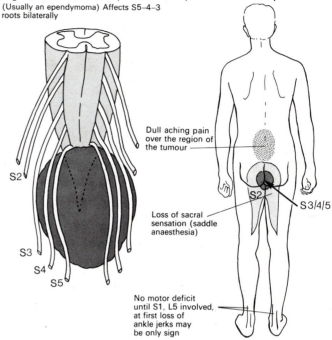

Figure 15.10. Midline (conus lesion) of the Cauda Equina
(Usually an ependymoma) Affects S5–4–3 roots bilaterally

Dull aching pain over the region of the tumour

S2

S3

S4

S5

Loss of sacral sensation (saddle anaesthesia)

S2

S3/4/5

No motor deficit until S1, L5 involved, at first loss of ankle jerks may be only sign

b. *Midline Cauda Equina Lesions from Within*
(Figure 15.10)

This is also known as a "conus lesion". The usual causes are an ependymoma, a dermoid tumour or a lipoma of the terminal cord. The roots are damaged from the inside i.e. S5→S4→S3 and so on. The initial symptoms include rectal pain, genital pain, micturition disturbances and loss of potency with no definite physical signs *unless* the perianal sensation and anal reflex are carefully tested. Later loss of the ankle jerks and weakness of the L5 and S1 muscle groups occurs. In the case of an ependymoma the patient may have a five-year history of dull backache *before* any other symptoms or signs appear.

An important benign cause of rectal pain that must be considered is the benign, but excruciating pain syndrome known as Proctalgia fugax. This can occur in either sex at any age, but seems to be more frequent in men. Attacks are mainly nocturnal and may accompany erection or ejaculation. The pain is an intense gripping sensation around the rectum about 2" inside the anal ring. Attacks typically last 15–20 minutes and then subside. Bearing down may relieve the pain slightly. It is thought to be due to cramp in the Levator ani muscles.

c. *Midline Cauda Equina Lesions from Outside*

The hallmark of this situation is bilateral lumbar and sacral root lesions. Root pain in unusual dermatomes (L2 or 3) (or

S2 or 3) should be regarded with great suspicion, but pain in L4, L5 or S1 may be readily and not unreasonably ascribed to simple disc disease. Severe pain not relieved by appropriate measures, and the detection of neurological signs indicates the need for myelography, not just to confirm a disc lesion but to exclude alternative pathology. In the adult the alternatives are extremely unpleasant and include primary sacral bone tumours (chordomas) metastatic disease (especially prostatic disease), reticulosis, leukaemia or direct seeding from malignant tumours in the C.N.S. notably medulloblastomas, ependymomas or pinealomas.

CASE REPORT

A 20-year-old female was admitted as an emergency with severe headaches of one month's duration and papilloedema. She gave a five-year history of left S1 root pain ascribed to a disc lesion. On physical examination there was papilloedema, neck stiffness, a positive Kernig test and absence of the left ankle jerk. An ependymoma with a spinal subarachnoid haemorrhage was suspected but at operation a piloid astrocytoma was found, with evidence of recent haemorrhage. This case emphasises the danger of diagnosing a disc lesion in a 15-year-old and the surprisingly slow clinical course of lesions in this situation.

Although low backache and various aches and pains in the legs are one of the most frequent reasons for hospital referral the importance of detecting *unusual* features in the history and a *careful* neurological examination in all cases cannot be over-emphasised.

TUMOURS AND THE SPINAL CORD

Now that the anatomy of the spinal cord in relation to the vertebra has been fully described it is appropriate to consider tumours and the spinal cord. This subject has been deferred until this stage because from an investigational and pathological point of view the relationship of the tumour to the vertebral column is of great importance. Furthermore, the relationship of the tumour to the cord and its coverings often provides a pre-operative clue to the pathology and to some extent governs the surgical approach.

As so often in neurological disease, we have to consider cord tumours in children and adults separately as there is a dramatic difference in the pathological possibilities in different age groups, and for certain tumours a marked difference in the sex incidence. As was the case in regard to cerebral tumours there is also a significant risk of a spinal tumour being due to a metastasis from malignant disease elsewhere. In children fifty per cent of spinal tumours are metastatic usually by direct spread from retroperitoneal neuroblastomas, ganglioneuromas and sarcomas. In adults some twenty to thirty per cent of all spinal tumours are metastatic. Metastases from carcinoma of the breast in the female (68 per cent) and prostate in the male (40 per cent) account for the majority. Lung (25 per cent), thyroid (15 per cent), uterus and cervix (10 per cent) and direct spread of Hodgkin's Disease and Multiple myeloma are the other major causes. In all these instances plain films will often show evidence of either the primary lesion or of the bone involvement and often the site of the primary can be guessed from the plain film changes.

Tumours in both groups are defined as extradural, intradural/extramedullary and intramedullary if actually in the substance of the cord.

The striking difference between childhood and adulthood is best seen in the following classification:

When a patient presents with symptoms and signs suggesting a cord lesion (see Chapter 13) the initial clinical evaluation should enable a distinction to be made between an intrinsic (intramedullary) lesion of the cord and a compressive (extradural or intradural) lesion. Considering the age, sex and site of the damage the probable nature of the lesion can be deduced but operative diagnosis and histology is always required.

The following brief profiles of different tumours may be used as a guide:

Neurofibromas: Sex incidence equal, 30–50 years age, 60 per cent above L1 causing spastic paraparesis, 30 per cent below L1 causing root pain and mimicking a disc lesion (16 per cent are sarcomas).

Meningiomas: Female/male ratio 9:1, nearly all mid-dorsal (D3–D6). Few in foramen magnum; female/male ratio 2:1 at this site.

Ependymomas: Male/female ratio 2:1, average age 30 years, either intrinsic in cord at C6–D2 (mimics syringomyelia) or on filum terminale (central cauda equina syndrome). Very high incidence of associated syringomyelic cavity, making the lesion seem much more extensive than its actual size.

Gliomas: Sex incidence equal, average age 35–45, nearly all in cervical cord.

Dermoids: All sacrococcygeal, usually associated with spina bifida; present at 15–20 years of age.

Chordomas: Slight male predominance, 80 per cent sacrococcygeal, 12 per cent in sphenoid. Considerable bone destruction and pain are features.

Vascular tumours affecting the cord are discussed in Chapter 14.

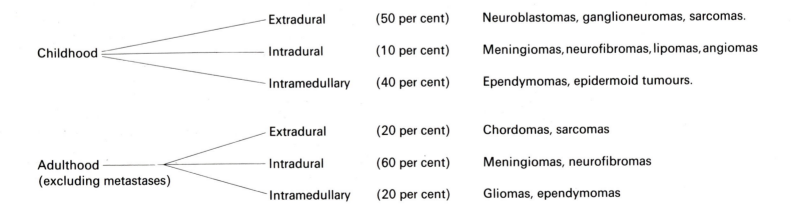

Childhood	Extradural	(50 per cent)	Neuroblastomas, ganglioneuromas, sarcomas.
	Intradural	(10 per cent)	Meningiomas, neurofibromas, lipomas, angiomas
	Intramedullary	(40 per cent)	Ependymomas, epidermoid tumours.
Adulthood (excluding metastases)	Extradural	(20 per cent)	Chordomas, sarcomas
	Intradural	(60 per cent)	Meningiomas, neurofibromas
	Intramedullary	(20 per cent)	Gliomas, ependymomas

Figure 15.11. Plain Film X-ray Appearances of Intra-Spinal Tumours

Spinous process

Pedicle

Vertebral body

Pedicle

Spinous process

Erosion of pedicle

Erosion of vertebral body

In the A.P. view the pedicles should be compared from side to side, and asymmetry of size and shape should be sought

Transverse process

In the lateral view the disc space does not erode, but the back of the vertebral body may, producing a scalloped appearance

Note. These appearances take some time to develop and in many patients no abnormality may be seen. It is always worth comparing the size of exit foraminae as these may be enlarged by a neurofibroma

The Investigation of Spinal Tumours

Routine physical examination and chest x-ray to exclude a primary neoplasm is essential. A rectal examination is particularly important in the male to detect carcinoma of the prostate. In the absence of any focal signs or symptoms to indicate the level of the tumour the cervical spine, including the foramen magnum and thoracic spine, including L1, should be x-rayed *if* the clinical picture is that of a spastic paraparesis.

If the picture is one of low backache, lumbar root pain and mixed upper and lower motor neurone signs in the legs the region D10–L3 is the most important from a radiological point of view.

If the symptoms started with rectal or genital pain the sacrum should be included in the x-rays but the importance of including the spinal column up to D10 must be stressed.

The correct investigation is a myelogram and this can be easily performed in most hospitals. However, the temptation to use this facility should be resisted *unless* neurosurgical help is available and under *no* circumstances should a simple lumbar puncture be performed. The reason for this advice is that often a highly delicate haemodynamic situation exists by the time cord compression is evident. Myelography or an L.P. by upsetting these dynamics, particularly if Queckenstedt's test is performed, may lead to acute worsening of the situation, requiring immediate neurosurgery. Furthermore, a simple L.P. may make it impossible to perform myelography for several days as well as worsening the clinical situation. In some patients myodil must also be put in through a cisternal puncture to demonstrate the upper limit of a tumour that is completely blocking the canal. This investigation should be performed only in a neurosurgical unit immediately prior to operation.

The plain film and myelographic appearances of the different types of tumour are shown in Figures 15.11 and 15.12.

Figure 15.12. Diagram to Show Myelographic Appearances of Intraspinal Tumours

A. Extradural tumour

B. Intradural tumour

C. Intramedullary tumour

Ghost of spinal cord

The tumour lifts the dura away from the vertebrae producing a smooth sloping effect

The tumour sits in the myodil column and produces a meniscus-shaped defect

The expanded cord occupies the canal and attenuates the myodil column on either side

MICTURITION AND NEUROLOGICAL DISEASE
(Figure 15.13)

Micturition disturbances are a common feature of spinal cord disease and cauda equina lesions and it is therefore most appropriate to discuss micturition disturbances at this point.

The normal anatomy and physiology of micturition are not well understood and hence the mechanisms of micturition disturbance in disease remain rather speculative. Males have a very considerable advantage over the females in both the length of urethra and additional sphincter mechanisms designed to isolate the bladder and contract the urethra

Figure 15.13. Schematic diagram of the Neural Control of Micturition

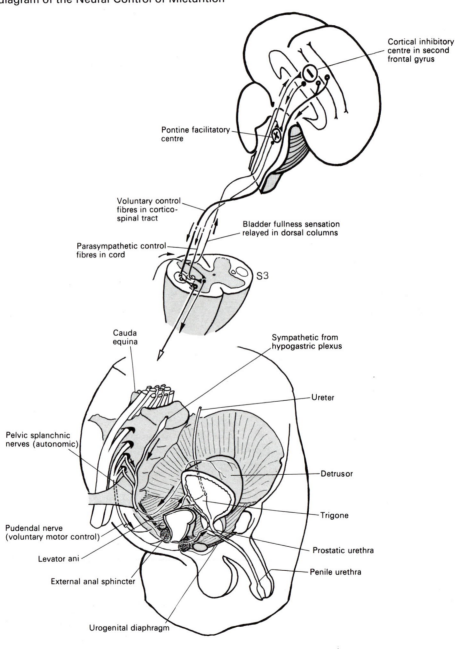

Cortical inhibitory centre in second frontal gyrus

Pontine facilitatory centre

Voluntary control fibres in cortico-spinal tract

Bladder fullness sensation relayed in dorsal columns

Parasympathetic control fibres in cord

S3

Cauda equina

Sympathetic from hypogastric plexus

Ureter

Pelvic splanchnic nerves (autonomic)

Detrusor

Trigone

Pudendal nerve (voluntary motor control)

Prostatic urethra

Levator ani

Penile urethra

External anal sphincter

Urogenital diaphragm

during erection and ejaculation. In neither sex is there a true internal sphincter mechanism; there are arrangements of smooth muscle that produce a "sphincteric" action complete with a condensation of elastic tissue that keeps the urethra in a collapsed state. The angle the bladder makes with the urethra is important and in both sexes collapse of the pelvic floor, allowing the bladder to flop back or gross faecal impaction, by tilting the bladder forward, may have some effect on bladder function for purely mechanical reasons. These possibilities should always be explored. There is a true external sphincter muscle under voluntary control at the uro-genital diaphragm. It is not capable of completely controlling continence—a fact well known to examination candidates!

The anatomy of the bladder and pelvis is shown schematically in Figure 15.13. It is important to notice that part of the urethra lies *in* the abdomen and is subject to the same external pressure alterations as the bladder itself, so that a high pressure differential is not created by coughing or sneezing.

The neural control of the bladder is extremely complicated.

The following details are essential to an understanding of pathological bladder function:

1. The bladder is basically a hollow bag of smooth muscle containing stretch receptors and contracting under the influence of parasympathetic nerves. This constitutes an autonomic stretch reflex.

2. The parasympathetic reflex is based on the S3 roots and S3 segment of the cord. The sympathetic supply descends into the pelvis from the hypogastric plexus but has no certain role in micturition although sympathetic endings on both the detrusor and urethra have been demonstrated and pharmacological evidence suggests that at urethral level the sympathetic may have a major role in the urethral sphincter mechanisms.

3. The stretch receptors fire impulses proportional to the stretch and weight of urine in the bladder. Therefore, there is less afferent activity lying down than standing, hence the instant desire to pass urine on getting up in the morning. Any infection or inflammation of the bladder wall will heighten the sensitivity of the stretch receptors. Stimulation of the perineum and anal canal inhibits the discharge.

4. The basic sacral reflex arc controls micturition in infancy, senility, unconsciousness and following various lesions to the nervous system.

5. The voluntary mechanisms involve both inhibition of the conditioned reflex, volitional control over the hy-pothalamic and pontine facilitating centres and direct physical control over the rather weak external sphincter and pelvic floor. This is all controlled by an area in the second frontal gyrus and the main descending pathways lie in or adjacent to the cortico-spinal tracts. This accounts for the early disturbance of micturition control in patients with spinal cord compression.

Micturition involves complete relaxation of volitional control; the external sphincter and pelvic floor relax and the local reflex is allowed to take over. As the detrusor contracts the bladder neck is pulled open and this combined with inhibition of the weak internal sphincter allows urine to flow by a combination of rising intravesical pressure and gravity. If there is any mechanical obstruction to flow an additional voluntary increase in intra-abdominal pressure by a combination of the Valsava manœuvre and contraction of the abdominal muscles can be used. This is the main cause of the condition known as micturition syncope (see Chapter 22).

Neurological Disorders

There are four main types of neurological bladder:

1. *The Uninhibited Bladder*

This condition is due to a lesion affecting the second frontal gyrus. These include local lesions such as frontal lobe tumours, parasagittal meningiomas and anterior communicating artery aneurysms. It is also a feature of dementia and as stressed before, if dementia *starts* with a micturition upset a focal frontal lesion should be carefully excluded.

The features are:

Urgency at low bladder volumes.
Sudden uncontrolled evacuation.
No residual urine.
If intellectual deterioration occurs urine may be passed anywhere without concern.

2. *The Spinal Bladder*

This condition results from damage to the spinal cord by trauma, cord tumour or multiple sclerosis.

The features are:

Bladder fullness is not appreciated, but may cause sweating pallor, flexor spasms and rises in the blood pressure to very high levels.
The bladder empties suddenly and reflexly.
Evacuation may be incomplete but with training can be complete and at will if the bladder is massaged by suprapubic pressure.
The bladder is spastic and only holds a small volume (less than 250 mls.).

retinitis pigmentosa. The serum phytanic acid (hexadec-anoic acid) is markedly elevated but as in so many metabolic disorders the relationship of this chemical abnormality to the disease is not clear.

Amyloid Neuropathy

There are three varieties of amyloid neuropathy. The first type to be reported is almost exclusively confined to patients of Portuguese extraction. This produces a very unpleasant, relentlessly progressive and ultimately fatal neuropathy that starts in the legs in the third decade and runs its course over some ten years. The second variety has been reported in Swiss families and is a milder disorder usually starting in the arms with a carpal-tunnel like syndrome. Vitreous opacities are common in this variety. The third variety is not determined on an ethnic or familial basis but occurs in a sporadic form and has been increasingly recognised since peripheral nerve biopsies became a routine investigation.

Lipoprotein Neuropathies

Two neuropathies associated with disorders of lipoprotein metabolism have been reported. These are Tangier Disease and Bassen–Kornzweig syndrome. In both the serum cholesterol is very low ($<$80 mgm per cent). Tangier Disease is associated with a virtual absence of high density lipoprotein from the serum and massive deposition of cholesterol in the enlarged tonsils. Bassen–Kornzweig syndrome includes a malabsorption syndrome, red cells with tentacles (acanthocytes) and a virtual absence of beta-lipoproteins from the serum.

Cerebral Lipoidoses

Several of the cerebral degenerative diseases associated with the deposition of abnormal lipids in the brain (metachromatic leucodystrophy, Krabbe's leukodystrophy) although dominated by cerebral problems include a peripheral neuropathy as part of the picture. Nerve conduction studies and nerve biopsies will often confirm the diagnosis without resort to cerebral biopsy.

All the inherited neuropathic conditions produce signs of a peripheral neuropathy; basically loss of all reflexes. The routine evaluation of all patients with neuropathy should include a careful family history, palpation of the peripheral nerves, examination of the eyes for vitreous opacities and retinitis pigmentosa and examination of the tonsils. A routine blood film, serum cholesterol and lipoprotein determination, and blood phytanic acid level should be included in the screening investigations.

In genetically determined and metabolic neuropathies a frequent finding is marked slowing of nerve conduction, which may be in the 10–20 m/sec. range (normal 38 m/sec. and higher). In other types of neuropathy slowing to the lower range of normal occurs but with the exception of Guillain–Barré syndrome this extreme slowing is rarely found.

2. Metabolically Triggered Neuropathy (Acute Intermittent Porphyria)

This rare and potentially fatal condition is due to a disorder of haemoglobin metabolism. Acute attacks may occur spontaneously but are particularly likely to be triggered by certain drugs listed in Table 5. The onset of an attack is usually marked by vomiting and severe abdominal pain, a condition easily misdiagnosed as an intra-abdominal emergency and worsened if barbiturate anaesthesia or sulphonamides are administered to the patient. The illness then affects the nervous system producing an acute psychosis or a rapidly progressive neuropathy or a combination of both. The weakness may be found mainly in the proximal muscles and the sensory loss may occur in a bathing suit distribution rather than peripherally. When these rather "non-organic" signs are coupled with the psychiatric complications the ease with which an attack can be misdiagnosed as hysteria is apparent and understandable. A careful history of drug ingestion should be taken routinely in *all* patients with *any* disorder of the central nervous system. There may be no family history until the first case is detected. Full family screening may reveal other members who have yet to have an attack and who may even have taken provocative drugs *without* developing an episode.

Table 5

DRUGS PRECIPITATING ATTACKS OF PORPHYRIA

Barbiturates
Sulphonamides
Alpha-methyl-dopa
Laevodopa
Griseofulvin
Dichloralphenazone (Welldorm)
Glutethimide (Doriden)
Phenylbutazone
Oestrogens (including the birth control pill)

The diagnosis is made by the detection of excess porphobilinogen and delta-amino laevulinic acid in the urine. Porphyrins, which are a deep red in colour, form when porphobilinogens are exposed to light and oxidation. The urine may not change colour for several hours.

Treatment is supportive and although cases occur too infrequently for controlled observations, consensus opinion suggests that chlorpromazine has a beneficial effect, possibly by an effect on liver function.

3. Infective Neuropathies

There are four neuropathies related to infective organisms. Leprosy, which is a direct infection of the nerves, diphtheria via a toxin produced in the body, Guillain–Barré syndrome possible due to an abnormal immune response to viral infections and botulinum poisoning in which the toxins produced by the organism are ingested.

Leprosy

Leprosy is probably the single most important cause of peripheral neuropathy on a world-wide scale. Fortunately it is now rare in Europe but is endemic throughout Africa and the Middle East. It is not very infective and travellers are unlikely to contract the disease, but contract workers who live in these areas for prolonged periods are at some risk. The nerves are directly infected and patches of numbness appear all over the body, but particularly on the extremities and the face. If the patient is coloured the affected patches become pale. The main nerve trunks are thickened and become pressure sensitive so that sudden pressure palsies of particularly vulnerable nerves (i.e. the ulnar and peroneal nerves) punctuate the slow development of a diffuse neuropathy. The patient therefore develops "mononeuritis multiplex" (the other causes of this condition being diabetes and polyarteritis nodosa). Pain and temperature sensation are specifically affected and severe trophic changes may occur with ulceration and necrosis of the extremities. One patient seen by the writer discovered his neuropathy when he accidentally shut his hand in the door of a Land-Rover. This was quite painless and later that day he found he could hold the injured hand in a fire without discomfort but devastating effect on his injuries! He had been completely asymptomatic until that time.

Diphtheria

In most civilised countries this disease has become a rarity due to mass immunisation. Occasional outbreaks still occur and reveal that the disease remains a very serious and often lethal infection of childhood. The neuropathy occurs in most patients to a minor degree as paralysis of accommodation and palatal weakness frequently occur in the third week of the illness. At any time up to two months after the onset an explosive neuropathy may occur with rapidly ascending paralysis, and respiratory problems. With intensive care recovery should occur, the limiting factor often being the myocarditis which complicates the illness.

Guillain–Barré Syndrome

This condition is thought to be a single response of the central nervous system to a variety of infective processes. It often follows acute upper respiratory tract or gut infections and specifically complicates glandular fever in a few cases. It may occur in association with a remote carcinoma. It can occur at any age, and the clinical findings may be very variable and hysteria is often suspected. The first symptoms are usually peripheral painful paraesthesiae but rarely accompanied by definite sensory findings. Weakness may come on quite explosively and a patient may become extremely weak over as short a period as thirty minutes, although more typically the period of advancing weakness in an acute case is some twelve to forty-eight hours. The weakness is often most marked in the proximal muscles, so that the patient may be unable to sit or stand at a time when peripheral strength is quite normal; it is this combination that may lead to a diagnosis of hysteria. In most cases the main clue, and in the writer's opinion almost diagnostic finding, is the total abolition of reflexes, even at the stage when the weakness has not become generalised. Bilateral facial weakness is quite common but easily missed unless eye closure, cheek blowing and lip pouting are routinely tested. If present this is another virtually diagnostic sign of Guillain–Barré syndrome—it is extremely rare in other forms of neuropathy.

Some twenty-five per cent of patients have significant respiratory problems and the ten per cent mortality rate is a measure of the potential danger of this disease. Patients should be moved to a unit where respiratory facilities are available. Dramatic deterioration may occur in an hour and transfer should not be delayed once the diagnosis is established.

The C.S.F. protein is typically elevated, but this may take several days to occur, and in the very acute stages of a severe attack some lymphocytes may be found in the C.S.F. raising diagnostic possibilities such as poliomyelitis.

Guillain–Barré syndrome is one of a few conditions that the writer regards as an acute neurological emergency, and yet it is often casually treated and regarded as a benign condition by those who see the occasional case that runs a mild course with recovery over a few weeks.

At the opposite extreme there is a variant of this disorder of slow onset, often over several weeks, with a tendency to persist or even slowly progress over a period of years with severe disability, and occasionally responding to steroids. In the acute type of attack ACTH may be of some benefit. In the

Figure 16.1.

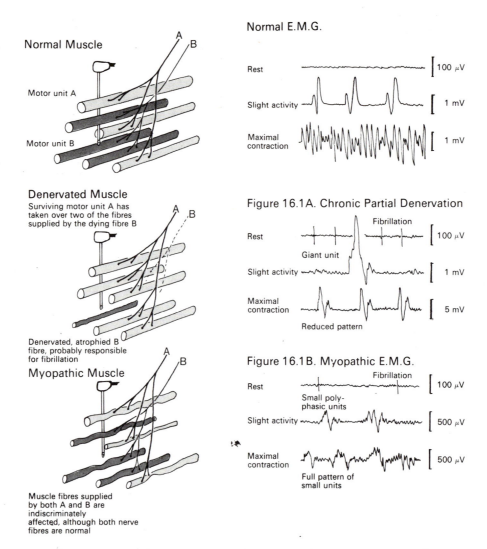

Normal Muscle

Motor unit A

Motor unit B

Normal E.M.G.

Rest — 100 μV

Slight activity — 1 mV

Maximal contraction — 1 mV

Denervated Muscle

Surviving motor unit A has taken over two of the fibres supplied by the dying fibre B

Denervated, atrophied B fibre, probably responsible for fibrillation

Figure 16.1A. Chronic Partial Denervation

Rest — Fibrillation — 100 μV

Giant unit

Slight activity — 1 mV

Maximal contraction — 5 mV

Reduced pattern

Myopathic Muscle

Muscle fibres supplied by both A and B are indiscriminately affected, although both nerve fibres are normal

Figure 16.1B. Myopathic E.M.G.

Rest — Fibrillation — 100 μV

Small polyphasic units

Slight activity — 500 μV

Maximal contraction — 500 μV

Full pattern of small units

d. The patient then contracts the muscle as hard as possible against resistance. In a normal muscle the activity is continuous as units contract and rest as others take over. The baseline sweep is completely obliterated. This is known as the interference pattern. In a denervated muscle gaps appear in the pattern marking the former position of a damaged unit in the sequence and the surviving units are often large and polyphasic. From their identical appearance it is often clear that it is the *same* giant unit repeating at regular intervals. This is known as a reduction in the interference pattern.

These findings may be patchy and in some diseases the fastest conducting fibres seem to be affected first so that the maximal findings of denervation are in the periphery of the muscle. This is a particular feature of motor neurone disease.

It must be stressed that these findings only indicate damage to the nerve fibres or ventral horn cell—the level at which the damage has occurred must be deduced from the clinical features and nerve conduction studies. Chronic partial denervation does *not* automatically indicate ventral horn cell disease.

2. *Myopathic Changes* (Figure 16.1b)

In muscle disease the situation is quite different. The disease process affects all or some muscle fibres in an entirely random way without regard to motor units. The only exception to this is in polymyositis in which the changes may be extremely patchy and full depth sampling in several areas of a muscle may be necessary before an area of typical damage is detected.

The following features are found in muscle disease:

a. Damaged muscle fibres, particularly in necrotic myopathies such as polymyositis and in Pompé's disease (see

Chapter 17), (in which glycogen storage disease affects both the muscle fibre and the ventral horn cell) may be irritable and show fibrillation which may lead to an incorrect diagnosis of denervation.

b. As the process is often patchy in individual fibres there is delayed or blocked conduction along the fibre, both dispersing the unit and reducing its size. The end result is a small (200–500 μV) polyphasic action potential. The interference pattern is usually full as part of all units survive but the small polyphasic potentials produce a very characteristic "crackling" noise on the E.M.G. amplifier.

c. In muscle disease associated with myotonia, the prolonged discharges that produce the typical stiffness of the muscles are audible as decrementing bursts of potentials that were formerly likened to "dive-bomber" noises, but in the author's view a more accurate and contemporary description would be the sound of a highly tuned Japanese motor-cycle engine. The bursts often superimpose on one another, quite unlike the brief "pseudo-myotonic" runs provoked by needle movement in irritable partially denervated muscles.

d. E.M.G. techniques have a limited place in the diagnosis of myasthenia gravis as the muscles typically affected are often inaccessible to EMG techniques.

Nerve Conduction Studies

1. The basic requirements for motor nerve conduction studies are that a suitable muscle is available and that its nerve supply can be stimulated at two points along its course. The time taken from the stimulus nearest the muscle is known as the distal latency and includes not only the time taken for the impulse to travel down the nerve but also the delay at the end plate and initiation of contraction. If the nerve is then stimulated higher up a second latency can be obtained, the difference in the time taken being an accurate measurement of the time taken for the impulse to traverse a measured length of nerve. From this the conduction velocity in metres per second is easily calculated. Very carefully documented velocity ranges for all the nerves that can be studied in this way have been reported. These are the median and ulnar nerves in the arm and the peroneal and tibial nerves in the leg. Nerves such as the radial and femoral can only be readily stimulated at one point and a latency to an appropriate muscle is all that can be measured.

In general if a muscle is denervated and it can be shown that the lesion responsible is above the proximal stimulus it is probably affecting the nerve root or ventral horn cell.

Figure 16.2. Nerve Conduction Studies in the Arm

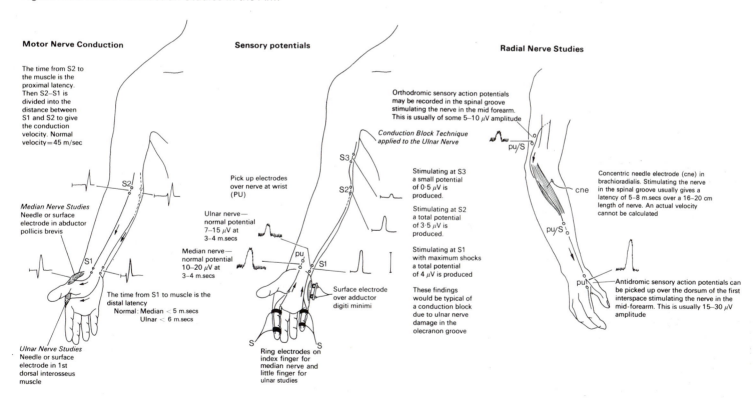

Motor Nerve Conduction

The time from S2 to the muscle is the proximal latency. Then S2–S1 is divided into the distance between S1 and S2 to give the conduction velocity. Normal velocity=45 m/sec

Median Nerve Studies Needle or surface electrode in abductor pollicis brevis

The time from S1 to muscle is the distal latency
Normal: Median < 5 m.secs
Ulnar < 6 m.secs

Ulnar Nerve Studies Needle or surface electrode in 1st dorsal interosseus muscle

Sensory potentials

Pick up electrodes over nerve at wrist (PU)

Ulnar nerve– normal potential 7–15 μV at 3–4 m.secs

Median nerve– normal potential 10–20 μV at 3–4 m.secs

Surface electrode over adductor digiti minimi

Ring electrodes on index finger for median nerve and little finger for ulnar studies

Conduction Block Technique applied to the Ulnar Nerve

Stimulating at S3 a small potential of 0.5 μV is produced.

Stimulating at S2 a total potential of 3.5 μV is produced.

Stimulating at S1 with maximum shocks a total potential of 4 μV is produced

These findings would be typical of a conduction block due to ulnar nerve damage in the olecranon groove

Radial Nerve Studies

Orthodromic sensory action potentials may be recorded in the spinal groove stimulating the nerve in the mid forearm. This is usually some 5–10 μV amplitude

Concentric needle electrode (cne) in brachioradialis. Stimulating the nerve in the spinal groove usually gives a latency of 5–8 m.secs over a 16–20 cm length of nerve. An actual velocity cannot be calculated

Antidromic sensory action potentials can be picked up over the dorsum of the first interspace stimulating the nerve in the mid-forearm. This is usually 15–30 μV amplitude

Figure 16.3. Nerve Conduction Studies in the Leg

Motor Nerve Conduction

Standard conduction velocity
measured while stimulating
peroneal nerve at S1 and S2
Normal: +35 m/sec

S3

S2

cne

Conduction Block technique
Stimulating at S1, a potential of 4 mV
obtained
From S2 a potential of less than 1 mV
is obtained, and the same from S3.
This confirms damage at fibula neck

4mV

S1

Either a needle or
a surface electrode
over extensor
digitorum brevis

pu

Sensory Nerve Conduction

Orthodromic potential (Peroneal nerve)
Stimulate anterior tibial nerve at the
ankle and pick up potential through needles
inserted adjacent to the nerve at the
fibula neck
Normal: 2–5 μV at 4–6 m.secs

pu

If E.D.B. wasted, a needle electrode in
midpoint of tibialis anterior is used
Normal latency: 4–6 m.secs over a
12–16 cm length

S

S

Antidromic potential (Sural nerve)
Stimulate nerve which is palpable just
behind and above lateral malleolus. Pick
up over the nerve below the malleolus
Normal: 5–15 μV at 2–4 m.secs

pu

The position of electrodes and velocities for the arm and legs are shown in Figures 16.2 and 16.3.

2. Nerve action potentials can be measured in two ways orthodromically or antidromically. Here the main requirement is a nerve near enough to the surface to be picked up by a surface elctrode or anatomically constant in position allowing needle electrodes to be inserted next to the nerve. Both the median and ulnar nerve action potentials can be detected at the wrist by stimulating the interdigital nerves of the appropriate fingers. Nerve action potentials in the leg present a great problem. The techniques are shown in Figures 16.2 and 16.3.

3. In the case of ulnar nerve lesions at the elbow or the peroneal nerve lesions at the fibula neck due to compression some patients do *not* demonstrate slowed conduction through the damaged area. A very useful ancillary test is the study of quantitative muscle action potentials. Using max-

imal shocks the full muscle potential produced from stimulation at the wrist or ankle is measured. The nerve is then stimulated just below the elbow or fibula neck. A slight reduction of potential of some ten per cent is normal. Then the nerve is stimulated *above* the elbow or in the popliteal fossa respectively. A dramatic drop in the potential is often seen indicating that some fifty to seventy-five per cent of fibres are *not* functioning in the damaged segments even though the velocity in the surviving fibres is normal (see Figures 16.2 and 16.3). Using this technique the actual point of damage may be detected at a position where the nerve is almost inexcitable.

There is no standard examination for any patient referred for E.M.G. and nerve conduction studies. The clinical problem is considered and a combination of muscle sampling and nerve studies are performed appropriate to the situation.

Chapter 17

DISEASES OF MUSCLE AND THE MUSCLE END PLATE

Muscles are subject to a wide range of inherited, degenerative, metabolic and toxic disorders. There is a marked similarity to peripheral nerve disease in that a wide range of disorders produce a limited group of symptoms and signs. Differential diagnosis depends on a careful family history, careful documentation of the extent and distribution of the muscle abnormalities and an awareness of all the diagnostic possibilities.

1. MUSCULAR DYSTROPHY

Muscular dystrophy is characterised by an inherited degeneration of various muscle groups that begins after a period of apparently normal muscle development and function. In some varieties the onset is delayed until adulthood. Although still regarded as a primary muscle disorder clinical and electro-physiological evidence has suggested a neurogenic component. A full discussion of these controversial views is beyond the scope of the present text.

Although clinical features often allow a confident diagnosis to be made it is essential that full confirmatory studies including electrophysiological tests and muscle biopsy are performed. The diagnosis must be certain for prognostic purposes and to allow genetic counselling to be firmly based. Occasionally, patients are seen who have been given a lethal prognosis, and who are later shown to have a restricted form of myopathy or a neuropathic disease such as Kugelberg–Welander syndrome.

The muscular dystrophies include:

a. Duchenne muscular dystrophy—
  1. Sex-linked disease of males with dominant inheritance.
  2. Non-sex-linked autosomal recessive in males and females.
b. Beckers muscular dystrophy—
  1. A mild sex-linked form of muscular dystrophy in males.
c. Limb-girdle dystrophy—
  1. Pelvi-femoral type (Leyden–Mobius variety).
  2. Scapulo-humeral dystrophy.
d. Facio-scapulo-humeral dystrophy (Landouzy–Dejerine).

e. Dystrophia myotonica (Steinert's disease).
f. Myotonia congenita (Thomsen's disease).
g. Ocular dystrophies.

General Clinical Features of Muscular Dystrophy

1. There is usually a positive family history. It is always worth remembering that family histories can be unreliable or impossible to obtain. Only a *positive* family history has any significance.

2. The distribution and sequence of muscle damage will vary widely depending on the type of dystrophy. Indeed, these features form the basis of the classification of muscular dystrophy (see Figures 17.1–17.5).

3. In muscular dystrophy the muscles become weak *before* significant wasting is apparent. This is because the degenerating fibres are often replaced by fat, and the muscles may even appear hypertrophied. Such muscles have a stodgy, doughy feel. This is quite the reverse of neural disease in which the atrophy proceeds faster than weakness.

4. Reflexes are often depressed or absent very early in the course of muscular dystrophy and long before the muscle is significantly wasted. This is one of the features that has led to the suggestion that there is a neurogenic component.

5. In the terminal stages of muscular dystrophy it may be impossible to make a clinical diagnosis as the widespread muscle wasting, weakness and loss of reflexes could equally well indicate a diffuse neurogenic disorder.

The sequence and distribution of weakness in the various types of muscular dystrophy are indicated in Figures 17.1–17.5, and the other features are summarised in the legend of each diagram.

2. CONGENITAL MYOPATHIES

For many years the term "floppy infant" was used to describe a group of muscular disorders, present from birth in which the child was hypotonic and showed delayed motor activity and development. The disabilities may be sufficiently severe to threaten the child's survival. A wide range of disorders may be responsible. In some cases the condition is merely evidence of severe cerebral damage, as spasticity and choreo-athetoid movements *cannot* develop until 1–2 years

Figure 17.1. Clinical Features of Duchenne Dystrophy

Facial, extra-ocular muscle and sternomastoid rarely affected

Occasional macroglossia

Cardiac muscle affected

Pseudohypertrophy may also occur in deltoid and infraspinatus

Weakness begins in quadriceps, hip flexors and back extensors, and extends upwards

Neck extensors remain unaffected

Calves hypertrophied and strong ankle jerks intact

DUCHENNE (Pseudohypertrophic) MUSCULAR DYSTROPHY

1. Males, inherited as sex-linked recessive (very rare female cases reported).

2. Onset between 3 and 10 years of age.

3. No abortive cases, most die within ten years of onset.

4. Onset in proximal muscles of leg, especially quadriceps and lower trunk muscles; later shoulder girdle and then extends peripherally. Contractures occur early and are severe.

5. Important early signs include loss of reflexes except the ankle jerk which usually remains intact and excludes a neuropathy.

6. The diaphragm, neck muscles, extraocular and facial muscles very rarely involved.

7. Other features include macroglossia in some cases and pseudohypertrophy usually of the calves but occasionally of the deltoid and infraspinatus.

8. Bone thinning, scoliosis, pathological fractures, fatty infiltration of the heart and respiratory infections are important complications that may lead to death.

9. Thirty per cent of affected patients have an I.Q. of less than 75.

10. The carrier state may be detected by serum enzyme studies and E.M.G. In the patient early on enzymes are very high with a later fall into normal range when atrophy is severe.

of age. Werdnig—Hoffman disease may be so severe at birth that floppy paralysis is already present. Dystrophia myotonica may be another cause of the "floppy infant" syndrome; although the usual onset is in the second or third decade.

This leaves several other disorders that appear to be due to a myopathic process, ranging from a benign variety with delayed but normal motor development, to a progressive myopathy. The routine use of muscle biopsy including electron microscopy and histochemistry has revealed several different pathologies.

Currently four varieties of congenital myopathy have been identified.

1. Central core disease: (abnormal structure and absence of muscle enzymes in the central areas of muscle fibres).

2. Nemaline-rod myopathy: (thread-like structures are found in the muscle fibres).

3. Myotubular myopathy: (the muscle fibres have a tubular structure similar to foetal muscle).

4. Congenital fibre-type disproportion: (abnormal ratio of type 1 and type 2 muscle fibres).

All these conditions cause a slowly progressive proximal weakness usually more severe in the legs. The nemaline-rod-myopathy is associated with kyphoscoliosis, pes cavus and a long thin face. The myotubular type may affect the extraocular muscles and in some cases may be associated with a long thin face. Congenital fibre-type disproportion causes very severe floppy weakness easily misdiagnosed as Werdnig—Hoffman disease. Even in this latter disorder some degree of improvement begins after two to three years, and most patients with these disorders survive into adulthood.

Figure 17.2. Clinical Features of Limb-Girdle Dystrophy

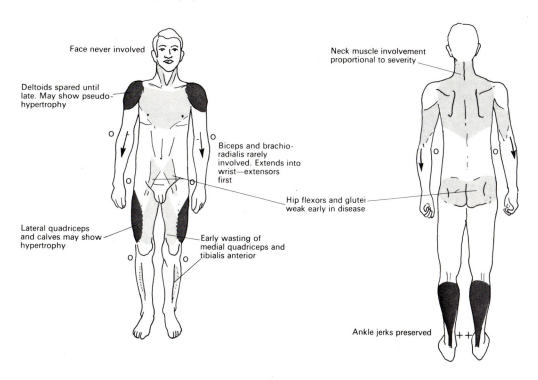

Face never involved

Deltoids spared until late. May show pseudo-hypertrophy

Biceps and brachio-radialis rarely involved. Extends into wrist—extensors first

Lateral quadriceps and calves may show hypertrophy

Early wasting of medial quadriceps and tibialis anterior

Neck muscle involvement proportional to severity

Hip flexors and glutei weak early in disease

Ankle jerks preserved

LIMB-GIRDLE DYSTROPHY

1. Males/females equally affected, autosomal recessive but occasionally dominant or sporadic.

2. Onset between 10 and 30 years of age.

3. Abortive cases with incomplete picture occur with mainly pelvic or shoulder girdle involvement. Usually causes disability over ten to twenty years after onset.

4. Onset may be in either pelvic or shoulder girdle and may remain confined to these areas or apparently static for years. In late cases considerable peripheral wasting and weakness may occur. Contractures are unusual.

5. Proximal reflexes are often impaired and as in Duchenne dystrophy the ankle jerks are usually preserved until late in the disease.

6. Cardiac involvement is extremely rare; and facial muscles are only slightly affected if at all.

7. Pseudohypertrophy may occur in the calves and deltoids and strikingly in the lateral quadriceps often associated with early and gross wasting of the medial thigh.

8. There are no special complications and life span is unaffected.

9. Intelligence is normal.

10. The serum enzymes are slightly elevated or normal.

Figure 17.6. Glucose-Glycogen Metabolism in Muscle

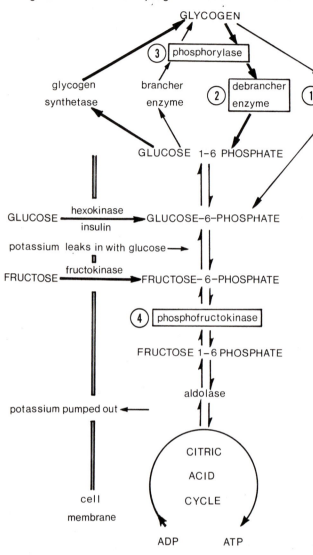

The following glycogen storage disorders produce muscle disease. The enzyme block is indicated on the figure

1. Pompé's disease (Type II glycogenosis)
2. Cori's disease (Type III glycogenosis)
3. McCardle's Syndrome (Type V glycogenosis)
4. Tarui's disease (Type VII glycogenosis)

Note also the leak of potassium into the cell during glucose uptake and the active pump mechanism which keeps the intracellular potassium down (see the periodic paralyses)

3. METABOLIC MYOPATHY

A complete discussion of muscle metabolism is beyond the immediate scope of the present text. For brevity discussion will be confined to generalisations which give an idea of the biochemical function of muscles on which discussion of the different types of myopathy can be based.

There are three main metabolic considerations:

1. Protein metabolism must be normal to maintain the contractile proteins. In some endocrine myopathies contractile protein abnormalities may contribute to muscle weakness.
2. The metabolism of energy production in the muscle must be intact. This basically means that glucose availability and the glycogen breakdown pathways must be normal. Several muscle disorders are based on either glucose assimilation disorders or enzyme deficiencies in the glycogen pathway.
3. The importance of normal sodium, potassium and calcium metabolism in maintaining resting membrane potentials and in the contractile mechanism is critical in the induction and cessation of contraction.

The metabolic pathways and inter-relationships of these metabolic activities are summarised in Figure 17.6.

The metabolic myopathies tend to cause chronic progressive muscle weakness, but in the initial stages episodes of sudden severe weakness during or following exertion are the most typical feature. The distinction can often be made on a typical history of the acute episodes.

Muscle Disease due to Abnormal Glycogen Metabolism

Although there are seven glycogen storage disorders only four are associated with muscle disease.

1. *Pompe's Disease (Type II glycogenosis)*

This is a disease of infancy and invariably fatal. In recent years however a few cases of a mild form of this disorder have been recognised in adults. In the infantile form the heart, liver, kidneys and the C.N.S. itself are also affected. Either cardiac failure or muscle weakness may be the first evidence of the disease. The neurological condition is very hard to distinguish from Werdnig–Hoffman disease including the fact that the E.M.G. shows profuse fibrillation—an indication of ventral horn cell disease or denervation. This is said to be due to co-existent ventral horn cell infiltration. The clinical clues lie in cardiac damage and often a very large tongue. These do not occur in Werdnig–Hoffman disease but the latter feature may suggest cretinism.

2. *Debranching Enzyme Disease (Limit dextrinosis) (Type III glycogenosis)*

In this variety the main infiltration and damage is to the liver causing hypoglycaemia. A mild proximal myopathy with hypotonia is present in infancy and a few adult cases have been reported—with a clinical appearance easily mistaken for motor neurone disease.

3. Myophosphorylase Deficiency (McArdle's Syndrome) (Type V glycogenosis)

The abnormality in this condition is confined to the skeletal muscles. The abnormality is apparent only on exertion as the defect blocks the glycogen-glucose conversion. Because the enzyme has no role in glycogen synthesis there is only a minimal excess of glycogen in the muscle. The disorder causes easy fatiguability and severe muscle cramping with breakdown of muscle proteins leading to myoglobinuria. As in all metabolic muscle disorders (see later) there is a tendency for the patients to develop permanent girdle muscle weakness later in life. The disease is inherited as an autosomal recessive. The classical investigation is to exercise the forearm muscles with a cuff on the arm so that the muscle is ischaemic. This increases the need for anaerobic glycolysis and the muscle promptly goes into severe cramp. If a venous sample of blood is taken from the exercised arm there is no rise in the blood lactate level and E.M.G. sampling of the muscles in cramp will reveal electrical silence—quite the reverse of normal muscle cramp.

The disorder is extremely rare. Few neurologists have seen more than two or three examples of the condition.

4. Phosphofructokinase Deficiency (Tarui's Disease) (Type VII glycogenosis)

The clinical details of this disease are virtually identical to McArdle's syndrome but in this case the block in the glycogen-glucose pathway is several stages lower down (see Figure 17.6).

4. MUSCLE DISEASE DUE TO ABNORMAL POTASSIUM HANDLING

These conditions are known as the periodic paralyses and are associated with alteration in serum potassium levels. The defect however probably lies in muscle membrane permeability, the serum potassium levels reflecting massive uptake or loss of potassium from the muscles. There are three types.

1. Familial Hypokalaemic Periodic Paralysis

This is inherited as an autosomal dominant affecting males more than females. The condition becomes evident between 10 and 20 years of age and tends to remit after 35 years of age. Attacks typically occur after rest, usually on waking in the morning. They specifically occur if a heavy carbohydrate meal or excessive exercise were taken on the previous evening. It is thought that an excess of potassium enters the muscle during the high rate of glucose uptake following a meal or after exercise. The serum potassium falls, weakness becoming apparent at a level of 3·5 mEq/L and maximal at 2·5 mEq/L, suggesting that it is the high intracellular potassium that causes the weakness rather than the serum level. It is extremely unusual for a patient to die in an attack as the diaphragm, respiratory muscles and eye muscles are normally unaffected. This is because the continual activity of these muscles even during sleep keeps pumping potassium out of the cells; further evidence that it is the intracellular potassium that is critical in causing weakness. Attacks usually last eight to twenty-four hours.

An attack may be relieved by 10 gms. of potassium chloride in water taken orally.

2. Adynamia Episodica Hereditaria (Gamstorp's Disease)

This disease is characterised by the sudden onset of weakness some thirty minutes after exercise. If the patient senses the stiffness and weakness coming on further exercise may delay the onset but the attack when it comes is then more severe. Proximal muscles are particularly affected and often become stiff and myotonic. Attacks start between 5 and 15 years of age and tend to remit after 20 years of age. Each attack lasts thirty minutes to two hours. A chronic proximal myopathy often develops after the disease itself has remitted.

The weakness is probably due to release of potassium from the muscles as it occurs when the serum level is only 5 mEq/L. In patients with potassium retention weakness does *not* occur until a serum level of 8 mEq/L.

Attacks may be prevented by the use of acetazolamide 50–100 mgs. daily and acute attacks terminated by 1–2 gms. of calcium chloride I.V.I.

3. Normokalaemic Periodic Paralysis

This very rare condition occurs in infancy between 2 and 10 years of age. The attacks consist of sudden episodes of flaccid quadriplegia, that may last from one to three weeks. They may respond to sodium chloride and can be prevented by the use of salt-retaining steroids such as fluorocortisone. The relationship of this disorder to potassium metabolism is obscure.

5. SECONDARY METABOLIC AND ENDOCRINE MYOPATHIES

Some features of endocrine myopathy are due to co-existent electrolyte disturbances so that some degree of overlap is necessary in discussing these problems.

Electrolyte Disturbance

Several disorders of sodium metabolism cause cerebral

symptoms that dominate the clinical features. Milder disorders contribute to muscle weakness in adrenal disease as discussed later.

Hypokalaemia

Hypokalaemia of less than 2·5 mEq/L causes severe flaccid tetraparesis. The most frequent causes are:

Conn's syndrome (aldosterone secreting adrenal tumour).
Renal disease (Fanconi syndrome, renal tubular acidosis).
Potassium losing enteritis and severe diarrhoea.
Excessive diuretic therapy (thiazide diuretics).
Carbenoxolone therapy (liquorice extract used in peptic ulcer disease).

An immediate serum potassium determination is indicated *in any* patient with acute or subacute flaccid paraparesis. One patient with Conn's syndrome was only diagnosed when a *third* attack of acute paralytic poliomyelitis was thought to be an unlikely diagnosis!

Hyperkalaemia

Hyperkalaemia greater than 7 mEq/L causes a severe ascending quadriplegia that may mimic Guillain–Barré syndrome. It is extremely rare for the extraocular muscles to be affected. The most frequent causes are:

Renal failure.
Excessive administration of potassium salts in I.V. infusions.
Aldosterone antagonists (spironolactone).

In these patients there is a much greater risk that the cardiotoxic effect of hyperkalaemia will kill the patient before the onset of paralysis.

Hypocalcaemia

Chronic hypocalcaemia causes attacks of tetany and muscle weakness. In infancy convulsions, papilloedema and calcification of the basal ganglia may occur. Hypocalcaemia should be carefully excluded in any young patient who is developing cataracts. Causes include primary or secondary hypoparathyroidism, renal disease or bladder diversion procedures, deficient diet or lack of Vitamin D.

Hypercalcaemia

Hypercalcaemia tends to cause striking cerebral dysfunction or psychosis of acute onset. A slower onset causes quite severe but variable proximal muscle weakness. This is usually combined with brisk reflexes which may raise the diagnostic possibility of motor neurone disease. The most frequent cause is primary hyperparathyroidism due to a parathyroid adenoma. It may also occur in patients with metastatic malignancy who have osteolytic metastases or occasionally as a primary disorder without bone metastases. Multiple myeloma in particular may cause diffuse bone destruction and hypercalcaemia. Sarcoidosis, excessive intake of Vitamin D, milk alkali syndrome and idiopathic hypercalcaemia of infancy are other possible causes.

Endocrine Disease

Thyroid Disease

There are several ways in which the thyroid gland may be associated with muscular disorders.

Myasthenia gravis is often associated with thyrotoxicosis (in ten per cent of cases) and routine thyroid investigations are indicated in any patient with myasthenia gravis.

Hypokalaemic periodic paralysis occurs in association with thyrotoxicosis particularly in the Japanese but also in other ethnic groups.

The most frequent complication is thyrotoxic myopathy which particularly affects the shoulder girdle (spinati, deltoid and triceps) or pelvic girdle (hip flexors and quadriceps). It often occurs as the only *overt* manifestation of the disease and more often in males (even though thyrotoxicosis occurs three times as commonly in females). The clue to this diagnosis is the retention of reflexes, which are often very brisk. The picture is similar to hypercalcaemic myopathy in this respect.

Extra-ocular muscle disease in thyrotoxicosis has been described in Chapter 5.

Myxoedema causes proximal muscle weakness as part of the general slowing down, but the more dramatic neurological complication of this disorder is cerebellar degeneration (see Chapter 11). Proximal muscle weakness also occurs in cretins.

Adrenal Disease

In Cushing's syndrome very striking wasting and weakness of the pelvic girdle and thigh muscles occurs. A similar picture is produced by the use of fluorinated steroids, especially triamcinolone.

In Addison's disease general lethargy, muscle cramps and weakness are an integral part of the disease. This is usually due to the hyponatraemia.

Conn's syndrome with hypokalaemic muscle weakness has been discussed above.

Parathyroid Disease

The effects of parathyroid disease on muscle have already been described in the section on disordered calcium metabolism.

6. MUSCLE DISEASE DUE TO DRUGS

Four drugs in general use may cause muscle disorders. Carbenoxolone (liquorice extract) used in the treatment of peptic ulceration and thiazide diuretics both cause loss of potassium and can cause very acute severe muscle weakness.

All steroid drugs, particularly fluorinated steroids and chloroquine may cause a progressive proximal myopathy. Even steroids used under occlusive dressings may cause systemic toxicity or wasting and weakness of the muscles under the dressing.

Within the last two years penicillamine has found increasing use in the treatment of rheumatoid and psoriatic arthropathy. Within recent months examples of both myasthenic syndromes and polymyositis apparently caused by the drug have been reported. The writer has had one patient with both anticholinsterase-sensitive weakness and polymyositis who had been on penicillamine for over a year, thought to be another example of this problem.

7. INFLAMMATORY MUSCLE DISEASE

Muscles are remarkably resistant to infection and with the exception of gas gangrene caused by Clostridium Welchii bacterial infection is rare. Sarcoidosis may also cause mild to severe muscle disease but the exact role of infection in this peculiar disease and its rarity do not justify more detailed consideration. Muscle inflammation in viral disease is exemplified by Bornholm disease (epidemic pleurodynia) and the general myalgia and listlessness of influenza may mimic acute poliomyelitis. Parasitic involvement is very rare in Great Britain with Trichinella spiralis (trichinosis— particularly affecting the extra-ocular muscles) and Taenia solium (cysticercosis—usually asymptomatic cysts in trunk muscles in a patient who has become an accidental intermediate host in the life cycle of the pork tape worm) are the only disorders worth mentioning. The latter condition usually causes epilepsy due to cerebral cysts, but plain x-rays of the trunk muscles to show the calcified cysts are important in establishing the diagnosis.

Muscle tenderness, severe aching and very severe deep burning, tearing pains in the muscles often described by the patient "as if the flesh were being torn from the bone" are the main symptoms of a peculiar disease known as "polymyalgia rheumatica". The E.S.R. is markedly elevated and an almost immediate response to indomethacin or steroids gives strong support for this diagnosis. The relationship of the disease to rheumatoid arthritis is uncertain but a special feature is that some forty per cent of patients go on to develop temporal arteritis. Prolonged observation is therefore necessary.

The most important inflammatory muscle disease is polymyositis.

Polymyositis

The importance of this disorder lies not only in the muscle problem, which may be considerable, but also in the possibility of serious underlying disease. There are several complicated classifications based on a combination of age and type of underlying disorder which includes malignant disease, collagen-vascular disease and Sjörgen's syndrome.

As with all neurological disorders the beginner's problem is less one of classification but more of recognising the condition in the first place. Polymyositis shares with porphyria and Guillain—Barré syndrome the distinction of being easily misdiagnosed as a functional disorder or hysteria.

Some of the difficulty stems from the name and usual descriptions which suggest that the muscles are very tender and weak and make the diagnosis obvious. This is unfortunately quite inaccurate as less than half the patients have demonstrable muscle tenderness and the weakness may be no greater than enough to make the patient feel rather listless with a tendency to fatigue easily; symptoms easily dismissed as due to depression or anxiety.

General Clinical Features

1. Muscle weakness is the usual presenting symptom and usually affects the pelvic girdle first. This causes difficulty climbing stairs or getting up from a chair.

2. This is followed by shoulder girdle weakness with difficulty reaching objects on shelves, washing the face or brushing the hair. Weakness of the neck muscles and dysphagia are very common at this stage but facial weakness and extraocular muscle weakness is extremely rare (an important distinguishing feature from myasthenia gravis).

3. Pain and tenderness of the affected muscles occurs in less than half the patients and is almost invariably found in the shoulder girdle muscles.

4. Systemic symptoms such as weight loss, anorexia, fever and lassitude occur more frequently in childhood polymyositis.

5. Atrophy of the affected muscles is late and mild and it is always difficult to detect atrophy in the plump pelvic area.

6. Evidence of collagen vascular disease such as Raynauds phenomenon, arthralgia, pneumonitis and renal damage are found in twenty-five to thirty per cent of cases.

7. Tendon reflexes are preserved until very late in the course of the disease.

Figure 17.7. Clinical Features of Progressive Ocular Myopathy

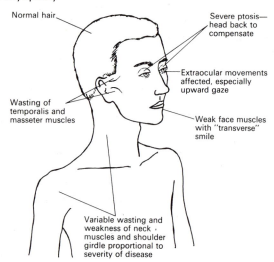

Normal hair

Severe ptosis—head back to compensate

Extraocular movements affected, especially upward gaze

Wasting of temporalis and masseter muscles

Weak face muscles with "transverse" smile

Variable wasting and weakness of neck muscles and shoulder girdle proportional to severity of disease

PROGRESSIVE OCULAR MYOPATHY (including oculo-pharyngeal muscular dystrophy)

1. Both sexes affected. Dominant or sporadic inheritance.

2. Clinical features range from ptosis alone to ptosis with eye movement disorder and facial weakness, and in some twenty-five per cent of cases shoulder girdle involvement.

3. Fifty per cent have dysphagia and the term oculo-pharyngeal muscular dystrophy has been proposed for this group.

4. Some families include retinitis pigmentosa, visual difficulties, endocrine abnormalities, cardiac involvement and cerebellar abnormalities. Electrical and histological studies confirm neuropathic rather than myopathic changes in some patients.

5. The disorder may lie somewhere between the muscular dystrophies and metabolic neuropathies such as Refsum's disease, and clinically must be distinguished from dystrophia myotonica.

8. The association with skin changes and its significance depends on the patient's age. The combination is known as dermatomyositis. The skin rash consists of a lilac-coloured rash over the cheeks and eyelids and thickened, reddened skin over the interphalangeal joints.

9. Dermatomyositis is the usual pattern of the disease in childhood but is *never* associated with underlying malignant disease in this age group. Systemic symptoms however, are very common in childhood, and the disorder may be associated with bowel perforation, intestinal obstruction and the deposition of calcium in the skin and subcutaneous tissues.

10. In adulthood only fifty per cent of patients show skin changes but the considerable risk of underlying malignant disease is almost confined to this group. There is also a marked sex difference. Over the age of 50, seventy per cent of males with dermatomyositis are eventually found to have underlying malignant disease. In females the risk is only twenty-five per cent. Underlying malignant disease occurs in the following sites; carcinoma of the stomach, breast, bronchus and ovary. Bowel tumours underlie some thirty per cent of cases and in contrast to the situation with peripheral neuropathy full bowel investigation *is* indicated in patients over fifty years of age with dermatomyositis, if no tumour in the breast or lung can be demonstrated.

CASE REPORT

A 58-year-old man returned from abroad to live with his family. He related that he had been slowing down physically for two years. This had been ascribed to depression following his wife's death and he had been on anti-depressants. On his arrival he showed marked physical inertia and had a persistent cough with profuse watery sputum. On examination he clearly had parkinsonism but the most dramatic finding was gross weakness and wasting of the proximal muscles. A chest x-ray revealed a cavitating carcinoma of the right upper lobe and E.M.G. studies showed findings consistent with polymyositis. He responded well to levodopa and prednisone but died a few weeks later while having radiotherapy.

This is almost certainly an example of malignancy-associated polymyositis although the good response to steroids was unusual.

All groups may be treated with steroids with the expectation of a good response in childhood and in the idiopathic cases in middle age but little or no response in patients with underlying malignant disease. In children a myasthenic syndrome may be superadded to the dermatomyositis and a tensilon test is indicated if the child's clinical status worsens or fluctuates.

8. MYASTHENIA GRAVIS AND MYASTHENIC SYNDROMES

Like many diseases *classical* myasthenia gravis is easy to diagnose; but in common with other disorders the *first* symptoms can be very difficult to recognise. In the case of myasthenia this is usually because the typical features of variability and fatiguability may *not* be obvious and the patient may present with a fixed mild ptosis or eye movement disorder that may be misdiagnosed as an incomplete extraocular nerve palsy. If the bulbar muscles are affected by a non-variable weakness motor neurone disease or a brain-stem vascular accident may be suspected. At the opposite extreme attacks of diplopia or dysarthria may be so brief that a breaking-down squint or a transient brainstem ischaemic attack may be considered. Finally there is the problem of the tensilon test. A basic requirement of the test is a measurable degree of weakness in a specific muscle that can be easily observed; this may not always be possible and in the early stages of the disorder myasthenic muscles may not respond to tensilon, or to longer acting anticholinesterases given as a clinical trial. One patient of the author's failed to respond to tensilon or prostigmine over a period of ten weeks. Quite suddenly the affected bulbar muscles became tensilon sensitive and good therapeutic control became possible.

As already indicated variable ptosis of one or other eyelid or variable diplopia are the most frequent presenting symptoms closely followed by weakness of chewing, dysarthria or difficulty in swallowing. In a severe case respiratory difficulty may occur, but the usual indication for tracheostomy in the management of myasthenia is to protect the airway from inhalation of food when swallowing is severely impaired. Limb symptoms are a late and relatively minor symptom in the majority of myasthenics. It is unusual for the reflexes to be altered, in fact they are often brisker than normal. The drug management of myasthenia is discussed in detail in Chapter 24.

Myasthenia may occur transiently in ten per cent of children born to myasthenic mothers. If the mother has needed large doses of anticholinesterases during labour the child may be born with cholinergic blockade. The latter is unusual as in general myasthenia tends to improve during pregnancy.

In childhood myasthenia is quite rare, but is invariably associated with severe generalised weakness quite unlike the adult form. Otherwise the clinical features are similar to the adult. In childhood myasthenia there is a good possibility that a spontaneous remission will occur. As noted above the condition may complicate dermatomyositis in this age group.

In adults with long-standing well-controlled disease a proximal "myasthenic myopathy" may supervene, and in most cases progressive atrophy of the maximally affected muscles with diminishing responsiveness to anticholinergic drugs occurs.

In all cases thyrotoxicosis should be excluded. This occurs in ten per cent of males and twenty per cent of females with myasthenia gravis. Routine and special x-ray investigations to exclude a thymic tumour are indicated, particularly in young patients with severe myasthenia in whom the possibility of thymectomy as a method of treatment is being considered.

Myasthenic Syndrome

This condition is also known as the Lambert–Eaton syndrome and usually occurs in association with an oat-cell carcinoma of the lung. The weakness is mainly found in the proximal muscles of the pelvic and shoulder girdles. Neck and trunk muscles are affected but involvement of the bulbar or extra-ocular muscles is unusual. Unlike myasthenia gravis repeated activity of the muscle leads to increasing strength rather than weakness. The condition sometimes responds to guanidine hydrochloride which is thought to act by releasing acetylcholine at the motor end plate. Although only half the patients have a detectable malignancy at diagnosis close follow-up is necessary as the syndrome may precede the identification of the underlying malignant disease by several years.

Chapter 18

DIAGNOSIS OF ROOT AND NERVE LESIONS AFFECTING THE ARM

Most clinical students and many doctors are reluctant to attempt to make an accurate diagnosis of nerve root or peripheral nerve lesions in the arm due to deficient anatomical knowledge. There is also a widely held misconception that plexus lesions are a frequent cause of disease affecting the nerve supply of the arms. The anatomy of the brachial plexus is intimidating enough to daunt anyone who encounters a patient with a suspected plexus lesion! In fact, plexus lesions are quite rare in most civilised countries with a frequency proportional to the deliberate or accidental misuse of fire arms and knives. There are few disease processes that primarily affect the brachial plexus.

In this chapter the anatomical and clinical difference between nerve root and peripheral nerve lesions will be compared and contrasted. A final section on plexus lesions is included containing a specially constructed diagram of the brachial plexus based on a functional approach.

The clinical problem can usually be reduced to a simple consideration; is the pain or weakness in the territory supplied by a single nerve root or a single peripheral nerve or one of its branches. Definitive diagnosis usually depends on a very careful evaluation of the motor system as in the arm motor findings are much more reliable than sensory findings for reasons to be discussed later. For this reason the comparative tables (see Tables 1 and 2) are based on a simple evaluation of the motor supply of the arm, tested by ten movements, which in all but the most exceptional cases should provide all the information required for accurate localising diagnosis.

THE VULNERABLE AREAS OF THE NERVE SUPPLY TO THE ARM

Figure 18.1 shows the entire course of each of the roots and peripheral nerves supplying the arm. Emphasis has been given to those areas where the relationship of the neural structures to bone or muscle may predispose to traumatic damage. Note that the radial nerve is vulnerable at three positions along its course, the ulnar nerve at two positions and the median nerve only at the wrist. In spite of this, damage to the median nerve at the wrist and the ulnar nerve at the elbow are the peripheral lesions most often encountered. When one considers the cervical roots; C5 and

C6 are those most often affected by cervical spondylosis, and C7 by acute disc lesions. Involvement of roots above and below these levels is relatively unusual and involvement of the C2, 3 or C8 and D1 roots requires careful consideration of other diagnostic possibilities. D1 root damage is quite a common consequence of altered anatomy in the area of the apical pleura, due to a cervical rib or invasion by neoplastic disease in the upper part of the lung.

CLINICAL EVALUATION OF SENSORY SYMPTOMS AND SIGNS

We have already noted the unreliability of sensory phenomena in the arms and this probably stems from the complex central representation of the limb and considerable overlapping of nerve territories at the periphery. Root pains may range from tingling paraesthesiae in a well-localised distribution to very severe pain which the patient cannot localise accurately (see Figure 18.2). Individual root irritation causes pain in the following distributions:

C5 root pain occurs across the shoulder and in the lateral arm and does not radiate below the elbow. A confirmatory clue is often an aching pain down the medial scapula border. (This scapula pain may also occur with C6 and C7 root irritation, but much less frequently.)

C6 root pain causes deep aching pain in the biceps muscle which spreads down the lateral fore-arm, involving the thumb and index fingers, on both the palmar and dorsal aspects.

C7 root pain is inherently diffuse as the C7 root supplies the periosteum of the bones of the arm with a long cutaneous distribution down the centre of both the front and back of the arm. There is usually deep aching in the triceps muscle with pain down the front and back of the central forearm, radiating particularly into the middle finger but often spreading into both the index and ring fingers. When C7 root pain is very severe patients often complain that the *entire* arm is hurting.

C8 root pain is relatively unusual. It radiates from just below the olecranon down into the little ring fingers.

D1 root irritation causes a deep aching sensation felt in the shoulder joint and axilla and occasionally down the medial side of the arm to the olecranon.

Table 6   COMPARATIVE DATA ON ROOT AND NERVE LESIONS IN THE ARM

ROOTS	C5	C6	C7	C8	D1
Sensory supply	Lateral border upper arm	Lateral forearm including thumb	Over triceps, mid-forearm and middle finger	Medial forearm to include little finger	Axilla down to the olecranon
Sensory loss	As above	As above	Middle fingers	As above	As above
Area of pain	As above and medial scapula border	As above esp. thumb and index finger	As above and medial scapula border	As above	Deep aching in shoulder and axilla to olecranon
Reflex arc	Biceps jerk	Supinator jerk	Triceps jerk	Finger jerk	None
Motor deficit	Deltoid Supraspinatus Infraspinatus Rhomboids	Biceps Brachioradialis Brachialis (Pronators and supinators of forearm)	Latissimus dorsi Pectoralis major Triceps Wrist extensors Wrist flexors	Finger flexors Finger extensors Flexor carpi ulnaris (thenar muscles in some patients)	*All* small hand muscles (in some thenar muscles via C8)
Causative lesions	Brachial neuritis Cervical spondylosis Upper plexus avulsion	Cervical spondylosis Acute disc lesions	Acute disc lesions Cervical spondylosis	Rare in disc lesions or spondylosis	Cervical rib Outlet syndromes Pancoast tumour Metastatic carcinoma in deep cervical nodes

Table 7

NERVES	AXILLARY	MUSCULO-CUTANEOUS	RADIAL	MEDIAN	ULNAR
Sensory supply	Over deltoid	Lateral forearm to wrist	Lateral dorsal forearm and back of thumb and index finger	Lateral palm and lateral fingers	Medial palm and 5th and medial half ring finger
Sensory loss	Small area over deltoid	Lateral forearm	Dorsum of thumb and index (if any)	As above	As above but often none at all
Area of pain	Across shoulder tip	Lateral forearm	Dorsum of thumb and index	Thumb, index and middle finger. Often spreads up forearm	Ulnar supplied fingers and palm distal to wrist. Pain occasionally along course of nerve
Reflex arc	Nil	Biceps jerk	Triceps jerk and supinator jerk	Finger jerks (flexor digitorum sublimis)	Nil
Motor deficit	Deltoid (Teres minor cannot be evaluated)	Biceps Brachialis (coracobrachialis weakness not detectable)	Triceps Wrist extensors Finger extensors Brachioradialis Supinator of forearm	Wrist flexors Long finger flexors (thumb, index and middle finger) Pronators of forearm. Abductor pollicis brevis	All small hand muscles excluding abductor pollicis brevis. Flexor carpi ulnaris. Long flexors of ring and little finger
Causative lesions	Fractured neck of humerus. Dislocated shoulder. Deep I.M. injections	Very rarely damaged	Crutch palsy. Saturday night palsy. Fractured humerus. In supinator muscle	Carpal tunnel syndrome Direct trauma to wrist	Elbow: trauma, bed rest, fractured olecranon. Wrist: local trauma, ganglion of wrist joint

Figure 18.1. Clinically Relevant Anatomy of the Nerve Supply to the Arm

The most frequently encountered causes of damage at the various sites are indicated

C7 Root
By far the most frequent "acute cervical disc lesion" occurs at this level. C6 and C5 less often. Other levels very rarely

C5 and C6 Roots
Most frequently involved roots in cervical spondylosis. C7 involved occasionally. Others very rarely

Axillary nerve
Fracture of humeral neck
Dislocation of the humerus
Intramuscular injections

Lower trunk of the brachial plexus
Cervical rib syndrome. Altered anatomy (outlet syndrome). Pancoast tumour of lung apex

Radial nerve in the axilla
Incorrect use of a crutch

Radial nerve in spiral groove
Direct blow laterally. During anaesthesia medially. While drunk medially ("Saturday night palsy"). Fractures of the humerus — immediate or delayed

Radial nerve (Posterior interosseus nerve)
Nerve enters forearm through supinator muscle. Occupational overuse of muscle may damage nerve. Also occurs idiopathically. Extensors of thumb and index finger mainly affected

Ulnar nerve
Damage from repeated minor trauma
Prolonged bed rest
Delayed following fractures

Median nerve (Anterior interosseous nerve)
Rarely damaged nerve lies very deep
Flexors of thumb and index finger are affected by damage to nerve

Median nerve (Carpal tunnel syndrome)
Nerve damaged by swelling or infiltration of tunnel it transverses. Transiently seen in pregnancy. Idiopathically in females using hands for washing or unaccustomed use. Complicates rheumatoid arthritis. Rarely seen in other systemic diseases

Ulnar nerve (Deep branch)
Trauma to heel of the hand. Idiopathically (often a ganglion found on exploration) No sensory loss in typical cases

Figure 18.2. Distribution of Root Pain and Paraesthesiae

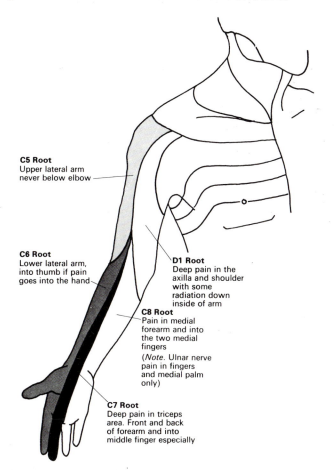

C5 Root
Upper lateral arm never below elbow

C6 Root
Lower lateral arm, into thumb if pain goes into the hand

D1 Root
Deep pain in the axilla and shoulder with some radiation down inside of arm

C8 Root
Pain in medial forearm and into the two medial fingers
(*Note*. Ulnar nerve pain in fingers and medial palm only)

C7 Root
Deep pain in triceps area. Front and back of forearm and into middle finger especially

Figure 18.3. Distribution of Pain and Paraesthesiae in Peripheral Nerve Lesions

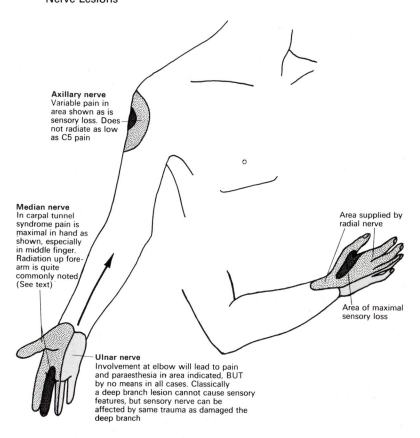

Axillary nerve
Variable pain in area shown as is sensory loss. Does not radiate as low as C5 pain

Median nerve
In carpal tunnel syndrome pain is maximal in hand as shown, especially in middle finger. Radiation up forearm is quite commonly noted (See text)

Area supplied by radial nerve

Area of maximal sensory loss

Ulnar nerve
Involvement at elbow will lead to pain and paraesthesia in area indicated, BUT by no means in all cases. Classically a deep branch lesion cannot cause sensory features, but sensory nerve can be affected by same trauma as damaged the deep branch

When one comes to consider the sensory symptoms due to involvement of peripheral nerves there are two special considerations (see Figure 18.3).

1. The area supplied by the radial nerve is so readily overlapped by other nerve supplies that detectable sensory loss is quite unusual and sensory symptoms may be confined to slight tingling over the dorsum of the thumb and index finger.

2. On purely anatomical grounds compression of the median nerve at the wrist should produce pain only in the lateral palm and three and a half fingers. In fact, many patients with carpal tunnel syndrome complain that the pain radiates up the central forearm to the elbow and occasionally to the shoulder. Many patients insist that at the height of the pain the fifth finger is also involved. The reasons for this are not clearly understood, but certainly the pain in all the fingers of the hand may well be related to the large number of sympathetic nerve fibres to the blood vessels of the hand, which are almost exclusively carried in the median nerve.

This probably accounts for the fact that most patients with pain in *all* fingers claim that at the height of an attack of pain, the fingers blanch and appear to be swollen, rather like Raynaud's phenomenon. In most patients with peripheral involvement of the median or ulnar nerves, appropriate sensory impairment may be found. Two-point discrimination sensation in the fingers is a particularly useful test to detect minimal sensory loss, but it must be realised that in many instances quite severe compression of either the median or the ulnar nerve may occur in the absence of any sensory symptoms or any sensory findings. It is this feature that can make diagnosis so difficult on occasions.

In the case of root involvement, although the pain may be exceptionally severe, it is very unusual to be able to document any definite sensory loss and extremely unusual for the sensory loss if found, to occupy the entire anatomical area supplied by a root. For example in the case of C6 some numbness over the dorsum of perhaps the index finger and thumb may be detected, even though the area in the forearm

Figure 18.4. Shoulder and Arm Movements

Shoulder abduction (C5) Second 90°
Deltoid. (Axillary nerve)

Shoulder abduction (C5) First 90°
Supraspinatus (Suprascapular nerve)

Shoulder adduction (C7)
Latissimus dorsi- (Nerve to lat. dorsi)
Pectoralis major (Dual innervation)
(See figure 18.6)

Shoulder external rotation (C5)
Infraspinatus (Suprascapular nerve)

Shoulder internal rotation (C5)
Subscapularis (Subscapular nerve)
Teres minor

Elbow flexion (fully supinated) C5 (6)
Biceps —(Musculo-cutaneous nerve)
Brachialis

Elbow flexion (half supinated) C(5) 6
Brachioradialis—(Radial nerve)

Elbow extension C7
Triceps (Radial nerve)

supplied by the root may appear to have normal sensation. In general, it should be stated that the failure to demonstrate sensory loss in any situation where there is pain in the arm should *not* be taken as evidence that the patient's symptoms are on a functional basis. It is for this reason that the motor findings are so important.

CLINICAL EVALUATION OF MOTOR FUNCTION IN THE ARM

For diagnostic purposes it is important to forget the multiplicity of roots contributing to the formation of individual peripheral nerves, particularly the radial and median nerves. One must think instead of the fact that each movement of the arm is controlled almost exclusively by a single root. It is not even necessary to remember all the muscles contributing to that movement. The only other consideration then becomes "which nerve carries the root to this or that muscle group?"

Thus for each of the basic movements of the arm there is a root value and a peripheral nerve value. These are indicated in Figures 18.4 and 18.5. It follows that each reflex in the arm also has a root value and a peripheral nerve value. If the reader will refer to the figures it will be noticed that the traditional methods used for testing arm function, the grip and opposition of the thumb and fifth finger are not included. A little thought will show that these movements involve several muscle groups, multiple nerves and multiple roots in their performance. Their diagnostic value is almost nil in terms of differentiating root and nerve lesions.

Special points that need to be emphasised in regard to testing of motor function in the arm are as follows.

1. A C5 root lesion will weaken all 180° of shoulder abduction. An axillary nerve lesion, affecting only the deltoid muscle, will weaken only the second 90° of movement. This should not be confused with the frozen shoulder syndrome in which severe pain prevents the second 90° of movement.

Figure 18.5. Forearm and Hand Movements

Elbow supination (C6)
Supinator—radial nerve

Wrist flexion (C7/8)
All fore-arm
muscles—median
flexor carpi
ulnaris—ulnar

Elbow pronation (C6)
Pronator Teres—
median nerve.
Pronator Quadratus—
(Anterior branch
of median)

Wrist extension C(6) 7
All extensor
muscles—radial
brachioradialis
group—Radial

Finger flexion (C8)
Flexor digitorum
profundus
Index/middle
finger—median
nerve
Ring/little—
ulnar nerve

Thumb abduction (D1)
Abductor pollicis
brevis—median
nerve

Finger extension (C8)
All extensors—
Radial

Finger abduction (D1)
Interossei and
abductor digitorum
minimi—ulnar nerve

Pinching movement (C8)
Long flexor of thumb
Long flexor of index
(Both anterior
interosseus nerve)

2. A C6 root lesion will produce weakness of elbow flexion in both the supine position (produced by biceps and brachialis) and in the half supinnated position (produced by brachioradialis muscle). A musculo-cutaneous nerve lesion (an extremely rare event) would only weaken the biceps and brachialis muscles. A radial nerve lesion will only weaken the brachioradialis muscle (as far as the elbow flexion is concerned).

3. A C7 root lesion causes weakness of shoulder adduction, elbow extension, wrist extension and wrist flexion because it contributes to both the radial and the median nerves. By contrast a radial nerve lesion cannot affect shoulder adduction or wrist flexion and in addition will also affect the brachioradialis muscle. This clinical distinction between a C7 root lesion and a radial nerve lesion is extremely important.

4. A C8 root lesion (relatively rare) will cause weakness of the long extensors and flexors of the fingers and many would add the small hand muscles. This latter feature is extremely controversial and it would appear that in some patients there is some contribution from C8 root to small hand muscles, but in the majority the small hand muscles are almost exclusively innervated by the D1 root.

5. A D1 root lesion will cause wasting and weakness of *all* the small hand muscles. An ulnar nerve lesion also causes wasting of the small hand muscles but spares the abductor pollicis brevis muscle as this is supplied by the D1 root but via the median nerve. Unfortunately, in some two to three per cent of otherwise normal persons *all* the small hand muscles are innervated by the ulnar nerve. This is a considerable diagnostic trap as in these instances *all* the small hand muscles will be wasted and a D1 root lesion or even more seriously, motor neurone disease may be diagnosed in error, when the patient has a simple ulnar nerve lesion.

It must be remembered that this is only a diagnostic guide; several movements have not even been considered. This is solely because their inclusion complicates the presentation without significantly improving the diagnostic value. In practice the information given will enable a confident conclusion to be arrived at in the majority of cases. To enhance the value of this approach we will now consider the different clinical conditions that should be considered after an initial history and examination has given some idea as to the diagnosis.

CLINICAL FEATURES OF CONDITIONS CAUSING ROOT AND NERVE LESIONS IN THE ARMS

Root Avulsion Syndromes

These conditions rarely cause differential diagnostic problems as the causative trauma is usually only too obvious. There are two basic syndromes:

1. Erb–Duchenne type of paralysis, which is due to avulsion of the C5 and C6 roots. This is usually the result of pressure applied to the shoulder, and may occur following motor-cycle accidents or in infancy during a forceps delivery, if the shoulders are stuck and the head is pulled too hard. This leads to loss of abduction of the shoulder and flexion at the elbow. This means that the arm hangs limply at the side and cannot be flexed, and therefore the hand cannot be placed into a useful, functional position, although hand function itself is perfectly normal.

2. The second type, known as Klumpke paralysis, occurs when the D1 and C8 roots have been avulsed. This tends to occur during falls when the patient makes an attempt to grasp something and the arm is pulled up while the body continues moving. A similar situation is sometimes encountered when the arm is trapped in a moving machine. In this instance there is gross loss of use of all the intrinsic muscles of the hand, and the long finger flexors and extensors so that although the arm can be moved normally into any position, there is no useful function in the hand itself. In both types severe causalgic pain in the affected areas often complicates root avulsion due to recent trauma.

Root lesions due to Cervical Spondylosis

Root lesions due to spondylosis have been discussed in detail in Chapter 15. We will mention them briefly in the present section. We have already noted that C5 and C6 are the two roots most likely to be affected. This leads to an almost diagnostic combination of reflex changes. The biceps and supinator jerks being carried by the C5 and C6 roots are usually depressed or absent and the triceps jerk is usually strikingly increased in a typical case. This is due to the local damage to the spinal roots at C5 and C6, blocking the reflex

arcs, and the narrowing of the canal at this level causing some degree of cord compression enhancing the triceps jerk which is passing through the C7 reflex arc just below the level of the compression. In some instances all three reflexes are absent in both arms. As already mentioned, root lesions apart from C5, C6 and C7 are relatively rare and if other roots are involved other diagnostic possibilities should be kept in mind. Cervical spondylosis is a physiological result of ageing and it is extremely dangerous to accept that root lesions or progressive problems in the cervical cord are due to spondylosis because of plain film changes, and careful investigation is indicated in the majority of cases.

Acute Cervical Disc Lesions

Acute cervical disc lesions are relatively uncommon compared to the very frequent occurrence of lumbar disc lesions. They fall into two main groups.

1. Those injuries occurring in an otherwise normal spine, usually the result of a sports injury in a young person. This is almost invariably strictly unilateral. The patient develops very severe neck pain with radicular pain in a typical root distribution, which may or may not be associated with weakness of the muscles innervated by the affected nerve root. The C7 root is most often affected by a traumatic disc lesion.

2. The second type of injury occurs in a person who already has an abnormal neck due to cervical spondylosis. In these patients sudden flexion or extension of the neck, following a simple trip or in a rear end collision in a car may produce acute root symptoms or even serious cord damage. In these instances root symptoms are often bilateral and may affect multiple roots and the cord damage may be so severe as to cause an acute tetraparesis. The potential seriousness of even minor trauma affecting the cervical spine in this way in patients with severe pre-existing spondylosis cannot be over-emphasised.

CASE REPORT

A 72-year-old man was given barbiturate sleeping pills. Under their influence he fell downstairs and became tetraparetic. He had the typical signs of acute C5/6 root lesions and a mild spastic paraparesis without sensory loss. His plain films showed very gross spondylotic damages and a very narrow canal at C4/5 level. In spite of skilled care he died of bronchopneumonia six days following the incident.

Brachial Neuritis (Serum Neuritis, Neuralgic Amyotrophy)

This is a classical neurological condition that was originally recognised as a sequel to immunisation procedures involving the injection of sera into the deltoid muscle. The condition is not due to any direct trauma to the peripheral nerves. It is believed to be an inflammatory process occurring in the roots. In a typical case very severe pain over the C5 dermatome is followed in two to three days by rapid wasting and weakness of all the C5 and C6 innervated muscles. In a particularly severe case there may also be involvement of the sterno-mastoid and upper trapezius and C7 innervated groups. Occasionally the condition may occur bilaterally simultaneously. In general the prognosis is extremely good. Cases showing definite evidence of recovery within five to six weeks usually make a full recovery over a period of three to six months. Those taking several months before any sign of recovery is apparent may take eighteen months to two years before maximal recovery is made and this is often incomplete. This seems to be a particular problem in patients who have severe co-existent cervical spondylosis.

The Cervical Rib Syndrome

Twenty years ago textbooks contained whole chapters devoted to what were known as the "outlet syndromes". At that time cervical spondylosis and carpal tunnel syndrome were not even recognised entities. With the recognition of the latter conditions the outlet syndromes have almost vanished from the diagnostic repertoire. The only unequivocal survivor is the cervical rib syndrome, and to this we may add the situation where a normal first rib is displaced upwards by distortion of the thorax. This may occur in patients with thoracic scoliosis or following artificial pneumothorax or thoracoplasty. The symptoms produced may be due to either neural or vascular damage.

The Neural Picture: The neural picture is extremely interesting. The sensory symptoms comprise a deep aching pain in the axilla and down the ulnar border of the arm, often into the hand, in other words, in the territory of both C8 and D1. The motor signs, however, are dominated by damage to the D1 root and in particular to those fibres destined to supply the abductor pollicis brevis muscle to the exclusion of the other small hand muscles. This leads to a situation where the main pain is in the ulnar innervated fingers, but the main wasting and weakness is in the median innervated abductor pollicis brevis muscle. Many patients have had their median nerve decompressed at the wrist for this syndrome, when in fact a careful evaluation of sensory symptoms should have made the diagnosis of carpal tunnel syndrome untenable. On electromyography the situation can be easily confirmed and the findings comprise an electromyographic "syndrome". This consists of evidence of denervation of the abductor pollicis brevis muscle with a normal median nerve action potential, coupled with normal ulnar innervated muscles in the hand, but an absent ulnar action potential at the wrist. On

these electromyographic findings alone, even if no cervical rib can be demonstrated on plain x-ray it is worth exploring the lower roots of the brachial plexus in the neck, as damage due to abnormal fibrous bands may be found in this situation.

The Vascular Syndrome: The vascular syndrome is a result of the fact that the abnormally high rib also displaces the axillary artery upwards. This causes an area of stenosis with the risk of the development of post-stenotic dilatation. Clot may form on the wall of the dilated vessel. Small fragments of clot then become detached and pass down the brachial artery into the hand. This causes acute embolic episodes resembling Raynaud's phenomena which may subsequently cause ischaemic changes in the fingers. In this situation there may be no abnormal neurological findings, but an incorrect diagnosis of carpal tunnel syndrome may be made when the patient relates the history of repeated attacks of severe pain in the hand, associated with blanching, and swelling of the fingers.

It is worth restating that the outlet syndromes described in the older books appear to be of doubtful validity. In fifteen years the writer has not seen a single example of a surgically proven lesion of the roots in the neck caused by simple muscle displacement. A cervical rib or an abnormal fibrous band associated with an unusually elongated transverse process of the C7 vertebra appear to be the only valid causes of the so-called outlet syndrome.

Lesions of the Radial Nerve

The radial nerve in the axilla is often damaged by the incorrect use of a crutch, in which the patient takes his weight on the axilla. It should be pointed out, however, that the correct use of the crutch, in which the patient takes his weight on the heel of the hand can damage the deep branch of the ulnar nerve in the palm!

Damage to the radial nerve in the axilla usually causes weakness of all the radial innervated muscles; the triceps, wrist extensors, finger extensors and brachioradialis.

Damage lower down may be produced in two ways. First by direct trauma to the radial nerve in the spiral groove on the lateral aspect of the upper arm. This may occur accidentally or be deliberately inflicted as in the schoolboy trick in which the outer aspect of the arm is punched hard, which causes an acute wrist drop. The nerve may be similarly damaged on the medial aspect of the arm in a "Saturday night palsy". This occurs in people who are inebriated or heavily sedated and go to sleep with their arm hanging over the back of a chair or over the edge of the bed. Fractures of the midshaft of the humerus may involve the nerve either acutely during the actual fracture or later if there is over-exuberant callus formation. In this situation, although the nerve palsy may appear to be progressive, it is unusual for permanent damage to result and rarely is surgical exploration of the nerve necessary. Lesions at mid-humerus level usually spare the triceps muscle, the weakness being confined to the wrist extensors, brachioradialis and the finger extensors. Damage to the nerve in the axilla or upper arm, although associated with aching, tingling or numbness in the radial nerve cutaneous distribution, very rarely causes detectable sensory loss as the territory is so readily overlapped by the adjacent ulnar and median nerves. If any sensory loss can be detected it is usually over the dorsum of the thumb and index finger. The terminal motor branch of the radial nerve is the posterior interosseus nerve and this enters the forearm by penetrating the supinator muscle. Damage to the posterior interosseus nerve causes weakness of the wrist extensors and in particular, the extensors of the index finger and thumb. This lesion may occur idiopathically or follow the unaccustomed use of a screw-driver. Cases involving damage to the nerve at this point have also been described following Indian bar wrestling in which the opponents rest their elbows on the table and try to force one another's hand over backwards, and in orchestral conductors, as a rather unique occupational hazard. Presumably, in these cases direct entrapment of the nerve by the contracting supinator muscle is the cause.

In older textbooks it is stated that lead poisoning specifically damages the posterior interosseus nerve. It may well be that the nerve was predisposed to damage by lead poisoning, but it seems probable that occupational over-use of the supinator muscle by house painters led to the localisation of the damage to this nerve.

Lesions of the Ulnar Nerve

The ease with which the ulnar nerve may be damaged at the elbow is well known from the common experience of hitting the "funny-bone". The fact that ulnar nerve palsies may result from repeated and apparently trivial trauma of this sort is less appreciated. Simple alteration in personal habits, such as the substitution of a modern wooden armed chair for a soft armchair may lead to the insidious onset of an ulnar nerve palsy. Driving with the arm resting on the door sill is another frequently encountered cause of an ulnar nerve palsy of this type. Patients confined to bed often use their elbows to shuffle about in bed and the insidious development of bilateral ulnar nerve palsies is a common sequel. Damage occurs idiopathically in women who have a larger carrying angle at the elbow than men and in whom repeated flexion and extension of the arm is more likely to stretch the nerve around the olecranon. A variant of this anatomical deformity

leads to the condition known as a "tardy ulnar palsy". In this situation the patient invariably suffered a supra-condylar fracture of the humerus in childhood, resulting in a slight developmental deformity of the elbow. As the years pass an insidious ulnar nerve palsy develops and it may be twenty to thirty years before its presence is recognised. In any situation in which insidious damage to the nerve has occurred there may be a remarkable absence of sensory phenomena. Although one would anticipate tingling and numbness in the ulnar fingers, quite severe and even complete loss of motor function in ulnar innervated muscles may occur in the total absence of any sensory symptoms. If one remembers that in two to three per cent of people *all* the small hand muscles are innervated by the ulnar nerve there is a real possibility of motor neurone disease being diagnosed when the patient is merely suffering from a simple painless ulnar nerve palsy. Lesions at the elbow ought theoretically to produce weakness of flexor carpal ulnaris and the medial part of the flexor digitorum profundus. For reasons that are far from clear it is quite unusual for these muscles to be affected and even more complicated is the fact that damage to the nerve at the elbow seems specifically to affect fibres destined to innervate the first dorsal interosseus muscle. Therefore, the patient may present with striking weakness and wasting of the first dorsal interosseus muscle with almost complete sparing of the abductor digiti minimi muscle on the medial side of the hand. In this situation the possibility of an ulnar nerve lesion at the wrist is suspected but this is rarely the case.

At the wrist the nerve divides into a superficial sensory part and a deep motor branch. Repeated trauma to the heel of the hand (using the heel of the hand to shut a sticking car door, or the use of a chuck key by a lathe worker etc.) will crush the nerve against the carpal bones. This usually produces wasting and weakness of all the ulnar innervated small hand muscles in the absence of sensory involvement. Again if the patient has an all ulnar innervated hand total wasting and weakness of *all* the intrinsic muscles of the hand may be found and an incorrect diagnosis of motor neurone disease made. Occasionally, the nerve may also be affected at the wrist by a ganglion arising from the joint and if there is no history of trauma to the heel of the hand it is worth exploring the nerve to exclude this possibility. In general whenever the intrinsic muscles of the hand are involved early exploration and attempts to decompress the nerve should be made as if wasting is allowed to persist delayed surgery produces very unsatisfactory results.

Lesions of the Median Nerve

The median nerve is well protected from trauma in the arm itself. Rarely the anterior interosseus nerve, given off from the median nerve just below the elbow, may be damaged in forearm fractures or dislocations of the elbow. An anterior interosseus nerve lesion (Kiloh–Nevin syndrome) causes weakness of the long flexors of the thumb and index finger. At the carpal tunnel, however, the nerve is extremely vulnerable and probably the commonest peripheral nerve lesion encountered is the carpal tunnel syndrome. It is difficult to realise that this condition was first recognised in the mid 1940s and only put on a firm electro-physiological basis in the mid 1950s. It is instructive to remember that some physicians denied the existence of this condition for a whole decade after its original description and insisted that all pain in the hand was due to "outlet syndromes". The striking clinical feature of carpal tunnel syndrome is that the pain is particularly severe during the night. The patient typically wakes with severe pain in the median innervated part of the hand and the symptoms are fairly readily relieved by swinging the arm or flexing and extending the wrist. Both these features are important diagnostic clues and however atypical the description of the pain may be, night pain in the arm should be assumed to be due to carpal tunnel syndrome until proved otherwise. Conversely, pain that is primarily present on waking in the morning is usually due to a cervical root irritation from spondylosis. The peculiarities of the distribution of sensory symptoms in carpal tunnel syndrome have already been pointed out in the introductory part of this chapter.

Sensory findings may be quite marked with total loss of sensation in the median innervated area of the hand or may be normal in spite of quite severe pain. Motor involvement is usually confined to the abductor pollicis brevis muscle as the other muscles supplied by the median nerve either have dual innervation from the ulnar nerve or can be readily substituted by long forearm muscles and it is usually only the wasting and weakness of abductor pollicis brevis that can be easily and convincingly demonstrated.

From a clinical point of view it is sufficient to test abductor pollicis brevis correctly as shown in Figure 18.5 and then to be certain that the ulnar innervated muscles are functioning normally.

Lesions of the Long Thoracic Nerve of Bell

A unique problem in the arm is the long thin nerve that supplies a solitary but important muscle; the serratus anterior. This muscle normally holds the scapula flat against the back, and stabilises the shoulder joint during abduction of the arm.

Patients notice they cannot hold the arm on the affected side up straight and have difficulty combing their hair and putting on clothes. Relatives notice the striking protrusion of the shoulder blade.

There are no specific causes; recent cases seen by the author, occurred after log cutting, exposure to cold and as a consequence of an episode of neuralgic amyotrophy. Recovery seems to be slow and incomplete.

The diagnostic problems presented by root and nerve lesions affecting the arm have been outlined. The wide disparity between what actually happens and what ought to happen on purely anatomical grounds has been emphasised. A simplified method of evaluating the arm directly applicable to these circumstances has been outlined. In most instances electro-diagnostic studies can be of considerable value and details of the techniques used and the results to be anticipated are described in Chapter 16.

Brachial Plexus Lesions

As noted in the introduction to this chapter pathological processes affecting the brachial plexus are rare. Traumatic lesions are certainly the most frequent cause and the only non-traumatic condition presenting a diagnostic problem is damage to the plexus caused by radiation of the axillary area for carcinoma of breast, the decision required usually being whether the problem is due to metastatic disease requiring more radiotherapy or due to radiotherapy itself. In the writer's experience there are four main sites of plexus damage producing fairly typical clinical pictures (see Figure 18.6).

a. *Lesions of the Upper Trunk*

Damage to this area which is the most superficial part of the plexus, often occurs with stab or bullet wounds in the neck. C5 and C6 are destroyed leaving the patient with numbness of the lateral arm, forearm and hand with loss of abduction, internal and external rotation of the shoulder, elbow flexion and radial wrist extension due to weakness in the extensor carpi radialis longus and brevis. The biceps and supinator jerks are absent. Note that the lesion is distal to the roots and spares the rhomboid muscles which are supplied by a branch from the C5 root and serratus anterior which is supplied by branches from C5, C6 and C7 roots.

b. *Lesions of the Lower Trunk*

Damage to this area has already been described to some extent in connection with cervical rib syndrome. This is also the area of the plexus that is damaged by carcinoma of the lung apex extending through the apical pleura (Pancoast's syndrome) and metastatic disease in the axillary glands, from malignant disease from the breast or elsewhere. The clinical

Figure 18.6. Scheme of the Anatomy of the Brachial Plexus showing the eventual destination of all Root Components

Dorsal scapular nerve–rhomboids–C5

Suprascapular nerve–pure C5 to supraspinatus (abduction) and infraspinatus (ext. rotation) of shoulder

upper

trunk

C5

C6

A

5

6

7

8

1

C6

middle trunk

Lateral anterior thoracic nerve–pectoralis major (adduction)–C7

lateral cord

C6

C7

lower trunk

C7

C5

C8

C8

D

posterior cord

C7

C8

B

Musculo-cutaneous nerve–to biceps, brachialis and coraco-brachialis (elbow flexion) – C5 (C6 contribution variable)

C6

C7

Long thoracic nerve to serratus anterior (abduction of scapula)– ? mainly C5

medial cord

Medial anterior thoracic nerve– pectoralis major and minor– shoulder adduction – C8

5 6

Median nerve
C6–pronators in forearm
C7–wrist flexors
C8–long finger flexors. (1.2)
D1–small hand muscles (see later)

D1

6 7 8 1

Subscapular nerves (2)– subscapularis and teres major (shoulder inversion) – C5

Axillary nerve– deltoid and teres minor (shoulder abduction)–C5

8 1

Thoraco-dorsal nerve–latissimus dorsi–(shoulder adduction) – C7

5 6 7 8

C

Ulnar nerve:
C8–ulnar wrist flexion/long finger flexors (3.4)
D1–ulnar innervated small hand muscles (see later)

Radial nerve:
C6—supinators (brachioradialis, supinator)
C7—triceps (elbow extn.) and wrist extensors
C8—long finger extensors

picture consists of pain and numbness down the medial arm and forearm into the little and ring fingers of the hand. Weakness of finger flexors and extensors and the small hand muscles follows and as noted above, is particularly likely to affect the abductor pollicis brevis first. There may also be some wasting and weakness of pectoralis major but this muscle has dual innervation and this finding is variable.

c. *A Radial Nerve Lesion in the Axilla*

This has already been discussed under crutch injuries to the nerve in the lower axilla and radial nerve damage may also occur following stab wounds and neoplastic disease in the axillary glands. A complete radial nerve palsy including weakness of the triceps muscle is found.

d. *Lesions of the Posterior Cord*

Lesions of the posterior cord in the author's experience seem to follow small calibre, low velocity bullet wounds to the plexus. The bullet traverses the region of the plexus and impacts against the inner surface of the scapula and the posterior cord seems to be particularly likely to be damaged. The picture is often a transient one with later recovery. A posterior cord lesion is easy to diagnose as it is essentially a radial nerve palsy combined with an axillary nerve lesion. Therefore, there is inability to extend the elbow, extend the wrist and fingers and weakness of the second 90° of shoulder abduction due to paralysis of the deltoid muscle.

Radiation Damage to the Plexus

Patients who have received irradiation to the lymphatic nodes adjacent to the plexus as prophylaxis against metastasis from a carcinoma of the breast, sustain damage to the C7 root with lesser involvement of C6 and C8. The numbness and weakness is of sudden onset and is progressive over a few weeks only. There is no pain and this is quite an important point against the diagnosis of malignant infiltration of the plexus. Three weeks' observation to establish that the lesion is static confirms that the damage is probably due to the irradiation and not due to malignant infiltration; although prolonged careful observation is necessary.

Chapter 19

DIAGNOSIS OF ROOT AND NERVE LESIONS AFFECTING THE LEG

In the previous chapter dealing with root and nerve lesions affecting the arm three points were emphasised:

1. Anatomical features that place nerves in vulnerable positions in fibrous tunnels against bone or traversing muscles.
2. Bizarre sensory disturbances that defy anatomical explanation and make sensory symptoms somewhat unreliable.
3. The reliability of motor signs, both the reflexes and muscle weakness in assessing nerve and root injuries.

When we come to consider the situation in the leg there are some striking differences:

1. The peripheral nerves are much less vulnerable to everyday trauma, and with the exception of the peroneal nerve at the fibula neck, are infrequently damaged compared with the nerves in the arm.
2. In root disease sensory symptoms are extremely reliable in indicating which root is affected. Furthermore, the two common peripheral nerve lesions, both the lateral cutaneous nerve of the thigh and the peroneal nerve produce pain and discomfort in an anatomically accurate area, making for easy diagnosis.
3. In general, motor signs in lumbar and sacral root disease are extremely unreliable due to the fact that most muscles have a nerve supply derived from two roots, making wasting and weakness extremely difficult to detect.

There are also several anatomical features that require re-emphasis at this stage. All the nerve roots supplying the leg arise from the spinal cord above L1 vertebral level and each root then traverses several inches in the spinal canal before reaching its exit foramen. It is therefore obvious that even if there is evidence of a single nerve root being affected, one cannot be certain at which level in the canal the damage has occurred, and the L5 root, for example, could be damaged anywhere over a six-inch intra-dural course. In practice the root is most commonly damaged in the region of its exit foramen by disc lesions but it is the failure to recognise the possibility that the damage could be higher if no local lesion can be demonstrated that occasionally leads to diagnostic errors.

The problems of the diagnosis of intra-dural lesions of the lumbar and sacral roots are fully discussed under cauda equina lesions in Chapter 15.

The clinical term "sciatica" also requires definition. It must be realised that "sciatica" is a symptom and not a disease. It is *not* inevitably due to disc disease and may be the presenting symptom of *serious* intra-pelvic disease. The cutaneous distribution of the sciatic nerve does not extend up the posterior thigh or on to the buttock. "Sciatica" means pain in the leg and is no more specific than that.

ANATOMICAL FEATURES OF THE NERVE SUPPLY OF THE LEG

The highest components of the nerve supply to the leg arise from roots L2, L3 and L4, and emerge from the vertebral canal just below the diaphragm to enter the fibres of origin of the psoas muscle (see Figure 19.1). These three roots form the lumbar plexus and the branches of the plexus have to reach the front of the leg. The first branch, the lateral cutaneous nerve of the thigh, does so by skirting around the pelvic brim and exits under the lateral part of the inguinal ligament. The femoral nerve remains on the lateral side of psoas muscle and passes with the muscle under the inguinal ligament into the anterior part of the thigh. The obturator nerve lies on the medial side of the psoas muscle and comes into close relationship with the uterus in the pelvis before emerging through the obturator foramen. Here it is subject to damage during obstetric procedures. The lumbar plexus therefore supplies the hip flexors, thigh adductors, knee extensors and skin over the anterior medial and lateral thigh and via the saphenous branch of the femoral nerve a long promontory of skin down the medial side of the leg including the medial surface of the ankle.

The rest of the leg is supplied by the sacral plexus which is derived from L4, L5, S1 and S2 roots. This plexus is formed over the sacro-iliac joint and almost immediately leaves the pelvis via the greater sciatic foramen. Its main branches, the gluteal nerves, the sciatic nerve and the posterior cutaneous nerve of thigh, then lie directly behind the hip joint. It is obvious that fractures of the upper femur, particularly those involving the acetabulum, represent a considerable threat to

Figure 19.1. Anterior View of the Pelvic Cavity Showing the Course of the Nerve Supply to the Leg

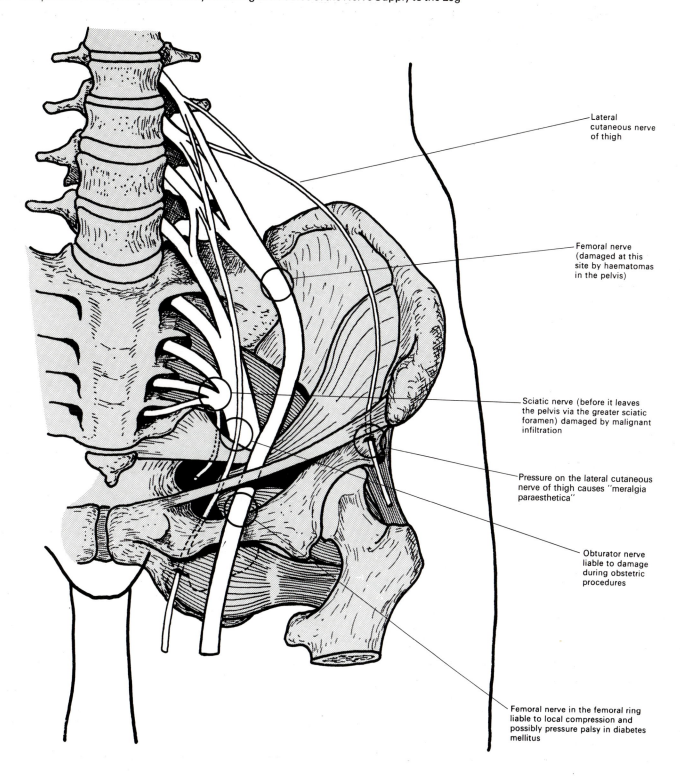

Lateral cutaneous nerve of thigh

Femoral nerve (damaged at this site by haematomas in the pelvis)

Sciatic nerve (before it leaves the pelvis via the greater sciatic foramen) damaged by malignant infiltration

Pressure on the lateral cutaneous nerve of thigh causes "meralgia paraesthetica"

Obturator nerve liable to damage during obstetric procedures

Femoral nerve in the femoral ring liable to local compression and possibly pressure palsy in diabetes mellitus

Figure 19.2. Posterior View of the Pelvis Showing the Nerves to the Posterior Part of the Leg

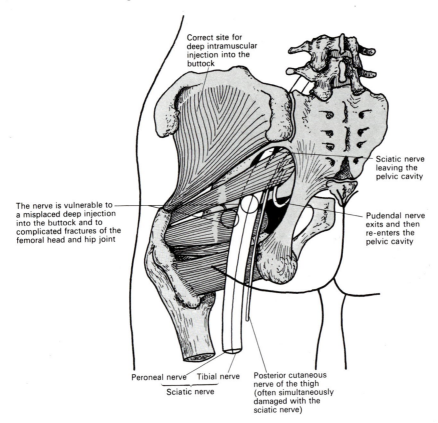

Correct site for deep intramuscular injection into the buttock

Sciatic nerve leaving the pelvic cavity

The nerve is vulnerable to a misplaced deep injection into the buttock and to complicated fractures of the femoral head and hip joint

Pudendal nerve exits and then re-enters the pelvic cavity

Peroneal nerve   Tibial nerve

Sciatic nerve

Posterior cutaneous nerve of the thigh (often simultaneously damaged with the sciatic nerve)

these nerves. They are also liable to damage from a misplaced intra-muscular injection in the buttock. The correct position for such an injection is shown in Figure 19.2.

The sciatic nerve is formed of two discrete components—the peroneal (lateral popliteal) and the tibial (medial popliteal) nerves. Even when the whole nerve is traumatised the peroneal component is much more likely to be damaged than the tibial component. The reason for this is not entirely clear, but this feature has considerable clinical significance. Following the separation into individual nerves in the lower thigh the tibial nerve remains deep and is very rarely damaged (Figure 19.3). The peroneal nerve, however, has to gain access to the anterior and lateral compartments of the leg, and in doing so becomes extremely vulnerable as it crosses the fibula neck. The subsequent division of the peroneal nerve into the anterior tibial and musculocutaneous nerves has little practical significance as damage to the nerves below the fibula neck is extremely rare. The terminal digital branches of the tibial nerve are subject to trauma as they lie under the metatarsal heads, leading to the condition known as Morton's metatarsalgia.

CLINICALLY IMPORTANT FEATURES OF THE SENSORY SUPPLY TO THE LEG

The Peripheral Nerve Supply

The area supplied by the lateral cutaneous nerve of the thigh is indicated in Figure 19.5; note that the area does not cross the midline of the thigh and compare this with the area supplied with the L2 root, shown in Figure 19.4. Secondly, note the long promontory of skin supplied by the saphenous branch of the femoral nerve. This is important as sensory loss following sciatic nerve injuries cannot produce complete stocking sensory loss below the knee, and one should always look for an area of preserved sensation on the medial side of the leg. The sciatic nerve itself supplies a relatively small area of the skin of the leg. Unless the posterior cutaneous nerve of the thigh is simultaneously injured the patient will not have numbness over the back of the thigh. A peroneal nerve pressure palsy at the fibula neck has many similarities to a radial nerve palsy in the arm, as it causes a foot drop, and the similarity extends to the fact that sensory loss is also relatively unusual with peroneal nerve lesions.

Figure 19.3. Diagram to Show the course and Bony Relations of the Nerve Supply to the Leg

Femoral nerve

Lateral cutaneous
nerve of thigh

Obturator nerve

Sciatic nerve

Tibial nerve (medial
popliteal nerve)

Saphenous nerve—cutaneous
branch of the femoral nerve.
Subject to damage during
varicose vein surgery

Peroneal nerve (lateral
popliteal nerve).
Subject to trauma at
the fibula neck

Musculocutaneous nerve

Anterior tibial nerve

Medial and lateral
plantar nerves

The area normally involved if such loss is present is shown on the figure.

The Root Supply

Refer to Figure 19.4. Note that the distribution of lumbar roots L2, L3 and L4 is in a spiral across the front of the thigh and down on to the medial side of the leg. This should be contrasted with the distribution of the cutaneous nerves of this area, which are essentially straight up and down the thigh. When one considers the rarity of disc disease above L4 level it is immediately apparent that pain in the anterior thigh should *not* be ascribed to disc disease. This point has been amplified further in the section on cauda equina lesions in Chapter 15. The L4 root is the highest root that may be affected by disc disease and even this is relatively rare. The pain produced radiates across the front of the knee on to the medial side of the leg down to the medial malleolus. L5 is the root most commonly affected by disc disease and the typical radiation of the pain is across the buttock, down the back of the thigh on to the lateral side of the leg and on to the dorsal and ventral aspects of the foot. Pain in the big toe seems to be particularly typical of an L5 root lesion. S1 root irritation produces pain down the back of the leg on to the side of the leg as L5, but the pain in the foot is confined to the lateral side. In either case, it is exceptional to find definite sensory loss although slightly altered perception of sensation over the dorsum of the foot in the case of the L5 root lesion or behind the lateral malleolus with an S1 root lesion may be found. The lower sacral roots S2 to S5 supply the skin of the inner posterior thigh, the inner buttocks and the genitalia. Sensation over these areas should be carefully checked in all patients complaining of pain in the posterior thigh or genitalia, and in patients with sphincter disturbances.

Figure 19.4. Cutaneous Distribution of Nerve Roots in the Leg

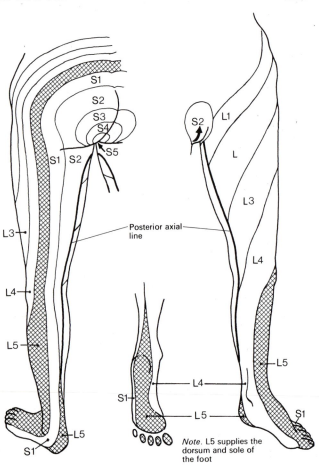

Note. L5 supplies the dorsum and sole of the foot

Figure 19.5. Cutaneous Nerves in the Leg

Table 8   COMPARATIVE DATA ON ROOT AND NERVE LESIONS IN THE LEG

ROOTS	L2	L3	L4	L5	S1
Sensory supply	Across upper thigh	Across lower thigh	Across knee to medial malleolus	Side of leg to dorsum and sole of foot	Behind lateral malleolus to lateral foot
Sensory loss	Often none	Often none	Medial leg	Dorsum of foot	Behind lateral malleolus
Area of pain	Across thigh	Across thigh	Down to medial malleolus	Back of thigh, lateral calf— dorsum of foot	Back of thigh, back of calf— lateral foot
Reflex arc	None	Adductor reflex	Knee jerk	None	Ankle jerk
Motor deficit	Hip flexion	Knee extension	Inversion of the foot	Dorsiflexion of toes and foot	Plantar flexion and eversion of foot
		Adduction of thigh		(latter L4 also)	
Causative lesions (in order of frequency)	Neurofibroma Meningioma Neoplastic disease Disc lesions very rare (except L4 <5 per cent *all*)			Disc lesions Metastatic Malignancy Neurofibromas Meningioma	

Table 9

NERVES	OBTURATOR	FEMORAL	SCIATIC NERVE	
			PERONEAL DIVISION	TIBIAL DIVISION
Sensory supply	Medial surface of thigh	Antero medial surface of thigh and leg to medial malleolus	Anterior leg, dorsum of ankle and foot	Posterior leg, sole and lateral border of foot
Sensory loss	Often none	Usually anatomical	Often just dorsum of foot	Sole of foot
Area of pain	Medial thigh	Anterior thigh and medial leg	Often painless	Often painless
Reflex arc	Adductor reflex	Knee jerk	None	Ankle jerk
Motor deficit	Adduction of thigh	Extension of knee	Dorsiflexion, inversion and eversion of the foot (+lateral hamstrings)	Plantar flexion and inversion of foot (+medial hamstrings)
Causative lesions	Pelvic neoplasm Pregnancy	Diabetes Femoral hernia Femoral artery aneurysm Posterior abdominal neoplasm Psoas abscess	Pressure palsy at fibula neck Hip fracture/dislocation Penetrating trauma to buttock Misplaced injection	Very rarely injured even in buttock Peroneal division more sensitive to damage

CLINICALLY IMPORTANT FEATURES OF THE MOTOR SUPPLY TO THE LEGS

The correct methods of testing leg movements and their root and nerve values are show in Figures 19.6 and 19.7.

The Peripheral Nerve Supply

The femoral nerve is partially responsible for hip flexion as it innervates the iliacus muscle and wholly responsible for knee extension as it innervates the entire quadriceps muscle. A lesion affecting the femoral nerve in the pelvis will weaken hip flexion as well as knee extension. Unfortunately, lesions in the abdomen will often interfere with psoas muscle contraction directly and may make hip flexion too painful for the patient to attempt. However, if psoas is weak, or attempts to use it cause severe pain, either is a strong indication that the lesion causing the femoral nerve palsy is intra-abdominal

so that from a strictly practical point of view no distinction as to the cause of the hip flexor weakness need be made.

The obturator nerve supplies the obturator externus muscle (lateral rotation of the thigh) and the adductor muscles of the thigh. Its function can be simply tested by the patient's ability to hold the legs together against resistance.

The peroneal nerve supplies part of the biceps femoris (the lateral ham-string muscle), the muscles in the anterior and lateral compartment of the leg and extensor digitorum brevis of the dorsum of the foot. This is the small muscle that can be detected just below and anterior to the lateral malleolus when the toes are dorsiflexed.

The tibial nerve supplies the bulk of the ham-string muscles, the muscles of the posterior compartment of the leg and all the small foot muscles with the exception of extensor digitorum brevis.

Figure 19.6. Movements of the Leg

Hip Flexion
(Ilio-psoas) (L2.3)
(Direct nerve supply and Femoral twigs)

Knee Extension
(Quadriceps) (L2.3.4) Femoral Nerve

Hip Abduction
(Glutei and tensor fascia lata) (L.4.5)

Hip Extension
(Glutei) (L4.5)
Gluteal nerves

Knee Flexion
(Hamstrings) (L5, S1)
Tibial nerve. Peroneal nerve
(Lateral head of biceps femoris only)

Hip Adduction
(Adductor group) (L2.3.4)
Obturator nerve

The Root Supply

The L2 root is predominantly responsible for hip flexion. Knee extension is usually unaffected even though it is generally stated that the quadriceps receive a contribution from L2, L3 and L4.

L3 root lesions cause weakness of both knee extension and thigh adduction, and it would appear clinically that the main motor innervation of the adductor muscles and the quadriceps is derived from L3.

L4 root lesions, although causing depression or absence of the knee jerk, rarely seem to lead to definite weakness of the quadriceps muscle. Clinically it would appear that its main importance in respect of the quadriceps is conveying the reflex arc. The important point about the L4 root is that it is the exclusive root supply to the inverters of the foot (tibialis anterior, in the anterior compartment of the leg and tibialis posterior, in the posterior compartment of the leg).

The L4 contribution to these muscles reaches them via the peroneal and tibial nerves respectively. Therefore, although in an L4 lesion a little weakness of dorsiflexion and plantar flexion of the foot may be apparent, there is striking weakness of inversion of the foot. A patient with a bilateral L4 root lesion walks in a most peculiar way, with the feet flapping on the ground, as if extremely flat footed.

In an L5 root lesion *if* any weakness is detectable, it is usually maximal in the toe extensors, particularly the extensor of the big toe. Because both L4 and S1 contribute to the innervation of the muscles responsible for plantar and dorsiflexion of the foot, it is unusual to be able to detect any weakness of these movements. Both L4 and L5 roots contribute to the nerve supply of the gluteal muscles, but wasting and weakness in these very powerful and bulky muscles may be extremely difficult to detect. In the case of an S1 root lesion the ankle jerk is usually abolished. Again,

Figure 19.7. Movements of the Foot

Plantar Flexion

S1, S2
Tibial nerve
(Gastrocnemii)
(Tibialis posterior)

Inversion of the Foot

L4
Tibial and peroneal nerves
(Note that tibialis anterior, an anterior compartment muscle, and tibialis posterior, a posterior compartment muscle, work together)

Dorsiflexion

L4, L5
Peroneal nerve
(Tibialis anterior)
(Long extensors)
(Peroneus tertius)
(Extensor digitorum brevis)

Eversion of the Foot

S1
Peroneal nerve
(Peronei longus and brevis)
(Long extensors assist)
(Extensor digitorum brevis)

weakness may be extremely difficult to detect and eversion of the foot is the best movement to test. In a severe S1 lesion there may be weakness of plantar flexion and of the ham-string muscles. The ham-strings present much the same problems as the glutei—they are such large powerful muscles that weakness and wasting may be extremely difficult to detect in the early stages of an S1 root lesion.

When examining power in the legs in any patient who has either back or abdominal pain it is necessary to make considerable allowances for inhibition caused by the pain. In general, if the patient is encouraged to make one maximal effort, however severe the pain, it is usually possible to establish whether or not strength is normal, and most patients will make this effort if they are told how important it is from a diagnostic point of view. In patients with leg pain it is not permissible to dismiss the motor examination as "impossible due to pain", as important localising evidence may be missed if the examination is incomplete.

SPECIFIC CLINICAL CONDITIONS AFFECTING THE NERVES AND NERVE ROOTS OF THE LEG

Meralgia Paraesthetica (lateral cutaneous nerve of the thigh)

This common condition produces a peculiar numb, tingling sensation in the upper lateral thigh. In the male it may be noticed when the hand is placed in the pocket because of the peculiar sensation that is provoked. The condition is most often encountered in obese patients who have lost a lot of weight (it is theorised that the sagging anterior abdominal wall pulls on the nerve) or may occur spontaneously without clear reasons. The writer has seen two examples of the condition in young males as a consequence of a young lady sitting on their laps! The condition quite often remits spontaneously and surgery should be deferred for three months in most instances to give it time to do so.

Femoral Nerve Lesions

The femoral nerve may be damaged in the upper abdomen by primary or secondary neoplasms or a psoas abscess. In the lower abdomen it may be damaged by an intra-pelvic haematoma. Direct trauma to the nerve during arterial catheterisation or by a femoral aneurysm can occur. Diabetics appear to be particularly prone to develop a femoral neuropathy. This condition is sometimes known as diabetic amyotrophy of Garland. It is characterised by the onset of very severe pain in the front of the thigh, which may radiate down the medial side of the leg to the medial malleolus. Within a few days or weeks of the onset of pain, which may require narcotics for its control, the patient suddenly develops complete weakness and wasting of the quadriceps muscle, making walking impossible. Usually as the weakness appears the pain tends to remit. The condition almost invariably eventually improves although four to six months may elapse before any recovery is apparent. Occasionally it is not the femoral nerve itself but the L2, L3 and L4 roots which seem to be affected, producing a picture of more widespread weakness and wasting including the hip flexors. With the exception of these diabetic patients femoral nerve lesions are extremely rare.

Sciatic Nerve Lesions

The sciatic nerve may be damaged in the pelvis by the direct spread of neoplasms of the rectum and genito-urinary tract. The nerve may also be compressed in the later stages of pregnancy. In the buttock, complicated hip fractures, penetrating trauma, especially by gunshot or knife wounds, and misplaced deep intra-muscular injections are the most frequent causes of sciatic nerve damage. An unusual feature of damage at this site, already mentioned earlier, is that the peroneal division is six times as likely to be damaged as the tibial division in spite of non-selective trauma to the whole nerve trunk. The practical importance of this may be seen in the following example.

A patient with severe traumatic damage to the hip may be impossible to examine initially and open joint surgery is performed. Subsequently it is discovered that the patient has a foot drop. The question will then arise as to whether this occurred as a result of pressure on the peroneal nerve during surgery, or as a result of any plaster casting that has been carried out or whether it was primarily injured in either the trauma or the subsequent surgery.

The marked difference in prognosis both in time and potential degree of recovery is extremely important. Clinically, the writer has found that the most useful sign is the detection of wasting and weakness in the biceps femoris. This is the part of the ham-string muscle supplied by the peroneal nerve and is unaffected by a peroneal nerve lesion at the fibula neck. Furthermore, one can elicit both medial and lateral ham-string reflexes by tapping the appropriate tendons and the lateral reflex invariably disappears in this situation.

Misplaced injections into the sciatic nerve are especially disastrous, as not only is there weakness of dorsiflexion and plantar flexion of the foot, but often very severe causalgic pain results, making it impossible for the patient to tolerate the leg splints necessary to compensate for the weakness.

Peroneal Nerve Lesions

This is probably the commonest nerve lesion in the leg and is due to compression of the nerve at the fibula neck. This may occur in quite normal persons following a sharp blow to the nerve, or while sitting with the legs crossed for a prolonged period. However, in all cases care should be taken to exclude any possible cause of impaired nutrition of the nerve. In Great Britain diabetes is probably the commonest cause, but polyarteritis nodosa should also be excluded and other collagen vascular diseases such as rheumatoid arthritis. In all these situations other peripheral nerves may be damaged by compression, particularly the ulnar nerve, and when multiple palsies occur in this way the condition is known as mono-neuritis multiplex. Leprosy is the commonest cause of this situation in appropriate areas of the world. Pressure on the peroneal nerve may occur while resting in bed, particularly if there has been marked weight loss or from a leg plaster. The patient complains of inability to dorsiflex or evert the foot. There is little or no sensory loss in most cases. It is important to distinguish the condition from a painless L5 root lesion and this may be extremely difficult unless one can detect weakness or wasting in the calf muscles. Electromyography is extremely useful in this situation.

Nerve lesions in the legs are relatively rare compared with the arm. Root lesions occur with a much greater frequency and are often related to serious intra-pelvic or abdominal disease, and it is quite wrong and extremely dangerous to assume that all leg pain is due to a simple disc lesion. It is essential to have a clear grasp of the anatomy of the lumbar and sacral nerve roots to be aware of the clinical clues that suggest the more ominous pathological possibilities. In the writer's view, the single most ominous symptom in a patient with back pain radiating into the leg is that the pain is worst at *rest*, particularly in bed at night. This is in marked contrast to simple disc disease in which rest is the main relieving factor.

Chapter 20

HEADACHE

Many student texts contain long classifications of the causes of headaches that seem to indicate that the differential diagnosis of headache is a mere formality.

With the exception of all but the most classical cases of migraine, this implication is certainly unjustified. The degree of overlap between both the aetiological factors and some of the features of the headache may make differential diagnosis extremely difficult. For example, many patients with headache who are referred as "diagnostic problems" are suffering from migraine headaches, the diagnostic difficulty usually having arisen because the headache was not frontal, strictly unilateral or throbbing in nature. All these features do occur in classical migraine, but none of them need to be present for the diagnosis of migraine headache to be made. When we consider aetiological factors, the main problem is the role played by tension in an individual case. Just because the patient is tense, it does not automatically follow that he had tension headache. Migraine is often precipitated by tension, and any patient who has had a series of bad migraine headaches soon becomes tense. Failure to appreciate the nature of the headache will lead to prolonged ineffectual therapy with tranquilisers, and deny the patient the possible symptomatic relief he could obtain with ergot preparations.

There are considerable similarities in the diagnostic approach and aetiological factors in patients with headache and face pain and the reader is strongly recommended to read this and the subsequent chapter in sequence.

General Considerations Concerning Headaches

There is a widely held misconception, not confined to the general public, that the most common causes of headache are eye strain and sinus disease. Very few patients are referred who have not already had their eyes tested and many have also had their sinuses x-rayed.

Refractive errors cause pain in and around the eye when the eyes are used for unusually long periods or in poor light. Refractive errors cannot cause intermittent severe headaches *not* linked to the use of the eyes for close work or reading. Occasionally serious delays are caused by referral to opticians, as it takes several weeks for the patient to obtain new glasses and discover that they do not relieve the headache.

Many patients complain of life-long "sinus headache" often abbreviated to the more colloquial "sinus". Close questioning usually reveals a typical history of migraine. Sinus disease causes pain in the affected sinus. The pain may be referred to other areas of the face and head, but the underlying pain in the sinus is identifiable. The suggestion that chronic *sub-clinical* sinus infection can cause recurrent severe headaches over decades is no longer acceptable.

The term "ordinary headaches" is also often used by patients. This term seems to mean headaches that have been sufficiently infrequent or so short-lived that the patient has never bothered to seek advice. It is essential to try to establish the nature of such headaches, and not accept the patient's own diagnosis.

The possibility that a headache is due to something serious does *not* increase in proportion to the severity of the headache. In fact, the most severe headaches are usually due to migraine, and many of the patients who are harbouring cerebral tumours complain of a "dull" or "muzzy" head, only on direct questioning. It is not often that the headache itself prompts the patient to seek medical advice.

X-rays of the skull, although greatly respected by patients, rarely give help in the investigation of headache. The views taken can be restricted to an AP and a lateral skull and often even these can be dispensed with if a confident clinical diagnosis has been made. Normal skull x-rays do not exclude anything. The most important investigation in the evaluation of headache is the history.

MIGRAINE HEADACHE

In the introductory paragraphs the emphasis placed on the recognition of migraine headache will be apparent. This is because migraine or migraine variants are responsible for the headache in a majority of patients referred to hospital.

The difficulty in making the diagnosis may be due to atypical features of the headache, and this cannot always be avoided. However, it is frequently due to the uncritical acceptance of the patient's history that he has only had "sinus" or "ordinary" headache previously. Headache apparently starting at the age of 55 years may create a diagnostic problem, but when seen in the setting of life-long migraine (hitherto called "sinus") the diagnosis is easy. Ascribing a causal role to tension, when the tension is secondary to the headache itself, is another error. Although

Figure 20.1. Classical Migraine (Hemicrania)

The headache starts in the temple on one side and spreads to involve the whole side of the head. It is a pulsatile headache, and any or all of the common migraine concomitants may occur. It usually remains strictly unilateral but may occur on either side on subsequent occasions. Usually self limited lasting from 30 minutes to several hours

Figure 20.2. Occipital-Orbital Migraine

This is the type of headache most often requiring hospital referral. The onset is less dramatic, often a dull ache in the occipital area which extends forward around the temple, or deep into the area behind the eye. A dull bursting ache behind the eye is an important diagnostic clue. The pain may also be bilateral in this type, although the pain on one side is usually worse than the other
Other migraine concomitants may not be present and the headache may last several days

Figure 20.3. Orbital Migraine

This is a minor variant of migrainous neuralgia. The pain is predominantly a deep nagging ache behind the eye with occasional stabs of pain "like a needle in the back of the eye"
Photophobia is common and light or sudden movement provokes the pain. This variety is seen (in the author's opinion) as a common variant of the vascular headache produced by the birth control Pill (see text)

the tension component may well require appropriate therapy with valium, it is unlikely that this will succeed, if the underlying headache is due to migraine, as the concomitantly prescribed simple analgesics *will not* relieve the headache that is causing the tension. This is because in the majority of migraine sufferers simple proprietary analgesics and even narcotics do *not* significantly alleviate the pain.

Several features of migraine that are rarely stressed are the tendency for attacks to be present on waking in the morning, especially at weekends. This often seems to be related to relaxation and "lying-in" and may be aborted by following a normal working day routine at weekends. The ultimate expression of these relaxation migraine attacks is found in patients who only get headaches during their holidays!

Site of the Headache (Figures 20.1, 20.2 and 20.3)

Classical migraine is frontal-temporal in site and usually unilateral. There should be little difficulty in diagnosis with this type of headache. The headache site shown on Figure 20.2 causes most difficulty. Such stress is laid on the tension in neck muscles that is held to be responsible for tension

headache that it is assumed that occipital headache is invariably due to tension. In fact many cases of otherwise typical migraine start in the occipital area and radiate forward to the "classical" frontal site. The variant shown in the figure is less typical, and creates a diagnostic problem. The pain starts sub-occipitally and radiates forward to the temple or deep in behind the eye. It is usually bilateral, although one side is more severely affected than the other. The most severe pain may be indicated by the patient clutching both temples and describing a "bursting" feeling. Throbbing may not occur, or may only be felt deep in the eye, and may be provoked by exertion or bright lights.

The third variety (Figure 20.3) is often ascribed to sinus disease. The pain is essentially confined to a position deep in behind the eye. It may be bilateral, and is aggravated by bright light. It is more or less continual over weeks with periodic exacerbations. It is usually referred to as migrainous neuralgia. It often supervenes in a patient with a previous history of migraine, and is more frequently seen in females (unlike cluster headache which is almost confined to males). This type of headache seems particularly to be produced by the birth control Pill. These patients may complain of a

Chapter 21

FACE PAIN

In the previous chapter the problem of headache was discussed and special emphasis was given to the importance of the history in the differential diagnosis. This is also the situation when we consider the symptom of pain in the face but unlike headaches, several of the conditions causing facial pain are nearly always "typical" in their historical features. This is particularly true of trigeminal neuralgia. Unfortunately, there are several popular misconceptions about facial pain. Prominent among these is the feeling that any pain that is not identifiable as trigeminal neuralgia is automatically due to the condition called "atypical facial pain". In fact in many ways "atypical facial pain" is just as "typical", historically, as trigeminal neuralgia. This underlines the importance of the history. In the case of headache no anatomically discrete areas of involvement are demanded, and the "headache" is allowed to spread on to the neck or well on to the face without much concern as to the anatomical substrate. In considering face pain an accurate knowledge of the anatomy of the fifth cranial nerve is essential, and this information is provided in Figure 21.1.

A brief discussion of the role of disease of the teeth and the sinuses in the context of face and head pain is necessary. A diseased tooth in the upper jaw can cause headache on the same side, that is not in direct continuity with the pain in the tooth. A diseased tooth in the lower jaw may cause considerable pain in the mandibular division of the nerve including pain felt deep in the ear. In both cases it must be stressed that the pain in the involved tooth dominates the picture—there is no difficulty in recognising that the pain is coming from a tooth. A similar situation exists in respect of sinus disease. Experimental work has shown that the lining of the sinuses is relatively pain insensitive, and that the bulk of the severe pain in sinus disease is due to the congestion of the nasal mucosa and the turbinates. As such involvement produces symptoms of nasal congestion and discharge the diagnosis should be obvious. This means that in the absence of such symptoms the time-honoured search for evidence of chronic sub-clinical sinus infection as the explanation for attacks of pain in the face is unnecessary.

On the premise that there was such a thing as chronic sub-clinical sinus infection causing face pain, various aetiological hypotheses were suggested. The most popular of these held that various autonomic nerves and ganglia were "irritated" by such infection and caused pain. Entities such as vidian neuralgia, ciliary neuralgia, spheno-palatine neuralgia, and petrosal neuralgia were described, and a variety of surgical procedures were designed to ablate the offending nerves. All these conditions are now known to be variants of facial migraine and we can add cluster headache and Sluder's lower-half headache to the list. As these conditions are subject to runs of attacks with long remissions the apparent success of surgical treatment is explained. Critical evaluation of these treatment methods has failed to substantiate the claims made for them.

In spite of the recognition of facial migraine and the psychological aetiology of atypical facial pain many patients with chronic facial pain are still subjected to extensive dental work and sinus drainage procedures, showing that these discredited theories of facial pain die hard, and that belief in their existence is not confined to the laity.

The Anatomy of the Fifth Cranial Nerve (Figure 21.1)

The central representation of the fifth cranial nerve is extremely complex and has been described in Chapter 15. The

Figure 21.1. Trigeminal Nerve Supply to Face

Note that the scalp back to the vertex is supplied by V_1

V_3 also supplies the tragus, the anterior wall of the auditory canal and the tympanic membrane

This area is supplied via the greater auricular nerve (C2.3)

The cornea is supplied by V_1

V_1 supplies the upper passages and the nasal septum

V_2 supplies the lateral nasal wall, the floor of the nasal cavity, the upper jaw, upper teeth, and the roof of the mouth

V_3 supplies the lower jaw, the lower teeth, the floor of the mouth and the tongue (not taste)

exact distribution of the peripheral fifth nerve is of some importance. The important points are as follows:

1. The upper limit of the territory supplied by the nerve is the vertex, and a line drawn from here to the top of the ear on each side indicates the posterior boundary.

2. The lower border of the territory supplied by the fifth nerve is not indicated by the line of the edge of the jaw, but by a line as shown. Notice the large area supplied by the cervical roots, covering the angle of the jaw and the lateral cheek.

3. The boundaries between the three divisions are not horizontal but sweep up towards the temple as shown. The large area of the temple that is supplied by the mandibular division accounts for the spread of toothache from the lower jaw into this area as mentioned in the introduction.

4. The distribution to the mucous membranes of the nasal cavity and the oral cavity is indicated on the diagram. Attention is drawn to the fact that pain inside the nose and in the tongue can and does occur in trigeminal neuralgia. Taste sensation is conveyed from the tongue in the lingual branch of the mandibular division, but the fibres, from the chorda tympani, join the nerve so far peripherally that they are rarely affected in fifth nerve lesions.

5. The second (Maxillary) and third (Mandibular) divisions of the nerve lie in the soft tissues of the nasopharynx

as they emerge from the skull base and are particularly likely to be involved by neoplasms arising in this area (see also Chapter 6).

TRIGEMINAL NEURALGIA (TIC DOULOUREUX)

Although great stress is quite rightly placed on the fact that the pain in this condition *never* extends outside the territory of the fifth nerve, it is not sufficiently appreciated that it is unusual for the pain to involve a whole division at any one time, let alone the entire territory of the nerve. It is also worth pointing out at this stage that the first (Ophthalmic) division is involved in *only* five per cent of cases. The practical point that emerges from this is that one of the least likely causes of pain in the eye or forehead is tic douloureux.

The main pain occurs in two zones. These are the mouth-ear zone (affected in about sixty per cent of cases) and the nose-orbit zone (affected in thirty per cent of cases). In the case of pain in the mouth-ear zone (Figure 21.2) the pain spreads from the region of the lower canine tooth back to a position felt deep in the ear (less frequently the pain may go from the ear to the jaw). Quite often the pain also spreads around the hinge, as shown, into the upper jaw, and therefore is along the line of the boundary between the second and third divisions and is not confined to the third division. The second, nose-orbit zone (Figure 21.3), is

Figure 21.2. Mouth-ear zone Trigeminal Neuralgia
This is the distribution of the pain in almost 60 per cent of cases

Figure 21.3. Nose-orbit Trigeminal Neuralgia
This is the distribution in 30 per cent of the cases

The pain radiates from A to B and is a deep sensation. It may also involve C at the heights of the pain. Less frequently it may shoot from B to A or C
Chewing, smiling, or hot and cold fluids in the mouth are the main triggering factors
The ophthalmic division (V_1) is involved in less than five per cent of cases

The pain shoots from A (the upper canine) to around the eye to B and or C. The areas B and C may also be 'trigger points'
The main trigger areas for this distribution are touching the alar of the nose, the outer 1/3 of the upper lip, and hot and cold fluids in the mouth

condition affecting the temporal artery may be accompanied by visible swelling, and tenderness of the artery. This may be misdiagnosed as temporal arteritis, unless the age of the patient is taken into account. Carotidynia, an episodic throbbing pain in the neck, is probably due to swelling and tenderness of the carotid artery. Slight pressure on the vessel causes pain but firm pressure may completely relieve the symptoms. In all the facial migraine syndromes the important clues are retro-orbital pain of stabbing type or a dull bursting feeling in the mastoid bone. These syndromes occur in both sexes, mainly between the ages of 25 and 45 years. Ergotamine may give some relief, and methysergide maleate is extremely effective in bringing a series of attacks to an end.

POST-HERPETIC NEURALGIA (Figure 21.6)

This rarely presents a diagnostic problem as the causative herpetic lesion is usually obvious. However, at the onset of Herpes Zoster, in the three to five days between the onset of the initial pain and the eruption of the vesicles, there is a considerable diagnostic problem. Ophthalmic herpes occurs in the elderly and the initial pain in the forehead may mimic temporal arteritis. The E.S.R. is not too helpful as in several cases seen by the author the E.S.R. was elevated, even though the subsequent diagnosis proved to be Herpes Zoster. A daily examination for vesicles seems the correct approach to this problem in the absence of an obviously swollen, tender temporal artery. As the vesicles appear the pain may diminish. If it does not do so it is essential to use the strongest analgesics necessary to control the pain. There is a strong suspicion that inadequate pain relief at this stage predisposes in some way to the subsequent development of the post-herpetic neuralgia syndrome. As the patients are often old and lonely the administration of anti-depressants with the analgesics to prevent a depressive reaction probably has some merit. When the condition develops, as it does in about ten per cent of patients with ophthalmic herpes, the pain alters to a continual dull burning sensation with exacerbations provoked by touching the eyebrow or brushing the hair. It is not the scars that are sensitive, it is the normal skin between them. The scars are anaesthetic. The pain may remit after twelve to eighteen months, but this is by no means certain, and those patients with persistent pain present a

Figure 21.6. Post Herpetic Neuralgia

Most frequently seen in the very elderly. It occurs mainly with first division herpes; although the whole zone hurts, the pain in the eyebrow and around the eye is especially severe
The thin papery white scars are anaesthetic. The tender areas are the patches of intact skin between the scars. Pain is continual and burning, with severe pain added by touching the eyebrow or brushing the hair
The condition shows a tendency to spontaneous remission

Figure 21.7. Costen's Syndrome
(temporo-mandibular arthritis)

Pain is mainly in the temporo-mandibular joint, spreading forwards onto the face and up into the temporalis muscle
The joint is tender to touch and pain is provoked by chewing or just opening the mouth
The pain ceases almost entirely if the mouth is held shut and still

distressing and formidable therapeutic problem. The suicide risk is high, and in the absence of effective therapy the use of narcotic analgesics may be necessary. Occasionally an excellent response even after years of pain may be obtained by using a combination of Imiprimine 25 mgs. t.d.s. and Phenytoin 100 mgs. t.d.s., even when narcotics have failed.

COSTEN'S SYNDROME (Temporo-mandibular Osteoarthritis) (Figure 21.7)

This condition causes pain in the temporo-mandibular joint which is maximally and often only present when the patient is chewing. The joint itself is usually tender to palpation, although it is possible to mistake this for tenderness of the temporal artery. The pain may radiate forward into the face or upward into the temporalis muscle. The condition can be relieved by prosthetic devices that prevent overclosure of the bite. The problem arises, as with tooth and sinus disease, when it is assumed that disease of the joint can cause pain in

the face without the joint itself being painful. Patients with atypical facial pain and the migrainous facial pain syndromes are often suspected of having this condition on this invalid premise.

OTHER CAUSES OF FACIAL PAIN

Although temporal arteritis has already been mentioned several times we must add the situation where the arteries to the muscles of mastication, including the tongue, are involved in the process. In these cases the patient may present with "intermittent claudication" of the masseter muscles, or in the tongue. The age of the patient is always a clue to this condition, and the diagnosis must always be considered in any patient over the age of 60 years who has headache or face pain.

Anginal pain is known to radiate up into the neck and lower jaw, in addition to the more typical radiation down the arms.

Table 11 | | | QUESTIONNAIRE APPROACH TO FACIAL PAIN | | |

TYPE OF PAIN	TRIGEMINAL NEURALGIA	ATYPICAL FACIAL PAIN	MIGRAINE FACE PAIN	POST HERPETIC NEURALGIA	COSTEN'S SYNDROME
Age/sex	Female male 3:1 R>L 5:1; over 50 years old	Females>males aged 30–50 years	Any age males> females	Very elderly females >males over 70 years old	Elderly females
Site	Lower jaw→ears Upper lip→nose Eye. Strictly unilateral	Maxillary area whole face, often other side also	May be anywhere but clue is deep eye pain or a feeling as if the mastoid swollen	Over V1 distribution usually most severe in eyebrow	In or just anterior to temporo-mandibular joint
Nature	Pain like hot needles —for seconds followed by severe pain	Described as continual, unbearable, intolerable	Throbbing pulsatile quality, lacrimation and conjunctival injection may occur	Very severe pain of non-stop type	Severe aching pain in joint radiating forwards
Special features	Unilateral nature of pain Occurs in isolated attacks	Extensive/bilateral Continual nature Interferes with sleep	Very sporadic attacks with clear gaps between	Tender area between the white scars of herpes	Over T.M. joint Only present on eating
Aggravating factors	Hot/cold fluids in mouth. Blowing nose. Chewing, smiling, talking	None, *but* may complain of triggering after many consultations	Alcohol	Touching affected area Cold draughts	Chewing Yawning
Relieving factors	Tegretol (Carbamezepine) Epanutin (Dilantin U.S.P.) (diphenyl-hydantoin) Surgical treatment	Antidepressants	Ergot derivatives Methysergide Maleate (Deseril G.B.) (Sansert U.S.P.)	Epanutin (Dilantin U.S.P.) (diphenyl-dantoin) Antidepressants Narcotics if necessary	Bite correction Surgery

CASE REPORT

A 73-year-old lady was seen with quite severe bilateral pain in both upper and lower jaws, which came on while walking, especially on cold days. Shortly after the onset of this pain a gripping feeling in the chest was noticed. The pain in the jaws was the presenting symptom and the seat of the worst pain. Cardiological advice was sought, and the diagnosis of cardiac pain referred to the jaws was confirmed.

Malignant disease in the skull base, often due to direct extension from a carcinoma of the nasopharynx, tends to involve the fifth nerve. Pain in the second and third division, or a patch of numbness on the face should be regarded as due to nasopharyngeal carcinoma until proved otherwise.

Tumours in the cerebello-pontine angle will invariably damage the root of the fifth nerve. This may produce a picture like tic douloureux but this is decidedly unusual. Careful examination in such a case will usually reveal other signs, such as a depressed corneal response, which are incompatible with the diagnosis of tic. However, tic douloureux does complicate two structural conditions in this area: Paget's disease, and basilar impression (due to senile osteoporosis). Both conditions alter the anatomy of the tip of the petrous bone which may irritate the trigeminal nerve root.

Aneurysmal dilatation of the carotid artery in the cavernous sinus will damage the first division of the fifth nerve causing severe pain in the forehead and eye. This is accompanied by multiple extraocular nerve palsies and a bloodshot eye and the diagnosis is quite obvious. It occurs mainly in hypertensive elderly females (see Chapter 5).

In this chapter, as in the case of headache, with the exception of the E.S.R., the whole diagnosis is based on the history—there are no special investigations that indicate the diagnosis. There is *no* alternative to sitting back and taking an accurate history even if it takes half an hour or more to do so.

Chapter 22

ATTACKS OF ALTERED CONSCIOUSNESS

This deliberately all-embracing title has been used to empha-sise the fact that loss of consciousness is not synonymous with epilepsy. From the patient's point of view the diagnosis of epilepsy has far-reaching implications both for employ-ment and social activities and in some instances the inability to drive a motor vehicle may lead to loss of employment. In some countries there are still laws denying an epileptic patient the right to marry and have children, based on Victorian concepts as to the cause and nature of epilepsy. While the protection of the patient and the public implicit in the restrictions placed on an epileptic have to be accepted by an epileptic patient, the tragic consequences of an incorrect diagnosis are obvious. Many patients are on anti-convulsant drugs quite unnecessarily because of misinterpretation of the history or the significance of an E.E.G. Too often the E.E.G. has been allowed to act as a final arbiter in cases of clinical uncertainty, with diagnostic errors in both directions. The diagnosis *must* be firmly based on the history and in this particular instance on any eye-witness accounts that are available. It is worth going to any lengths to get such an account if there is any chance of locating the eye witness to an attack. A long-distance phone call or even a detailed letter answering specific points can often completely alter the diagnosis.

As epilepsy is such an enormous subject coverage will be confined to fairly classical identifiable attacks, and a neuro-logical opinion is suggested for borderline cases rather than an E.E.G. The alternative possibilities will be covered in greater detail than is usual in a textbook of neurology—as the alternatives lie in the field of general medicine and should be diagnosed without recourse to neurological advice.

EPILEPTIC PHENOMENA

Epileptic phenomena fall into three main groups, petit-mal attacks, temporal lobe attacks and grand-mal epilepsy. There are considerable misconceptions about the meanings of these terms and serious therapeutic errors may result from this problem (see drug therapy of epilepsy, Chapter 24). The single most important error is an almost universal belief that "petit-mal" is a literal translation and merely means *any* short-lived attack or any attack in which the patient falls, but does not actually jerk or become incontinent.

Petit Mal

Petit mal describes the single most easily identifiable and constant variant of epilepsy. Attacks usually begin in child-hood between five and ten years of age. It is *very* unusual for attacks to start after twenty years of age. Episodes last three to twenty seconds and consist of a brief suspension of awareness. The only motor activity may consist of some fluttering of the eyelids or a jerk of the hands. The facial expression may remain quite normal and the colour does not alter. At the end of the episode there is no confusion and conversation or play will resume as if nothing had happened. The patient is usually unaware that an attack has occurred. If there is awareness it is normally because of the reaction of bystanders, and the child learns to sense that something has happened. An E.E.G. is usually diagnostic as a run of 2–3 c.p.s. spike wave activity during an observed attack confirms the diagnosis. The reverse is *not* true and this is the second serious cause of misdiagnosis. In any epileptic patient the most frequent epileptic event seen on an E.E.G. is a short run of spike-wave activity. This does *not* mean that the patient has petit mal *unless* the E.E.G. technician noted a clinical attack of petit mal *at the same time*. Non-neurologists reading an E.E.G. report frequently make this serious mis-take; serious because of the therapeutic problems that follow (see Chapter 24).

Temporal Lobe Attacks

A wide range of epileptic phenomena arise in the temporal lobe. Brief episodes of this type are those most often mistakenly diagnosed as "petit mal". There are many features to distinguish these "minor" temporal lobe attacks.

In a child the differentiation presents some difficulty, but a careful history will usually elicit the following pointers. The child will become pale and distressed. He may complain of abdominal pain, or just run and hold on to his mother's legs in a frightened way, but cannot describe what is happening to him. The episode may last several minutes and is often followed by drowsiness. In older patients an epigastric rising sensation may be followed by pallor, lip-smacking or chew-ing movements, and more complex "zombie-like" activity. Recurrent irrelevant sentences may be uttered but no formal conversation can be carried on with the patient. Afterwards the patient is usually aware that an attack has occurred as he feels confused, "washed out" or sleepy, but he is amnesic for events that occurred while his consciousness was impaired. Because of the amnesia and the complex motor activity, the patient may come to, to find himself in a different room, or if the attack occurs in the street, several hundred yards from his intended route. Occasionally, what starts as a temporal lobe or "psychomotor" attack ends in a major convulsion.

Major Seizures

Major episodes are those most generally recognised. One of the variants that is difficult to distinguish from a "faint" is the type known as an "akinetic seizure". In these episodes the patient falls suddenly and heavily, often seriously injuring his head or face, and then after a brief period of rigidity, comes round. The absence of prodromal symptoms and the injury are useful pointers to the diagnosis of epilepsy. More classical major attacks with tonic-clonic movements leave little doubt as to their nature, lasting two to five minutes with post-ictal confusion, drowsiness and headache. Fortunately, relatively few attacks occur in the street, as the majority of patients have their attacks in bed on awakening or shortly thereafter. For this reason even neurologists see surprisingly few actual seizures so much so that when a patient has a convenient attack in the clinic one immediately wonders whether it is organic!

Although incontinence of urine and injury are thought to be diagnostic of epilepsy, both can occur in other types of unconsciousness including "simple faints". These symptoms should always be very carefully assessed. Less than half the patients with epilepsy have ever been incontinent in an attack, and relatively few have ever sustained a serious injury.

When a patient is referred to a neurologist with the diagnosis of epilepsy the chance that it indicates that the patient has a cerebral tumour is *not* high. This does not indicate a lack of awareness but merely the appreciation that of all patients with epilepsy less than one per cent have a cerebral tumour. Even in the peak decade for cerebral tumours (45–55 years of age) prospective studies have shown that only ten per cent of this highly selected group— presenting with a first epileptic seizure in this decade— eventually prove to have a cerebral tumour.

In general cerebral tumours can present as epilepsy in all age groups and the writer has seen two children under 15 with gliomas in this category but the order of risk ranges from 0·02 per cent below 15 years of age to ten per cent at 50 years of age. Careful history taking and physical examination is important in selecting tumour suspects. In any age group a focal onset, residual weakness or numbness after an attack or

a focal abnormality on E.E.G. should certainly be taken into consideration. In children, however, focal attacks, focal E.E.G.s and a post-ictal (or Todd's paralysis) occur so often that these findings have minimal significance in this age group. In the adult *any* residual weakness after an attack has very ominous implications and it is perhaps wrong to use the expression "Todd's paralysis" with its benign connotation, in this group. If a focal E.E.G. abnormality is also found, full investigation is indicated. At this stage non-neurologists are usually quite happy if cerebral scanning and angiography reveal no abnormality. The neurologist is not—"once a tumour suspect, always a tumour suspect" is a useful rule. Quite often the patient develops permanent neurological signs some five to fifteen years later and re-investigation then reveals the tumour that has been there throughout. Some would regard this as a serious diagnostic failure, but when one considers the possible consequences of cerebral surgery if a patient can conceal his tumour for fifteen years, it is very much to his advantage! It is surgical accessibility and the potential physical defects resulting from surgery that govern operation in these situations, *not* the mere demonstration of a tumour. There is also a view not based on any published data that uncontrolled epilepsy indicates the presence of a tumour. This is certainly not so and one of the disarming features of epilepsy associated with cerebral tumours is that it is often easy to control. The only exception to this is the tendency for frontal tumours to cause status epilepticus (see Chapter 9).

SYNCOPAL ATTACKS

Syncopal attacks, vasovagal attacks or simple faints are the main differential diagnosis in a patient who has had an attack of unconsciousness, or more colloquially a "black-out". A careful history will readily reveal the diagnosis. The attack is often postural and indeed it is very unusual for a faint to occur in any position other than standing. Hot, stuffy rooms, a hot bath, or severe abdominal pain may all predispose to a sudden drop in blood pressure, Syncopal attacks seem to occur more frequently in young females and often in association with their periods. In Victorian times, "swooning" was an everyday part of female life to judge from contemporary novels. In males at any age "fainting" is almost invariably associated with emotional pressures, such as examinations, pending divorce, etc. In a few cases, when the circumstances are appropriate, a faint may occur almost instantaneously. These situations would include the sight of blood, severe emotional shock, or extreme fear and the circumstances would lead to an automatic presumption that a faint had occurred. In a more typical faint there is quite a long prodromal period described as "feeling faint". This consists of a feeling of hunger, coldness with "goose-pimples", light-headedness, pallor and sweating. A dizzy feeling with noises seeming to become louder and louder is usually the prelude to the loss of consciousness. This often happens when the patient unwisely gets to his feet to "get some fresh air". Almost as soon as the patient falls to the ground he becomes conscious as cerebral blood flow is restored. If he attempts to get up immediately, a further period of unconsciousness may occur. Fainting can only occur in the supine position in a few rare pathological states. These include, diabetic autonomic neuropathy, tabes dorsalis, Shy–Drager syndrome (autonomic neuropathy and parkinsonism), late pregnancy and during severe blood loss. Occasionally cerebral anoxia during a faint may lead to an epileptic seizure, especially if the patient is held in the upright position and not allowed to fall. There is no doubt that with increasing age there is a greater risk of a simple syncopal attack terminating in an epileptic seizure. This is presumably because the brain is less able to tolerate the period of cerebral anoxia that is the cause of loss of consciousness. In this situation it is best to defer diagnosis and the use of anti-convulsants as such attacks usually prove to be isolated episodes. During a faint, even though the prolonged warning usually allows a fairly graceful fall, the patient will sometimes injure himself. Similarly if the patient has a full bladder at the time, incontinence may occur.

An E.E.G. is rarely of help in this situation. Many neurologists, if they are certain that a faint occurred, do not order an E.E.G. This is because some twenty per cent of non-epileptic patients have abnormal E.E.G.s and such a finding may lead to diagnostic confusion. It is best to rely on clinical judgement in this situation and await further developments. Whenever a patient, either a child or adult has a series of syncopal attacks the commonest underlying cause is a stress situation, and this possibility should always be explored.

Specific Types of Syncopal Attack

There are three special varieties of syncopal attack, all likely to occur in elderly males. These are carotid sinus hypersensitivity (also known as vasodepressor syncope), cough syncope and micturition syncope. Carotid sinus hypersensitivity causes abrupt fainting whenever the patient touches the side of the neck. This may occur when he turns his head, wears a tight collar or while shaving. It may easily be mistaken for arterial diseases such as carotid artery thrombosis or vertebral-basilar ischaemic attacks. Cough syncope occurs at the end of a protracted bout of coughing, which is in effect a prolonged Valsava manœuvre, impairing venous return and reducing the cardiac output. Micturition syncope is an unpleasant and dangerous syndrome. The attacks mainly occur when the patient has had to get up from a warm bed to pass urine. While standing and straining against a hypertrophied prostate gland the patient inadvertently performs the Valsava manœuvre. There is also speculation that the sudden emptying of the bladder has a reflex effect. In any event, syncope is the result, and in a toilet or bathroom this can be disastrous. What started as a faint may end up as a serious head injury, with the additional concern that the patient may have seizured or suffered a cerebral vascular accident. Elderly males with nocturia are well advised to pass urine in a sitting position!

HYPERVENTILATION ATTACKS

These episodes are also called hyperventilation syncope, although it is unusual for the patients actually to lose consciousness. Vision is blurred and may "blackout" but actual loss of consciousness is rare. These episodes are well recognised in the U.S.A. but are very underdiagnosed in Britain. Many anxious patients referred with "dizziness" are suffering from this condition. The patient is usually anxious and in a great many cases a phobic situation exists that provokes episodes. One patient had an attack every time she had to cross the road where her mother had been knocked down and killed.

The condition occurs almost exclusively in females and attacks occurring in supermarkets are such a constant feature that the writer now calls this the "supermarket syndrome". The patient typically develops the episode while queueing at the checkout desk. Many relate either placing everything back on the shelves or just leaving their basket and hurrying from the shop. Many patients suffering from various phobic situations seem to respond well once the mechanism of their "phobic" attacks are explained to them, often after long periods of ineffectual psychotherapy. Although the attacks are determined by anxiety the severity and frightening nature of the physical symptoms should not be underestimated.

The fully developed picture can only develop in a state of anxiety with elevated blood catecholamines. It is impossible to reproduce a full attack merely by hyperventilating. The patient feels hot and stuffy and finds the surroundings oppressive. Friends advise taking deep breaths. This gradually causes a lightheaded feeling, increasing the patient's fear of passing out. As the blood becomes alkalotic the ionised calcium falls producing fine tingling sensations in the limbs and around the mouth. The muscles become weak and the patients nearly always use the expression "my legs turn to jelly". By this stage the chest muscles become tired at first sight would appear to be straightforward vasovagal episodes.

HYPOGLYCAEMIA

Although special charts distinguishing between diabetic and hypoglycaemic coma are included in many texts the differentiation is usually easy. The patient going into diabetic coma becomes progressively obtunded over a period of hours, whereas hypoglycaemia can be truly "syncopal" in onset. The cause is usually excess insulin or an inadequate diet in a known diabetic. Primary hypoglycaemia is extremely rare, although frequently suspected. In the patient who is becoming hypoglycaemic the prodomal symptoms are very similar to the prodrome of a syncopal attack. (In both cases these symptoms are produced by adrenaline release in response to falling blood pressure and falling blood sugar respectively.) However, in the premonitory phase of hypoglycaemia there is often a personality alteration with aggression as a common feature which may be homicidal in degree. Increasing pallor and sweating and finally yawning are the physical clues to the diagnosis. In fact, any pathologically drowsy patient who yawns continually should be quickly checked for hypoglycaemia. Once consciousness is lost, there is a real risk of the patient having an epileptic fit. Immediate intravenous injection of glucose is indicated. There is a considerable risk of brain damage and every minute counts. In spite of adequate replacement if the coma has been prolonged and particularly if a fit has occurred, the patient may take several hours to regain consciousness. If the diagnosis is suspected and there is likely to be delay in getting the patient to hospital, it is essential to give intravenous glucose or glucagon even though pathological confirmation may be prevented. The considerable danger of prolonged hypoglycaemia cannot be over-emphasised.

CASE REPORT

A girl of 22 was referred because of frequent syncopal attacks and had been admitted in coma to several hospitals over four years. She had gradually developed a spastic dysarthria and a spastic tetraparesis. Her blood sugar during an attack was 8 mgm per cent. She was subsequently shown to have an islet cell tumour. Her blood sugar had not been estimated on any of her previous admissions.

In any unconscious patient the blood sugar and serum drug levels should be estimated immediately however obvious the clinical diagnosis may seem to be.

CASE REPORT

A 30-year-old Civil Servant collapsed by a post-box. When the ambulance arrived he was dead. He was rescusitated in the ambulance and extensive investigations were performed to try to determine the cause of his collapse. Three days later the suicide note that he had posted to his brother, just as he died, arrived. At no stage had the possibility of a drug overdose been considered. Unfortunately, in spite of intensive care the patient subsequently died from irreversible brain damage.

One of the most frequent reasons for referring a patient to the neurological clinic is for the investigation of an attack of altered consciousness. Almost invariably there are no physical signs between the episodes and the E.E.G. does not always give diagnostic information. The diagnosis depends on the history and the eyewitness account. Too often the patient attends without the eyewitness. The referring doctor could make a very helpful contribution if whenever he referred such a patient, he could advise him to find, question and if possible bring the eyewitness to the clinic with him.

Table 12 — DIFFERENTIAL DIAGNOSIS OF EPILEPTIC VARIANTS

	PETIT MAL	TEMPORAL LOBE EPILEPSY	GRAND MAL	AKINETIC GRAND MAL
Age	5–15 years	Any age	Any age	Any age
Onset	Instantaneous	Prolonged prodrome	Very brief warning, if any	None at all
Duration	5–20 seconds	5 seconds to hours or days	2–5 minutes	1–2 minutes
Type of attack	Brief suspension of awareness	Prolonged altered behaviour may culminate in major attack	Period of rigidity with cyanosis (the tonic phase) then generalised jerking (the clonic phase) and then sleep	Unheralded sudden fall. Very brief attack—little or no jerking but injury risk high
Facial features	Eyelids may flutter—"day-dreaming"	Pallor, anxious bewildered expression—lip smacking or chewing movements	Unconsciousness—eyes may roll upwards or to the sides	No particular features
Limbs	Slight jerking movements of arms—this is unusual	Rather ponderous "Zombie like" activity or fiddling with clothing	Generalised jerking—(look for *focal* jerking at onset)	Initially rigid then quite still
End of attack	Abrupt—no confusion	Confused and amnesic	Confused, drowsy, headache	Often severe headache
Continence	Very rarely incontinent	Rarely incontinent	Occasionally incontinent	Occasionally incontinent
E.E.G.	Invariably abnormal and diagnostic	Often normal—sphenoidal recording may increase value	Normal in 40 per cent patients	Often normal

Table 13 — DIFFERENTIAL DIAGNOSIS OF NON-EPILEPTIC ATTACKS

	VASOVAGAL	HYPERVENTILATION	DROP ATTACKS	STOKES-ADAMS ATTACKS	HYPOGLYCAEMIA
Age/sex	Young males/females	Females>males	Elderly females	Any age or sex	Any age or sex
Prodromal symptoms	Feeling "faint", hot, stuffy, "swimmy", sweaty, vision blurred, noises distant	Prolonged "dizziness", tingling, paraesthesiae in limbs and around mouth, legs feel like "jelly"	None—typically very sudden	None	Personality change confusion, aggressive hunger, sweating, yawning
Consciousness	Briefly unconscious	Rarely unconscious	Conscious throughout	Unconscious	Unconscious
Duration of attack	Seconds	Prolonged symptoms often hours *but* rarely unconscious	Seconds only	Up to thirty seconds or fatal arrest	Minutes to hours if diagnosis not established
Colour change	Very pale	Pale	Normal	Pale initially. Cyanosed during attack. Flushed on recovery	Pale and sweating
Recovery	Abrupt but often sick	Slow, ? from exhaustion	Abrupt and complete	Abrupt and complete	Slow and confused
Precipitating features	Anxiety, pain especially visceral pain. Blood loss. Heat	Anxiety and phobic states	Unknown—almost invariably occur while walking along	Complete heart block with ventricular standstill	Excess insulin dose Hypoglycaemic drugs Islet cell tumour Retroperitoneal sarcoma
Risk of seizure	Small, but occasionally does lead to a fit, especially in the elderly	Slight risk if patient is epileptic	No risk	High risk due to cerebral anoxia	High risk and often prolonged recovery phase
Special types	Micturition Syncope Cough Syncope Carotid sinus hypersensitivity	"Supermarket" syndrome			

Figure 23.3. Longitudinal fractures of the Petrous Temporal Bone
(Right half of skull base seen from behind)

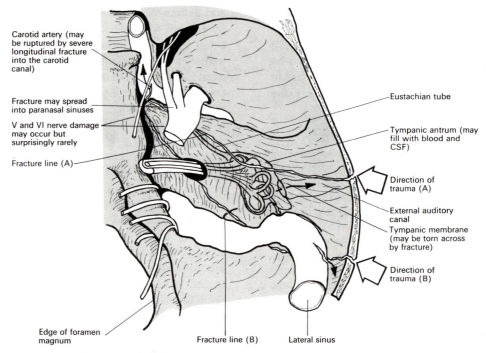

Carotid artery (may be ruptured by severe longitudinal fracture into the carotid canal)

Fracture may spread into paranasal sinuses

V and VI nerve damage may occur but surprisingly rarely

Fracture line (A)

Eustachian tube

Tympanic antrum (may fill with blood and CSF)

Direction of trauma (A)

External auditory canal

Tympanic membrane (may be torn across by fracture)

Direction of trauma (B)

Edge of foramen magnum

Fracture line (B)

Lateral sinus

head injury. This need not necessarily indicate that the patient will suffer from post-traumatic epilepsy (see later).

In the first forty-eight hours following injury the main risk to the patient is the development of an acute extradural haematoma. This risk is virtually confined to those patients with a demonstrable fracture of the temporal bone crossing the middle meningeal artery. A fracture across the vertex may tear the superior sagittal sinus, and the haemorrhage can strip up the dura and lead to an acute extradural haematoma over the vertex. In either instance the diagnosis is not difficult if the patient recovers consciousness and then becomes drowsy again, the so-called "lucid" interval. Problems arise when the patient does *not* recover consciousness and goes steadily downhill. This may be caused by serious brain laceration and oedema, but exploratory burr holes should be made in such a situation.

A special group of complications and problems are based on the fractures of the skull base that traverse the petrous temporal bone. These fractures complicate some thirty per cent of all head injuries. Even in patients without a demonstrable fracture of the bone, damage to the contained structures may occur. The organ of Corti may be affected by blunt trauma to the petrous temporal bone, causing a transient perceptive deafness. The vestibular apparatus is less easily damaged, but many cases of the condition known as benign positional vertigo appear to be related to mild head

trauma. This causes transient giddiness whenever the position of the head is altered, especially as the head is put back on to a pillow. This symptom may persist up to eighteen months after the injury but eventually subsides.

Fractures of the petrous temporal bone occur in two directions. Blows from the temporoparietal or frontotemporal direction, tend to cause longitudinal fractures which may extend across the midline into the opposite middle cranial fossa, occasionally causing fatal laceration of the carotid artery (Figure 23.3). These fractures often tear the tympanic membrane and dislocate the auditory ossicles. Although the fracture line extends to the petrous tip it is very unusual for the fifth or sixth nerve to be clinically involved. However, in some twenty per cent of patients with this type of fracture a seventh nerve palsy appears. Even without therapy of any sort seventy-five to ninety per cent of these will recover fully. Recently, evidence has been presented that the use of ACTH improves the prognosis further. If the onset is delayed until a few days after the injury, the prognosis is excellent in any event. The acute damage to the ossicles and the blood and C.S.F. in the middle ear cavity causes conductive deafness that should improve. The degree of perceptive loss caused by concussion of the organ of Corti will be apparent later.

Blows to the posterior pole of the head tend to lead to fractures that traverse the occipital bone, continue across the foramen magnum and then extend up transversely across the

Figure 23.4. Transverse fractures of the Petrous Temporal Bone

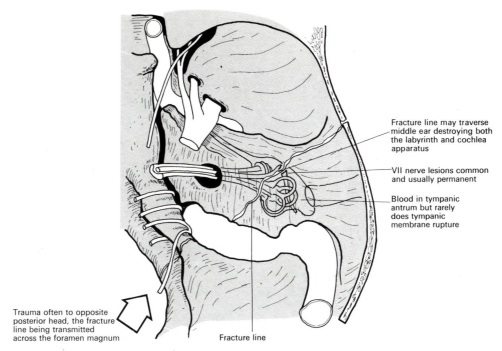

Fracture line may traverse middle ear destroying both the labyrinth and cochlea apparatus

VII nerve lesions common and usually permanent

Blood in tympanic antrum but rarely does tympanic membrane rupture

Trauma often to opposite posterior head, the fracture line being transmitted across the foramen magnum

Fracture line

petrous temporal bone (Figure 23.4). The fracture usually destroys both the cochlea and the vestibular apparatus. Occasionally one or other of these functions is spared. The severe vertigo produced by this injury disappears over a period of three to twelve weeks. The facial nerve is also frequently damaged by these fractures and with this type of fracture the nerve rarely recovers. The ear drum is usually intact. Occasionally lower cranial nerve palsies occur due to damage to the jugular foramen. This is relatively unusual as such fractures are almost invariably fatal.

The long-term implications of fractures that traverse the skull base is that whatever the immediate problems, i.e. loss of sense of smell, deafness or vertigo, the main risk to the patient is meningitis. In the days before antibiotics seven per cent of patients died of meningitis. The risk continues over many years and is a recurrent one. If the dural tear can be identified surgical closure is indicated.

Late Sequelae

1. Chronic Subdural Haematoma

This subject is dealt with first, *not* because it *is* the most frequent complication, but because it is the most frequently *suspected* complication of head injury. Subdural haematomas may be acute, subacute or chronic. Acute subdural haematomas occur over an area of lacerated brain and are

associated with a very bad prognosis for both serious residual disability or survival. Subacute subdural haematomas occur within a few weeks of the original injury and usually follow a fairly typical progression of symptoms. These include headaches, increasing drowsiness, confusion and finally the signs of tentorial herniation. Usually the history of recent trauma and the clinical course make the diagnosis obvious even if the clinical picture is not classical. The problem really arises when we consider the chronic subdural haematoma. Although this may follow head trauma the exact relationship is rather tenuous. As the patients are often elderly or alcoholic it may be difficult to elicit a clear history of trauma at all. A mild confusional state may develop over weeks and when a mild hemiparesis becomes apparent the picture is easily labelled "cerebral vascular disease" or "a small stroke". There is no typical clinical picture. Any patient with progressive intellectual impairment or a slow evolution of signs suggesting a stroke should be considered a subdural haematoma suspect.

CASE REPORT

A man, 67 years of age, was in hospital for the investigation of a gastric ulcer. On the day following a barium meal he was noticed to have a right facial weakness, and further examination revealed a mild right hemiparesis. This had appeared overnight. His C.S.F. was examined and showed an elevated protein. He gave a history of having been unconscious after being run over by a car seven years before. Investigation showed an enormous left-sided chronic subdural haematoma. At operation the capsule of the haematoma was nearly half an inch thick.

The reason for the sudden onset of physical signs, with a lesion that had clearly been the same size for many years, is not apparent. If this had not occurred while he was in hospital it would undoubtedly have been regarded as a mild stroke.

The typical site for these haematomas is shown in Figure 23.2. The leak is a low pressure venous ooze resulting from tearing of the veins bridging the veins of the cortex to the sagittal sinus. Why there is such a variation in the rate of development of the various types and the exact mechanism by which the contents change from blood to a thin yellow fluid in the chronic type is unknown. The latter are often called "subdural hygromas" as the evidence of previous bleeding is minimal or absent.

2. *The Post-Concussional Syndrome*

This is the most frequent complication of head injury leading to referral to the neurological clinic, and invariably the question is raised: Has the patient got a subdural haematoma?

The syndrome consists of a triad of symptoms—headache, dizziness and difficulty in concentration. The headache is described as a continual burning pain or a tight band or pressure on top of the head. This is similar to a patient's description of tension headache. It is exacerbated by noise, fatigue, mental stress and attempts to resume work. The dizziness is not accompanied by a sense of rotation but is more a feeling of lightheadedness. It is provoked by standing up, turning suddenly or indeed by any sudden movement. The difficulty in concentration prevents the patient working and is often ascribed to the headache.

As mentioned previously the syndrome is not encountered in children and occurs infrequently after serious head injuries. It usually follows very mild head trauma without loss of consciousness. Studies on service personnel have shown that an early return to full activities is the best way of improving the symptoms. Unfortunately as many civilian cases involve litigation the patient is very unwilling to return to work and is often aided and abetted in this by relatives and other advisers. Most studies reveal that the pre-morbid personality of the patient is critical to the development of the syndrome with hypochondriacal and depressive personality traits being of major importance. Hysterical features may also occur in some cases. The condition has no known pathological basis but constitutes a disabling complex of symptoms in persons of a certain pre-morbid personality.

3. *Post-traumatic Epilepsy*

When a patient has suffered injuries involving the dura of the skull (penetrating trauma), the risk of post-traumatic epilepsy is between thirty per cent and fifty per cent. The risk is much higher if the injury is to the central part of the brain in the frontotemporal area. In closed head injuries (no fracture demonstrated) the risk is about five per cent. If there is evidence of laceration of the brain with focal neurological deficit the risk is also about fifty per cent. In all cases there is a tendency for the attacks to become less frequent with the passage of time, although the longer the period after the injury when the first attack occurs the less likelihood there is of eventual remission. If the patient has not had a seizure by the end of the second year after the injury it is increasingly unlikely that he will do so. Standard anti-convulsant drugs are effective, but effective control may be difficult if the post-traumatic epileptic state is complicated by personality disorder. These patients are likely to be irregular attenders and do not take their medication regularly.

Patients with personality problems following head trauma are usually aggressive and paranoid and very difficult to manage. As in the case of children, in many cases, there is considerable evidence that the pre-morbid personality was abnormal and that their drinking and fighting and outbreaks of aggression towards their family are exaggerations of previous habits. As this situation and post-traumatic epilepsy often co-exist in the same patient much of the bad behaviour is incorrectly held to be caused by post-epileptic confusion or even part of the actual seizure. When closely questioned most patients will admit that they are not having an epileptic attack when these outbursts occur.

TRAUMATIC LESIONS OF THE SPINAL CORD

Although the cervical and lumbar spine are the least supported parts of the spinal column their mobility to some extent protects them from damage. The majority of serious spinal injuries occur in the dorsal area particularly between D6 and D12. In the absence of any pathological abnormality of the vertebra (osteoporosis due to steroids, metastatic cancer), considerable force is needed to fracture the spine. This may be either compressive i.e. falling from a height on to the feet or due to hyperflexion, when a weight falls on to the back. The force needed is so great that these fractures are frequently accompanied by cord transection. Cervical cord injuries, although less frequent, account for the majority of early deaths, due to respiratory paralysis.

Cervical Spine Injuries

1. The mechanism and results of fractures of the cervical

Figure 23.5. Diagram to show the Mechanism of Cervical Spine Injuries

A. Injuries to the atlanto-axial joint

Direction of trauma

Forward dislocation but adequate space posteriorly, so cord damage may be minor

Fractured odontoid or torn check ligament

B. Injuries to the lower cervical spine

Articular facets override and lock, causing permanent deformity. This requires reduction by traction

Forward rotation of neck causes crush fracture of vertebral body

Figure 23.6

Anterior arch of atlas fractured

Arch and odontoid displaced posteriorly

Spinal cord sharply angulated around dislocated odontoid, risk of fatal damage high

Disruption of apophyseal joint allows vertebra to dislocate backwards with severe cord damage

Following trauma vertebrae may come back into alignment leaving the cord destroyed but little visible abnormality on x-ray

spine are indicated in Figures 23.5, 23.6. These may result from trauma to the front or back of the head as shown.

2. Atlanto-axial dislocation may also occur in patients with rheumatoid arthritis due to ligamentous degeneration or absorption of the odontoid peg. This usually but not always occurs in patients on steroids.

3. Atlanto-axial dislocations occurring in childhood may produce an unusual delayed myelopathy. The injury often results from a fall on to the back of the head from a swing. An acute transient tetraparesis lasting less than thirty minutes may occur with complete recovery. Some twenty years later the patient develops a progressive tetraparesis punctuated by acute episodes of tetraparesis while flexing the neck, sneezing or when slapped on the back. This is presumably due to repeated mild trauma inflicted by the sliding dislocation on neck flexion. (The anatomical features of the foramen magnum region are shown in Figure 23.7).

CASE REPORT

A 38-year-old man was referred because of increasing clumsiness of gait. He was partially sighted due to retrolental fibroplasia. At the age of 4 he fell from a swing. He was unconscious and totally paralysed for about twenty minutes. Following recovery he was completely deaf, suggesting bilateral temporal bone fractures. He was otherwise well until four years before referral. Over that period he had developed stiffness of the limbs and clumsiness. He

frequently played touch football (the American Game) and his friends found that if he was running with the ball he could best be stopped by a sharp push into the middle of his back. This made him drop the ball and fall to the ground, temporarily tetraplegic! It was these repeated insults that probably led to his spastic tetraparesis. He was found to have a sliding atlanto-axial dislocation.

4. Mid cervical fractures at C3/4 level are potentially more serious as there is less room for the spinal cord to ride the blow and the risk of respiratory paralysis is maximal at this level. Fragments of vertebra are more likely to break off and compress the cord; and fractures of the transverse process may damage the vertebral artery. This may cause brainstem signs or further vascular damage to the cord below the level of the fracture (see cord blood supply, Chapter 14).

Clinical Features

The clinical features of damage at any level are dominated initially by the stage of spinal shock with a total flaccid paralysis below the level of the lesion. At this stage the sensory findings provide the best evidence of the extent and severity of the damage. As soon as the cord settles down (the nature of spinal shock is *not* understood) tone returns to the limbs below the level of the injury and the extent of local damage becomes obvious, as the residual weakness and wasting of the supplied muscles becomes apparent.

245

Chapter 24

DRUG INTERACTIONS AND SIDE-EFFECTS IN NEUROLOGY

As might be anticipated, many of the drugs used in the treatment of neurological disorders are liable to produce neurological side-effects. Sometimes these side-effects are merely extensions of the therapeutic effect but in other cases serious new neurological phenomena are produced.

Many drugs in use for non-neurological diseases may also produce neurological side-effects which may be mistaken for neurological complications of the underlying disease. Drugs may occasionally worsen the situation for which they are being administered. For example, it is not widely appreciated that all anticonvulsant drugs can produce seizures in toxic doses and even in therapeutic dosage if used inappropriately.

To avoid the risk of the text becoming a bewildering list of complications we will consider the special problems encountered in the treament of various neurological disorders and then the neurological complications of drugs with similar therapeutic indications.

Two tables are included, one showing the drug groups and the side-effects likely to be encountered (Table 15) and the other specific neurological complications with a list of drugs that could be responsible (Table 14).

Although these lists are fairly comprehensive other drugs may be found to have similar side effects and a constant awareness of the possibility that drugs may be responsible for a patient's symptoms should always be maintained. A complete list of all drugs taken by the patient in the previous year is an essential part of the history, and it should be remembered that some patients who have taken a drug for years may completely fail to consider it a drug as it has become part of their daily routine!

One never ceases to be amazed at the attitude of the patient who is reluctant to take a prescribed "drug" and yet has been happily taking eight or more aspirins or compound analgesic tablets daily for many years, on the dubious premise that anything one can buy cannot be a "drug". The press publicity of the "drug problem" has also led to considerable difficulty in persuading elderly patients to take any medication for fear of becoming an addict, and a belief that all doctors are totally ignorant of drug side-effects.

There have been many papers and sociological surveys on the frequency with which patients fail to take the medication as prescribed or dispose of it down the drain as soon as they arrive home! This is *not* a failing of the patient but the responsibility of the doctor who has failed to explain to the patient the reason for prescribing the drug, its anticipated effect on the symptoms and the potential side effects. The latter feature is rather disputed but in an anxious patient the onset of even quite minor and predictable side-effects may lead to their stopping treatment. It seems sensible for the patient, who after all is the person using the medication, to be fully aware of these possibilities. It must be admitted that even the most painstaking explanation may fall on deaf ears and the writer will never forget the expression on the face of a Mexican-American patient as he left the clinic, after an explanation, including mime because of the language barrier, as to the correct use of an ergotamine suppository!

Occasionally the patient must be asked specifically to tolerate quite unpleasant side-effects in order to get the benefit of the drug. Perhaps the best example of this was in the early days of L-Dopa therapy when the patient had to tolerate nausea, vomiting, constipation and postural hypotension for several weeks before any improvement in the parkinsonian symptoms was apparent. The sedative effects of anticonvulsants are another very good example as the initial sedation wears off if the patient can be persuaded to persevere and this is best achieved if he is completely aware of the necessity to do this and the fact that eventually the side-effects will lessen or disappear.

GENERAL CONSIDERATIONS OF MECHANISMS OF DRUG TOXICITY

1. Every drug has inherent toxic potential. This is quantitative and varies from patient to patient in the exact dose required to produce the toxic effect.

2. The age of the patient influences the risk of an unanticipated toxic effect. The dangers of chloramphenicol in infancy, and the increasing risk of eighth nerve damage by streptomycin with increasing age are well known.

3. Toxic blood levels of a drug may be achieved with normal doses in the presence of renal failure. This risk is a particular problem of antibiotic therapy.

4. Similar side-effects of two drugs may summate if the drugs are used in combination. This is a problem of

Table 14
NEUROLOGICAL SYMPTOMS AND CAUSATIVE DRUGS

PERIPHERAL NEUROPATHY:	Thalidomide		Birth control pill
	Nitrofurantoin		Hypervitaminosis A
	Isoniazid	*DEPRESSION:*	Diazepam
	Vincristine/Vinblastine		Chlordiazepoxide
	Imiprimine		Reserpine
	Amitriptyline		Birth control pill
ACUTE MUSCLE WEAKNESS:	Diuretics—Potassium loss		Clonidine hydrochloride
	Carbenoxolone—Potassium loss	*CONFUSION AND HYPOMANIA:*	Antiparkinsonian drugs
			Steroids
	Neomycin—muscle blocking effect		Excessive penicillin/cephalo-sporins (prior to encephalo-pathy and coma)
	Penicillamine—myasthenic syndrome	*PARKINSONISM:*	Reserpine
CHRONIC MUSCLE WEAKNESS:	Steroids (especially fluorinated steroids)		Phenothiazines
			Tricyclic antidepressants (rare)
	Chloroquine		Lithium carbonate
EPILEPTIC SEIZURES:	Anticonvulsants	*DYSTONIC REACTIONS:*	Phenothiazines (especially anti-emetic group)
	Sedatives (especially meprobamate)		Metoclopromide (Maxalon)
	Triptylines		L-Dopa
	Phenothiazines	*VISUAL DISTURBANCES:*	Tricyclic antidepressants
	Amphetamines		Mono-amine oxidase inhibitors
	Mono-amine oxidase inhibitors		Streptomycin
	Amantadine hydrochloride		Chloramphenicol
	Cycloserine		Isoniazid
HEADACHES:	Indomethacin		Chloroquine
	Mono-amine oxidase inhibitors		Ethambutol
	Excessive doses of ergotamine		Birth control pill

anticonvulsant combinations where excessive sedation often becomes a major problem.

5. The possibility that the metabolic effect of one drug alters the action of another should always be considered. The onset of digitalis toxicity caused by hypokalaemia produced by diuretics is an example.

6. Individual variations in the ability of the patient to metabolise some drugs can occur and is based on inherited enzymic defects. Sensitivity to isoniazed and diphenylhydantoin (Epanutin or Dilantin U.S.P.) can occur on this basis.

7. One drug may interfere with the metabolic degradation of another. Phenylbutazone (Butazolidine) can block the metabolism of Tolbutamide (Rastinon) leading to hypoglycaemic reactions. Coumarin anticoagulants and sulthiam (Ospolot) block metabolism of diphenylhydantoin (Epanutin or Dilantin U.S.P.) and may lead to toxic blood levels.

8. Conversely some drugs may facilitate their own metabolism and that of other drugs by the process known as enzyme induction. Phenobarbital, glutethimide (Doriden) and meprobamate (Equanil) share this property and all can speed the metabolism of diphenylhydantoin—reducing the expected blood levels of this drug.

9. A drug may sensitise the body to otherwise innocuous endogenous substances. The potentially fatal rise in blood pressure or subarachnoid haemorrhage produced by dietary tyramine in patients receiving monoamine-oxidase inhibitors is well known.

10. Drugs may unmask a latent enzyme defect in the patient. This is an important factor in the precipitation of attacks of acute porphyria by a series of drugs listed in Chapter 16.

It is clear that in such a complex setting of possible mechanisms of drug toxicity that the simultaneous use of even innocuous and unrelated drugs requires careful consideration. As will be pointed out later, one of the dangers of drugs in combined capsules is that one of the agents in the combination may not be familiar to the user and could lead to

Figure 25.2. Correct position

Head in comfortable neutral position need not be forcibly flexed

Top shoulder square

Supporting pillows hold top leg up in the air

Back is straight and vertical

Back right to edge of bed for firm support

Vertebral position with patient correctly positioned

L3/4 disc

Target area lies in midline beneath spinous process

L3

L4

Note. Needle ideally angled slightly headwards

Figure 25.3. Correct position from above

One or two pillows pushed into abdomen and between legs

Shoulders kept square

Back should be vertical

Upper leg supported on a pillow to prevent rolling forward

Figure 25.4. Some common stilette problems

Stilette too small

Stilette too long

Correct stilette

Venus'' posture and the effect this has on the target area between the laminae of the two vertebrae and compare this with the correct position shown on Figures 25.2 and 25.3. The importance of repeatedly checking that the back is vertical (which keeps the target area directly beneath the spines) must be stressed.

Sterile Procedures

Meningitis after lumbar puncture is exceptionally rare. The author knows only of one example in the last fifteen years in hospitals with which he has been associated. Nevertheless, sterile precautions should be observed. The author prefers not to wear rubber gloves as they spoil the feel. This would seem to be quite safe provided the hands are correctly scrubbed and the shaft of the needle is not touched during the procedure.

Equipment

The equipment provided varies so much from hospital to hospital that no specific advice can be given. However, the most important thing is to check that all the needles, stopcocks and manometers fit each other. One may have to ''cannibalise'' several packs to get a suitable kit, but it is worth the effort. Then check that the stilette on the needle chosen fits flush to the end of the needle (Figure 25.4), if it does not, it becomes a very traumatic weapon. Check that the stilette is not stuck, check that the stopcock rotates freely, and check the flow direction in the different stopcock positions. Finally make sure that the manometer is not broken inside its pack. Having established that there are not going to be any holdups caused by equipment failure, the actual lumbar puncture can begin.

1. Select a sharp, medium-sized needle. (Needle sizes are 18, 19, 20 and 21—the higher the number the smaller the bore and length.) A number 19 is best for general use, a number 21 for small people and children other than infants.

2. Select the interspace between the spines of L3 and L4. This lies just below the line joining the anterior superior iliac spines. Mark the position of the spines with a ball pen for further reference if needed.

3. Clean the area with whatever skin cleansing agent is available, and finally with alcohol. Allow to dry. Then finally prepare the skin over an area about six inches square, centred on the chosen space, with either mercurochrome or iodine (Figure 25.5).

4. Arrange three towels as shown in Figure 25.6. The upper one should not hang down on to the needle, but it is very useful for moving the patient about and checking the position of the anterior superior iliac spine if the landmarks are lost. The writer prefers not to use the towel with a window in it that is sometimes provided. It makes it difficult to see where you are, is hard to keep in position and tends to fall down on to the needle.

5. While the skin preparation is drying, drawn up 1–2 cc. of two per cent lignocaine in a small syringe. There is no need to infiltrate the area with 5–10 cc. as some do. This usually causes a lot of bleeding and turns the entry route into a bloody mush that destroys the ''feel''. Warn the patient that the local anaesthetic will ''sting'' for about ten seconds. Raise a skin bleb about 1 cm. across as shown in Figure 25.7 and then inject another 0·5 ml just below the skin. Massage it in with a finger. If the skin is not held taut as in the diagram, you may find that the area you have anaesthetised is about one inch from the midline.

Check that the skin is anaesthetised with a small needle. Then check that the patient has not altered position and warn him that he will feel a pushing sensation against the back. Ask him to tell you immediately if he feels any sharp pain. Holding the skin as shown in Figure 25.7, push the needle through the skin. This may be difficult but do not lunge at it or you will suddenly plunge in too deeply. As soon as you are through the skin check that the position is correct and then penetrate the dense supraspinous ligament (Figure 25.8). Once you have done so, stop, let go of the needle and see that it is at 90 degrees to the back. A correct line through this ligament is vital; if the needle has been deflected off line start again.

7. Once the needle is correctly aligned push it gently inwards and slightly towards the head. Usually the interspinous ligament is quite easily penetrated and little effort is needed.

8. If the line is correct at about $1\frac{1}{2}$–2 inches deep a slight resistance will be felt. Check the needle line, and if it is in the correct position, give the needle a little push quite firmly but only for about $\frac{1}{8}$ inch. This will penetrate the ligamentum flavum with a slight ''pop''. As the same push often also penetrates the dura *do not* advance the needle any further without withdrawing the stilette from the needle. If no fluid emerges it is always worth rotating the needle slightly as a nerve root may be lying across the end. If no fluid emerges replace the stilette (*never* advance the needle without the stilette in position) and advance the needle another $\frac{1}{8}$ inch and repeat. Continue advancing in this way until fluid emerges, firm resistance is encountered or the patient complains of pain down either leg.

9. If firm resistance is encountered *do not* force the needle, it may be against the opposite intervertebral disc and this can be damaged. If a nerve root is hit, find out which leg was affected. If the pain was in the right leg, withdraw the

polymyositis complicating the use of the drug with improvement on withdrawal.

Considerable muscle atrophy occurs in long-standing cases and although much of this results from disuse, in five per cent of cases pathological evidence of inflammatory muscle disease has been found.

The most serious neurological complication is due to avulsion or absorption of the odontoid peg. This may happen acutely during a sneeze or a fall or be found on routine x-ray in patients complaining of neck pain. An acute or progressive spastic tetraparesis results and may prove fatal.

Polyarteritis nodosa

This is the most lethal of the collagen-vascular diseases and unlike systemic lupus erythematosus and rheumatoid arthritis occurs more frequently in males (eighty per cent of cases). The age incidence is similar, the majority of cases occurring in the 20–40 age group. A very similar disorder has been described as a reaction to sulphonamides, penicillin and diphenylhydantoin.

The main pathological lesion is a pan-arteritis with destruction of all layers of the arterial wall with local thrombosis and occasionally rupture of the vessel and microhaemorrhages.

The common neurological manifestations are due to peripheral nerve and nerve root infarction. The disease is one of the commonest causes of mononeuritis multiplex, but equally often infarction of multiple nerve roots occurs particularly affecting nerve roots C5–C7 and L2–L4. Once the patient is disabled the risk of further compression palsies is extremely high.

Although cranial nerve palsies and cerebral vascular accidents may occur they are uncommon.

The lethal nature of the condition is due to renal arteriolar disease often leading to uncontrollable hypertension. A few patients also develop polymyositis and the use of high doses of steroids to control the underlying disease may cause a steroid myopathy, adding to the diagnostic problems.

CASE REPORT

A 48-year-old aeronautical draughtsman had suffered from unexplained asthma for several years. Over a period of a few weeks he lost weight and felt very ill. Over a period of days he developed bilateral ulnar and median nerve palsies. His E.S.R. and eosinophil count were elevated. He was given steroids with complete remission of the systemic systems and a slow recovery of the nerve lesions. A few weeks later he became unable to walk because of gross weakness of both hip flexor muscles and the quadriceps. E.M.G. evidence confirmed an acute inflammatory myopathy. The dose of steroids was increased with a rapid improvement in muscle strength.

An unusual form of this disorder occurs in young patients which is known as "Cogan's syndrome". This consists of an association of interstitial keratitis, bilateral vestibular symptoms and deafness.

CASE REPORT

A 26-year-old housewife developed right-sided headache, felt increasingly unwell and lost weight. The headache was associated with vertigo. These symptoms partially remitted and then recurred on the left side. The clinical findings and oto-neurological studies suggested a left-sided cerebello-pontine angle lesion and the systemic illness suggested this might be due to metastatic malignant disease. During neurosurgical investigations she developed bilateral keratitis, the E.S.R. rose to 140 mm. and the eosinophil count rose to forty per cent. High dose steroids led to a prompt remission of symptoms although she remained partially deaf.

Although the E.S.R. is widely regarded as an old-fashioned and unreliable test it remains an important investigation for the neurologist. The speed with which the result is obtained and the almost invariable gross elevation in patients with collagen vascular disease cannot be matched by any other test.

Polymyositis

This acute inflammatory disease of muscle may complicate any of the collagen-vascular diseases already discussed. It also occurs as a primary condition and is sometimes a remote complication of malignant disease. It is discussed in detail in Chapter 17.

Scleroderma

Scleroderma is characterised by thickening of the collagen in the skin producing the typical skin changes of the disorder and similar changes in the bowel which may result in malabsorption. The condition may also occur in association with systemic lupus erythematosus and dermatomyositis.

Clinical presentations include Raynaud's phenomenon and rarely muscle weakness and evidence of cutaneous nerve damage in the thickened skin. Steroids are not helpful in this condition.

Sjögren's Syndrome

Sjögren's syndrome is now regarded as a collagen-vascular disease. The main features are a dry kerato-conjunctivitis, xerostomia (dry mouth) and a rheumatoid-like arthritis. In recent years an association with a progressive proximal myopathy has been recognised. Pathological and electromyographic evidence indicates that this is an inflammatory muscle lesion but there is rarely any response to steroids.

Polymyalgia Rheumatica

This disorder is also discussed in Chapter 17. It occurs in the elderly and is characterised by severe muscle pain in the limbs and girdle regions and is usually associated with a systemic illness and a high E.S.R. Some of these patients later develop temporal arteritis. The response to steroids is dramatic and diagnostic.

Thrombotic Thrombocytopenic Purpura

This is an extremely rare and usually ultimately lethal condition dominated by acute haemolytic anaemia and thrombocytopenia. The onset is usually acute with abdominal pain, fever, vomiting, headache and jaundice, quickly complicated by confusion, delirium and coma, with seizures, hemiplegia and almost any other acute cerebral vascular event.

The main pathological lesions are due to severe acute inflammatory changes in arteriolar walls with thrombosis and multiple petechial haemorrhages; throughout the substance of the brain but particularly in the cortex.

Very rarely the disorder may run a relapsing course over several years but is almost invariably eventually fatal. Steroids may occasionally prove beneficial.

The frequency with which collagen-vascular diseases present as an acute neurological disorder places considerable responsibility on the neurologist to recognise this group of diseases.

4. NEUROLOGICAL COMPLICATIONS OF ENDOCRINE AND METABOLIC DISEASE

Although there are some specific complications associated with changes in hormonal levels per se, in many instances the neurological involvement in endocrine disorders is really a reflection of alterations in electrolyte metabolism. These problems are discussed in greater detail in the chapters on muscle and peripheral nerve disease. Discussion in the present section will therefore be extremely brief and references to more detailed discussions are given.

1. Thyrotoxicosis

In thyrotoxic exophthalmos with ophthalmoplegia (Chapter 5), the exophthalmos is probably due to excessive T.S.H. production but the diplopia is not purely due to displacement of the globe. Pathological studies have shown inflammatory changes in the affected extraocular muscles.

A similar situation exists in thyrotoxic myopathy (Chapter 17). The muscle weakness usually recovers surprisingly rapidly once the euthyroid state is restored. Thyrotoxicosis also occurs in some patients with periodic paralysis (particularly in the Japanese) and in ten per cent of patients with myasthenia gravis.

Acute thyroid crisis with fever, delirium, epileptic seizures and coma has become rare now that quick control of the peripheral effects of thyroid hormone can be gained with guanethidine.

In addition to the typical fine tremor of the hands, a rare complication is the acute onset of choreiform movements due to hormonal effects on the basal ganglia (Chapter 12).

In the elderly "masked thyrotoxicosis" may occur, in which the classical signs of the disease may be easily overlooked. This is quite common in patients presenting with thyrotoxic myopathy. The other important group to consider are those patients in whom auricular fibrillation secondary to thyrotoxicosis has caused cerebral embolism.

2. Myxoedema

Carpal tunnel syndrome is a frequent complication of myxoedema (Chapter 18). Proximal muscle weakness is quite common in cretinism and adult myxoedema (Chapter 17). Although a great deal is made of myxoedema madness this is an extremely rare complication; complete mental and physical inertia usually dominates the illness. Cerebellar degeneration may also complicate myxoedema (Chapter 12) but is also exceedingly rare.

3. Hyperparathyroidism

The complications of hyperparathyroidism directly reflect the elevation of serum calcium. This may produce a variable proximal muscle weakness (Chapter 17) or profound personality change occasionally amounting to an acute psychotic state (Chapter 10).

4. Hypoparathyroidism

The lowered serum calcium level causes the complications although the mechanism in some situations is unknown. In children hypocalcaemia may cause convulsions and papilloedema which may direct investigations along purely neurological lines unless this unusual presentation is recognised. Extrapyramidal disorders may occur usually taking the form of choreiform movements associated with the deposition of calcium in the basal ganglia. Tetany may be provoked by minor hyperventilation or occur spontaneously. Proximal muscle weakness may occur (Chapter 17). Psychotic changes in personality have been reported but are much less frequent than in hypercalcaemia. In adults, cataracts are a common complication of unrecognised chronic hypocalcaemia.

5. Cushing's Syndrome

In the active stages of this disease mental changes due to high endogenous steroid levels may precipitate a "steroid psychosis". For the same reason a proximal "steroid myopathy" occurs and in combination with the typical deposition of fat over the back contributes to the "Buffalo Hump" shape of the patient who has the fully developed syndrome.

After adrenalectomy, or in those patients in whom the disease is due to a functional tumour of the pituitary gland bitemporal field defects (Chapter 3) or extra-ocular nerve palsies (Chapter 5) may be found.

6. Addison's Disease

The physical symptoms of this disorder are dominated by mental and physical lethargy and inertia. A mild proximal myopathy with easy fatiguability occurs and exertion is often accompanied by muscle cramping. Syncope due to the associated hypotension may also lead to neurological referral.

7. Acromegaly

In the early stages of this disorder there is a considerable increase in muscle strength, paralleling the dramatic changes in facial appearance and the size of the hands and feet. Later, as the pituitary gland is replaced by the enlarging eosinophil adenoma, weakness ensues as panhypopituitarism develops. The tumour may then compress the optic chiasm causing a bitemporal hemianopia.

The overgrowth of the hands frequently leads to carpal tunnel syndrome and peroneal nerve entrapment has also been reported.

Diabetes mellitus with all its neurological consequences occurs in some twenty per cent of patients with acromegaly.

8. Hypopituitarism

The features of panhypopituitarism, including the visual problems caused by pituitary tumours, are described in Chapter 3. The problems presented by the tumour itself may be combined with features of both myxoedema and Addison's disease.

9. Inappropriate Secretion of Antidiuretic Hormone

Hyponatraemia may occur for many reasons, but a variety of special interest to the neurologist is due to inappropriate secretion of antidiuretic hormone. The term "inappropriate" has been applied because normally when serum sodium and osmolarity are falling a hypotonic urine is secreted as ADH production falls. If ADH continues to be secreted a hyperosmolar urine is produced and the renal excretion of sodium continues, further compounding the situation. This is a very simple and incomplete explanation of an extremely complicated metabolic situation.

The neurological importance of the condition stems from the fact that the well-established syndrome may produce symptoms and signs suggesting intracranial disease *and* intracranial disease may cause the syndrome.

The neurological manifestations are due to water intoxication and typically include confusion, headache, nausea and vomiting. Later the patient may become comatose and epileptic seizures can occur. There may be considerable fluctuation in the symptoms on a day-to-day basis.

Most cases are due to an underlying oat cell carcinoma of the lung and in many instances the tumour itself secretes ADH. The difficulty in distinguishing the clinical picture from that produced by multiple cerebral metastases is obvious.

Meningitis, subarachnoid haemorrhage, cerebral tumours and head injury have all been responsible for examples of the condition. Myxoedema and acute porphyria have also been implicated and the possibility of the cerebral symptoms being ascribed to the underlying disease rather than to the potentially fatal disturbance of salt metabolism is obvious.

The condition is relatively easily treated by fluid restriction to less than 1,000 mls. daily. Salt loading does not help and is only indicated in patients who are comatose or convulsing in an immediate attempt to reduce the water intoxication.

The importance of routine electrolyte studies in confusion, comatose or convulsing patients cannot be overestimated.

CASE REPORT

An 18-year-old university student was admitted to hospital after having an accident on his motor-cycle. He was conscious on arrival but was remarkably confused. He insisted he was drunk and that it was 10 p.m. He was quite sober and it was 4 p.m. in the afternoon. He was bleeding from both ears but no fracture could be seen on x-ray. Far from improving he became increasingly confused over the next thirty-six hours; and his serum sodium fell to 119 mEq/L. He was secreting a concentrated urine (specific gravity 1030). An E.E.G. showed an alarming slow wave disturbance over the left frontal region suggesting contrecoup bruising of the left frontal lobe. His fluids were restricted immediately and osmolarity studies revealed a low serum osmolarity of 252 m osmoles/L and a urine osmolarity of 723 m osm/L. Within twenty-four hours he became rational and the E.E.G. became completely normal. The remarkably rapid onset of confusion in this patient suggests that he had cerebral bruising with oedema rapidly compounded by the simultaneous development of inappropriate ADH secretion with water intoxication.

10. Alcoholism

The neurological complications of alcoholism are considered here because they basically represent metabolic effects rather than a direct toxic effect of alcohol. In Great Britain this problem presents a minor, but unfortunately increasing, part of neurological practice. In the U.S.A. these complications are extremely common.

Alcoholic peripheral neuropathy, the complication most directly related to altered niacin metabolism, is the most common complication. It is described in Chapter 16. Acute compression palsies also occur due to the inebriated patient lying on the vulnerable nerves. The radial and peroneal nerves are usually affected.

Acute and chronic muscle changes due to alcohol have been reported. The symptoms of the acute form resemble the effects of sudden exertion on untrained muscles with muscle pain and tenderness on movement usually following a period of high alcoholic intake. The chronic form consists of a mild generalised myopathy.

Cerebellar degeneration may also occur in an acute reversible form and a chronic irreversible form with massive degeneration of the anterior lobe of the cerebellum (Chapter 12).

Acute haemorrhagic polio-encephalitis or Wernicke's encephalopathy is invariably associated with damage to the hippocampal-mamillary body complex, causing the abrupt memory deficit known as Korsakoff's psychosis. The brainstem features are described in Chapter 11. The immediate administration of massive doses of Vitamin B_1 will usually reverse the potentially lethal brainstem lesion but recovery of the memory disturbance is variable and always incomplete.

One very unusual and almost specific complication of alcohol abuse is acute auditory hallucinosis. In this condition a pure auditory hallucination, often musical in content is associated with paranoid thoughts.

Acute auditory hallucinosis and delirium tremens are alcohol withdrawal syndromes. Both conditions particularly tend to occur in alcoholics who have been admitted to hospital unless alcohol is being smuggled in to the patient to maintain the intake!

Delirium tremens often begins as a series of epileptic fits followed by severe confusion and agitation, sympathetic overaction and vivid visual hallucinations.

The condition is treated by heavy sedation with chlordiazepoxide or chlormethiazole and vitamin supplements. The majority of patients recover over a few days but the condition may be fatal.

Alcohol or sedative drug abuse should be suspected in any patient who has a fit after admission to hospital.

5. NEUROLOGICAL COMPLICATIONS ASSOCIATED WITH CARDIAC DISEASE

The most frequent cardiac disease is myocardial infarction. Because this is only one manifestation of diffuse vascular disease it is hardly surprising that some forty per cent of patients who suffer a cerebral vascular accident subsequently die of a myocardial infarct.

During and following acute myocardial infarction there are the immediate risks of impaired cerebral perfusion during the shock phase and the later risk of cerebral embolism when the circulation recovers and mural thrombus becomes detached from the damaged heart wall. In some series as many as thirty per cent of cerebral emboli were found to originate in the heart. Preventing these complications with anti-coagulants may lead to fatal subarachnoid haemorrhage. Fortunately anti-coagulants no longer play a major role in the management of myocardial infarction.

Congenital cardiac disease carries many risks. Coarctation of the aorta is associated with a high incidence of cerebral aneurysms almost certainly a direct consequence of the associated hypertension. The risk of subarachnoid haemorrhage is high and subarachnoid haemorrhage in children under 15 should always suggest this possibility.

Congenital cyanotic heart disease may cause complications due to chronic cerebral anoxia, polycythaemia or cerebral abscess as the blood bypasses the normal filtering effect of the pulmonary circulation.

Both congenital and acquired disease of the aortic and mitral valves predispose to subacute bacterial endocarditis. This may cause cerebral embolism, cerebral abscess or mycotic aneurysms.

Surgical treatment of valvular disease, although now much safer with cardiac bypass and an open heart approach, still carries the risk of operative or post-operative clot or air embolism with a tragic outcome in some instances with cortical blindness or hemiplegia.

Simple syncopal attacks always require careful auscultation of the heart to detect aortic or mitral valve lesions and in patients complaining of syncope occurring on exertion evidence of atrial septal defects and pulmonary valve disease should be sought. The stethoscope is an important part of a neurologist's diagnostic equipment.

6. NEUROLOGICAL COMPLICATIONS OF NEOPLASTIC DISEASE

The neurology of malignant disease is a subject in itself, and it is possible to make only some broad generalisations in the space available.

In spite of many extremely interesting but very rare remote

complications of malignant disease the fact remains that the majority of patients with malignant disease who develop a neurological disorder prove to have metastatic deposits.

These remote complications have been mentioned elsewhere and include peripheral neuropathy (Chapter 16), polymyositis (Chapter 17), Lambert–Eaton syndrome (Chapter 17), limbic encephalitis (Chapter 10) cerebellar degeneration (Chapter 12) and inappropriate secretion of A.D.H. (Chapter 26). A supposed relationship between motor neurone disease and visceral malignancy has not been substantiated.

Surprisingly, in view of their widespread nature and chronic clinical course, the malignant lymphomas produce few neurological complications other than by direct spread. Cord compression due to Hodgkin's disease and meningeal infiltration in the leukaemias are the main problem. Fungal meningitis due to cryptococcosis neoformans (cryptococcal meningitis) is occasionally encountered. An indian ink preparation of the C.S.F. is necessary to demonstrate the fungi. One of the rare complications of considerable interest is progressive multifocal leucoencephalopathy as there is now overwhelming evidence that this is due to an opportunist virus infection of the C.N.S. in patients with chronic diseases, particularly those leading to altered immune mechanisms. It produces a rapidly progressive illness in which brain stem and cerebellar signs are coupled with confusion and drowsiness. All patients with this condition have died, usually within a few months.

It should also be remembered that an altered immune state may predispose to the development of Herpes Zoster and herpes may complicate both malignant lymphomas, chronic lymphatic leukaemia and bowel carcinomas in particular.

In addition to metastasis (the source and location of metastases to the C.N.S. are described in Chapters 8 and 15), there are the additional problems posed by the neurological side effects of cytotoxic drugs (Chapter 24) and radiation damage (Chapters 14 and 18).

As a cautionary note it is important to remember that just because a patient has had malignant disease in the past it does not follow that any *new* disorder is necessarily a complication of that malignancy. An open mind is necessary until the diagnosis is established beyond doubt.

CASE REPORT

A 42-year-old female who had had a mastectomy for carcinoma of the breast four years previously developed diabetes insipidus and a bitemporal field defect. A metastasis seemed certain and steroids and other hormonal therapy were used without effect for several months. Further investigation and exploration were eventually undertaken and revealed a cystic craniopharyngioma which was successfully removed.

7. INFECTIOUS DISEASES AND THE NERVOUS SYSTEM

In general infection of the nervous system is a complication of infection elsewhere. For example, meningococcal meningitis can be regarded as a complication of meningococcal septicaemia, tuberculous meningitis is a complication of a breaking down tuberculous lesion or miliary tuberculosis and listeria monocytogenes or cryptococcal meningitis as opportunist nervous system infections in the presence of debilitating disease or altered immune status.

The meninges and subarachnoid space may be infected by viruses, bacteria, spirochaetes and fungi. The relative incidence of these causes varies enormously in different areas of the world and viral and bacterial infections sometimes show a seasonal variation.

A classical case of meningitis is unmistakable, but, as usual, there are many subtle presentations that may lead to a fatal delay in diagnosis. There are also several common disorders that can mimic "meningitis" to the extent that an immediate L.P. is desirable. These may include any febrile illness in childhood, acute influenza, a severe migraine attack or subarachnoid haemorrhage. There is also the very dangerous situation in which neck stiffness in a drowsy patient is due to coning. In these patients an L.P. may prove fatal (Chapter 25).

The diagnosis may prove difficult in infancy and senescence and the chronic types of meningitis may produce a "tumour-like" clinical picture in any age group.

In infancy the child may become unusually quiet or utter only occasional brief cries. Neck stiffness may be difficult to detect and one may be faced with a pyrexial, quiet, listless, limp infant. An epileptic fit is a common early feature of meningitis in infancy and may provide a clue to the diagnosis.

In senescence the features that may make the diagnosis difficult include an apyrexial course and neurological symptoms dominated by confusion, delirium or focal signs due to cerebral venous thrombosis, mimicking a cerebral vascular accident.

At any age focal inflammation of the brain, venous sinus thrombosis, cerebral arterial occlusions, blockage of C.S.F. circulation or cranial nerve palsies may lead to very focal presenting signs. If these complications develop later in the course of the illness, they may prompt reconsideration of the diagnosis and require definitive treatment in their own right. Many of these complications occur in incorrectly or inadequately treated meningitis.

Classical Features

In typical acute meningitis the features include a pyrexial

onset, considerable headache and photophobia and the development of neck stiffness and backache. The similarity to prodromal influenza is immediately obvious. If left un-diagnosed and untreated drowsiness, vomiting and even-tually coma may ensue. Different types of meningitis affect different age groups and produce some fairly specific fea-tures which may have diagnostic value.

Meningococcal Meningitis

Neisseria meningitides remains the commonest infecting organism, showing a seasonal variation (January to June) and an association with overcrowding. The illness invariably starts as a meningococcal septicaemia and this may prove to be the main problem and cause death. In some cases a chronic meningococcal septicaemia without meningitis may occur. The disease usually affects the under-12 age group and starts as an acute pharyngitis with fever which may rapidly worsen to include a petechial rash and in some cases a florid purpuric rash. In this group massive intravascular coagulation may occur with shock and circulatory collapse. This is known as the Waterhouse—Friderichsen syndrome and it has been suggested that Heparin may be of benefit. Previously steroids were used with little success, a use based mainly on the post-mortem finding of haemorrhagic necrosis of the adrenal glands. The onset of the meningitic com-ponent is usually fairly classical and is often associated with a herpes simplex eruption around the mouth. Metastatic infection of the eyes, joints and bones may occur and complicate the later course. From a neurological point of view late complications occur relatively rarely in correctly diagnosed and treated meningococcal meningitis.

Penicillin is the drug of choice although sulphonamide sensitive organisms are still responsible for the majority of cases in Great Britain. The dosage is 24–30 mega/24 hours in adults I.V. and 1 mega/Kg/24 hours in children I.V.

Haemophilus Influenzae Meningitis

Haemophilus meningitis occurs almost exclusively in child-ren under five years of age. It tends to have a more benign onset and the signs of meningitis may be minimal. The child may be merely drowsy and febrile.

The special complication of haemophilus influenzae meningitis is the development of a subdural collection of pus. This may lead to an apparent relapse or the late develop-ment of focal neurological signs. In the writer's experience this is often the result of inadequate treatment with ampicillin.

Chloramphenicol remains the drug of choice in a dose of 75 mgm./Kg/24 hours for at least ten days. If ampicillin is used very high dosage is necessary; 400 mgm./Kg/24 hours should be given by intravenous infusion.

Pneumococcal Meningitis

Pneumococcal meningitis is relatively uncommon. It is liable to occur when the dura is damaged or infected by a skull fracture, middle ear disease or sinus infections. The organism may also reach the brain via the blood stream in patients who have pneumococcal pneumonia. It is potentially the most lethal form of meningitis, a somewhat paradoxical situation considering that the organism is extremely penicillin sen-sitive. The danger arises from the rapid development of a thick basal exudate, cortical venous thrombosis and cerebral oedema. Total eradication may prove difficult and frequent recurrences may occur in patients with underlying sources of infection such as a basal skull fracture.

Penicillin in adequate dosage is the treatment of choice. The dose is 24–30 Megaunits/24 hours in the adult and 1 Megaunit/Kg/24 hours in children. Chloramphenicol is re-commended in patients who are allergic to penicillin in a dose of 100 mgm./Kg/24 hours.

Other organisms

Other gram positive and gram negative organisms may cause meningitis. For this reason it has been traditional to use a triple therapy regime in those patients who do not have clinical evidence to suggest a specific organism and in those cases in which the gram stain of the C.S.F. is uncertain. The tradi-tional regime included penicillin, chloramphenicol and sul-phadiazine, all three drugs being used until the organism was identified. Recently regimes which include kanamycin and gentamycin combined with penicillin have been sug-gested and many use a wide spectrum antibiotic such as ampicillin. In the writer's view the old regime still has much to commend it.

The only important point in the management of meningitis is that once the diagnosis has been made an *adequate* dose of the *appropriate* antibiotic must be given. Many thera-peutic failures result from the use of inadequate doses of specialised antibiotics such as cloxacillin or cephalosporin in the mistaken belief that the meningitis is due to a rare or antibiotic-resistant organism. Intrathecal therapy is rarely indicated in the treatment of meningitis. Therapeutic disas-ters have occurred as a result of intrathecal injections of antibiotics. The dosage of penicillin is 20,000 units in aqueous solution. This should be prepared by a pharmacist and no other dilution or diluent should be used. The intrathecal use of streptomycin is discussed in the next section.

Uncus 100
Uric acid
　　elevation in Lesch–Nyhan disease 128

Vagus nerve 53–55
　　central nuclei of 111
Vascular disease of the brain 86–98, 114–116
Vascular malformation of the orbit 38
Vasculitis
　　in callogen vascular disease 275
　　in temporal arteritis 221, 229
Ventral horn cell disease 173–175
Ventriculography—in posterior fossa tumours 85
Vernet's syndrome 56
Vertebral angiography
　　in brain stem disease 117
　　in cerebellopontine angle lesions 46
Vertebral artery 87, 113
Vertebral basilar ischaemia 113
Vertebral haemangiomas 155
Vertigo 52–53
　　in brain stem disease 114
　　in brain stem ischaemic attacks 53, 115
Vestibular nerve 47–53
　　caloric testing 48
　　central connections of 60, 113
　　hearing tests 51–52
　　influence on eye movement 58–60
　　neuronitis 52

Vibration sense 74, 143
Villaret's syndrome 56
Vincristine—causing peripheral neuropathy 179
Viral meningitis 282
Visual acuity 11, 13
Visual agnosia 78
Visual cortex 15
Visual evoked responses (V.E.R.) 14, 267
Visual fields 11–25
　　attention hemianopia 14, 78
　　binasal hemianopia 22, 23
　　bitemporal hemianopia 12, 13, 21, 22, 23, 278
　　confrontation tests 11
　　homonymous hemianopia 14, 91, 92
　　in chiasmal lesions 13
　　in hemisphere lesions 22, 91, 92, 93
　　in optic nerve lesions 18, 19, 20
　　in optic tract lesions 22
　　in retinal lesions 15
　　in visual cortex lesions 24, 78, 115
　　macular sparing hemianopia 13, 14, 15, 115
　　macular splitting hemianopia 13, 14, 15
　　non-organic defects 24
　　quadrantic hemianopia 13, 80
　　scotomata 12
Visual hallucinations 24
　　in parieto-occipital lesions 78
　　in temporal lobe lesion 79, 104
Visual pathways 11–25
Visual radiations 15–24

Vitamin B_1 therapy
　　in alcoholic neuropathy 178, 279
　　in Wernicke's encephalopathy 117
Vitamin B_{12}—deficiency of 19, 149
Vomiting in brain stem disease 114
　　in cerebellar disease 133
Von Economo's encephalitis 4, 105, 121

Wallenberg's syndrome 115
Waterhouse–Friderichsen syndrome 281
Weber's syndrome 114
Werdnig–Hoffman disease 173
Wernicke's encephalopathy 105, 117, 135, 279
　　abducens weakness in 34, 117
　　gaze palsy in 63, 117
　　memory disturbance 105
　　nystagmus in 67
　　pupil reaction in 4
　　vitamin B_1 therapy 117
Wilson's disease 127
Writer's cramp 128
Writing
　　in cerebellar disease 133
　　in parkinsonism 125

Zarontin—in petit mal 252
Zombie-like state in temporal lobe epilepsy 104